NATURAL PRODUCTS AND CANCER DRUG DISCOVERY

Edited by **Farid A. Badria**

Natural Products and Cancer Drug Discovery
http://dx.doi.org/10.5772/65205
Edited by Farid A. Badria

Contributors

Rosa Guzmán-Gerónimo, Edna Alarcón-Aparicio, Oscar García-Barradas, Jose Chavez-Servia, Tania Alarcón-Zavala, Newman Osafo, Yaw Duah Boakye, Prince Amankwaah Amankwaah Baffour Minkah, Judith Edem Foli, Christian Agyare, Samuel Obeng, Kazim Sahin, Sanda Vladimir-Knežević, Biljana Blazekovic, Maja Bival Štefan, Marija Kindl, Wim Quax, Christel L.C. Seegers, Rita Setroikromo, Corina Danciu, Codruta Soica, Diana Antal, Stefana Avram, Roxana Ghiulai, Ioana Zinuca Pavel, Alexandra Popescu, Cristina Dehelean, Fidele Ntie-Kang, Ludger Wessjohann, Conrad Veranso Simoben, Wolfgang Sippl, Aurelien F. A. Moumbock, Stefan Günther, Jackson Roberto Guedes Da Silva Almeida, Erica Lavor, Christiane Ferraz, Raimundo Oliveira-Junior, Mariana Silva, Julianeli Lima, Larissa Rolim, Audrey Fleury, Laurent Picot, Jullyana de Souza Siqueira Quintans, Lucindo Quintans-Júnior, Edwin Ogechukwu Omeje, Nneka Ibekwe, Joy Ahomafor, Sunday Onyeloni, Philip Monioro, Charles Chime, Pongtip Sithisarn, Piyanuch Rojsanga, Marius Mioc, Roxana Babuta, Mirela Voicu, Dorina Coricovac

Published by InTech
Janeza Trdine 9, 51000 Rijeka, Croatia

Notice

Publishing Process Manager Nina Kalinic
Technical Editor SPi Global
Cover InTech Design team

First published July, 2017
Printed in Croatia
Legal deposit, Croatia: National and University Library in Zagreb

Additional hard copies can be obtained from orders@intechopen.com

Natural Products and Cancer Drug Discovery, Edited by Farid A. Badria
p. cm.
Print ISBN 978-953-51-3313-1
Online ISBN 978-953-51-3314-8

For EU product safety concerns:
IN TECH d.o.o., Prolaz Marije Krucifikse Kozulić 3, 51000 Rijeka, Croatia,
info@intechopen.com or visit our website at intechopen.com.

Meet the editor

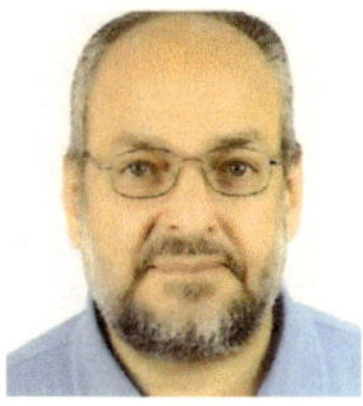

Professor Farid Badria received his PhD degree in Pharmacognosy (Microbial Transformation) from the University of Mississippi, USA, with a BSc degree in Pharmaceutical Sciences and two masters degrees of Science in Pharmacognosy and Cell Biology from Mansoura University and the University of Minnesota.TWAS-ARO (The World Academy of Sciences for the advancement of science in developing countries, Arab Regional Office, 2013) award; World Intellectual Property Organization Gold Medal, 2011 [the best inventor in Egypt]; State Recognition Outstanding Award in Medicine (Egyptian Academy of Science) 2001; Outstanding Arab Scholar, Kuwait (2000); and Khwarizmi International Award, Iran (2000), to mention a few, are just some of the awards he received.
He has also been a scholar of the Arab Development Fund, Kuwait (2000); ICRO-UNESCO International, Chile (1999); UNESCO Biotechnology Fellowship, France (1994); and Honorary Fellowship, University of Mississippi, USA (1987–1990).
Prof. Badria has submitted 44 patents to the Egyptian Academy of Sciences, of which 16 had been granted final certificates with intellectual protection for 20 years. With over 170 publications, 10 books, and other international contributions, he continues to lead research projects on developing new therapy for liver disorders, parasites, malnutrition, simple diagnostic tools, arthritis, skin disorders, and biomarkers for cancer.

Contents

Preface

"We have met the enemy, and he is us," a quote from the comic strip "Pogo" by Walt Kelly, summarizes the primary difficulty of treating cancer using chemotherapeutics, since cancer and normal cells are remarkably similar. Although cancer cells harbor mutated genes and resultant mutated proteins that affect cell division and/or contribute to oncogenesis, the tumor and normal cells share the same DNA and major metabolic pathways. Thus, currently used chemotherapeutic compounds that attack DNA replication or cell division in a cancer cell can also attack a normal dividing cell, resulting in serious side effects.

Linking scientific advances with clinical practice is one among many objectives in writing this book, so management of cancer must be based on sound evidence-based research. Therefore, this book is a book that everybody involved in the area of drug discovery, phytochemistry, cancer biology, and cancer patients must have and benefit from its contents.

This book, *Natural Products and Cancer Drug Discovery*, is written by leading experts in various fields relevant to the development and use of natural products in cancer therapy with up-to-date research in the prevention and treatment of cancer. **First section**, an extensive review on the use of Afro-Asian flora in combating cancer; **second section**, a contemporary survey on anticancer natural compounds from nutritional and herbal products; **third section**, a very interesting reviews of some of the most exciting areas for the development of new chemotherapeutics from *Cannabis* and endophytic fungi; **fourth section**, a special chapter on developing and formulating natural products for treatment of malignant melanoma; and, **fifth section**, a computational and tissue engineering approach to made-to-order new anticancer therapy from natural products are extensively discussed.

These various sections provide reviews of some of the most exciting areas for the development of new anticancer natural products. Hopefully, they may inspire the development of new compounds or approaches that will help reduce the suffering and toll from cancer.

It is our hope that this book may motivate readers to approach the evidence of anticancer natural products with an open mind and thereby spark an interest in making further contributions to the current scientific debate and cancer treatment efforts.

Farid A. Badria, PhD
Prof. of Pharmacognosy
Head of Drug Discovery Research Unit, FAB-Liver Research Lab
Faculty of Pharmacy, Mansoura University,
Mansoura, Egypt

Section 1

Afro-Asian Antiproliferative Medicinal Plants

Chapter 1

African Plants with Antiproliferative Properties

Newman Osafo, Yaw Duah Boakye,
Christian Agyare, Samuel Obeng,
Judith Edem Foli and
Prince Amankwaah Baffour Minkah

Additional information is available at the end of the chapter

http://dx.doi.org/10.5772/intechopen.68568

Abstract

Plant-derived compounds have been an integral component in man's quest to discover ideal anticancer agents. A number of new agents are currently in clinical development with promising selective activity against cancer cell lines and cancer-related molecular targets. This book chapter discusses 14 of such compounds isolated from African plants from 15 plant families. Also contained in this book chapter are compounds from African plants that hold prospect as potential anticancer agents as informed by their *in vitro* and *in vivo* preclinical studies. It is, therefore, worthwhile that researchers in the African continent and the world over should keep on working on identifying biomolecules with potential in cancer management.

Keywords: African plants, antiproliferation, clinical trials, preclinical studies, cancer

1. Introduction

Plant-derived compounds have been an important source of several clinically useful antiproliferative agents in the past half century [1, 2]. Compounds of natural origin such as vinblastine, vincristine, topotecan and irinotecan, etoposide, and paclitaxel have been some of the chemotherapeutic agents still in clinical practice. A number of new agents are currently in clinical development with promising selective activity against cancer cell lines and cancer-related molecular targets, while some agents that failed in earlier clinical studies are stimulating renewed interest.

The present chapter will consider plant-derived antineoplastic single chemical entities currently in clinical trials as oncology drugs. Lead compounds from plants showing promising *in vivo* antiproliferative activity will also be discussed in terms of their origin, possible mechanism of action, and their potential use in cancer management. Most importantly, natural products are generally believed to possess therapeutic potentials hence mostly pharmacologically relevant. This is coupled with the belief that they hold a significant advantage of them being the safer alternative to synthetic molecules [3–5].

Natural products hold a convincing prospect in the continual search for effective anticancer agents with tolerable side effect profile. These observations are well articulated in reviews that have unearthed the fact that about 47% of new anticancer agents that have been approved up to 2006 were either a natural product or their derivative [6]. Due to the labor-intensiveness of bioassay-guided isolation of natural products from crude extracts, more pharmaceutical firms tend to resort to a rapid high-throughput screening of molecular target-based pure compound chemical libraries. Nevertheless, the importance of identification of these bioactive molecules from natural origin is still very palpable in recent years with industries adopting screening procedures that maximize their output [7–9].

A substantial number of chemical moieties of plant origin are currently in various stages of clinical trials [10–12]. However, most of these plant-derived biomolecules are derived from the anticancer agents in clinical therapy which include paclitaxel [ABI-007, RPR-116278A, XRP9881 (RPR109881A)], camptothecin [exatecan mesylate, orathecin], vinblastine and vincristine (vinflunine ditartrate, vinorelbine, anhydrovinblastine, vincristine sulfate TCS), and epipodophyllotoxin (NK-611 and tafluposide 105) [10–12]. Such newer molecules based on the structures of these anticancer agents were not discussed in this book chapter. However, newly isolated compounds from African plants which show potential as possible anticancer agent based on their *in vivo* and *in vitro* studies were included in this book chapter.

2. Compounds of plant origins currently under clinical trial as potential anticancer drugs

2.1. Betulin, β-sitosterol, and betulinic acid

Parinari curatellifolia Planch. ex. Benth (Chrysobalanaceae) is a plant found widely distributed in Africa. Traditionally, it is used for the treatment of toothache (root infusion), pneumonia (hot fomentation of the bark), fevers (leaf decoction), and also as dressing agents for fractures, dislocations, wounds, sores, and cuts (crushed leaves) [13]. In Northern Nigeria, traditional healers use it for the treatment of cancer. Research has indicated that the bioactive constituents of the plant can decrease cancer risk through their antioxidant, antitumorigenic, and antimicrobial activity as well as their ability to directly suppress carcinogen bioactivation. Betulinic acid has been shown to be cytotoxic to neuroectodermal and brain tumor cells [14]. Its apoptotic property is through the regulation of the intrinsic pathway by changing mitochondrial membrane potential and activation of p38 MAPK and SAP/JNK by initiating reactive oxygen species (ROS) generation [15]. This compound can be semisynthesized by oxidation of betulin, which occurs more abundantly [16]. A betulinic acid-containing ointment is undergoing

Phase I/II clinical evaluation for the treatment of dysplastic nevi with moderate to severe dysplasia [17]. Halilu et al. after preliminary investigations also revealed that betulin, β-sitosterol, and betulinic acid were toxic to the cervical epithelial carcinoma (HeLa) cell line used in the assay using the XTT colorimetric assay and cell proliferation Kit II [18].

2.2. Curcumin (diferuloylmethane)

Curcumin, a polyphenol obtained from turmeric (*Curcuma longa* L., Family: Zingiberaceae), has been associated with a wide range of activities including potential antitumor effect, antimicrobial, antioxidant, anti-inflammatory, and immunomodulatory effect [19]. Turmeric plant is very common in Asia and Africa [20]. The plant is employed in traditional medicine for treating a wide range of communicable and noncommunicable diseases such as skin infections, worm infestations, diabetes, liver diseases, and gallstones [21]. A phase II clinical trial of curcumin in patients with advanced pancreatic cancer showed a brief but significant tumor regression with no toxicities observed. Also, clinical studies of curcumin alone or in combination with other chemotherapeutic agents (gemcitabine, 5-fluorouracil, and oxaliplatin) have been carried out in the United States and Israel for patients with colorectal and pancreatic cancers [22]. The mechanism of action was shown to be possibly due to its ability to downregulate expression of nuclear factor kappa-light-chain-enhancer of activated B cells (NF-κB), cyclooxygenase-2 (COX-2), and phosphorylated signal transducer and activator of transcription 3 (STAT3) in peripheral blood mononuclear cells. However, absorption was observed to be poor [22].

2.3. Lycopene

This compound is present in fruits and vegetables, notably *Solanum lycopersicum* L. (Solanaceae) and its processed products [23]. *Solanum lycopersicum* is widely distributed in Africa. It is used in folk medicine for treating burns, wounds, and toothaches. Nahum et al. reported that lycopene inhibits cell cycle progression via reduction of the cyclin D level and retention of p27 in cyclin E-cdk2, thus leading to inhibition of G1 CDK activities in breast and endometrial cancers [24]. Besides its antioxidant and anti-inflammatory activities, lycopene has been established to possess anticancer property in both *in vitro* and *in vivo* models. Its mechanism of action has been established to be via the activation of the electrophile/antioxidant response element (EpRE/ARE) transcription system, inducing the expression of phase II detoxifying enzymes, and arresting the cell cycle at the G0/G1 phase by regulating cyclin D1 and the PI3K/Akt pathway [25]. Lycopene is currently in Phase II clinical trials in the United States for the prevention and treatment of prostate cancer [26].

2.4. Resveratrol

Resveratrol (3,4,5-trihydrostilbene) is a phenolic compound found in several plants such as *Vitis vinifera* L. (Vitaceae), *Morus alba* L. (Moraceae), and *Arachis hypogaea* L. (Fabaceae). *A. hypogea* and *M. alba* are widely distributed in Africa. It is used in the treatment of infectious diseases. The cardioprotective property of red wine has been attributed to resveratrol [27, 28].

A number of studies have reported on the antioxidant, anti-inflammatory, anticancer, and anti-aging activities of resveratrol [27–29]. Its mechanism of action entails the enhancement of apoptosis by acting at multiple cellular targets, including activation of p53, inhibiting cyclo-oxygenase and cytochrome P450 enzymes, and activating AMP-activated kinase (AMPK) [27–29]. Also, it exhibits sensitization effects on drug-resistant tumor cells and results in a synergistic cytotoxicity when combined with established anticancer therapies [30]. This compound is now undergoing Phase I/II clinical trials for the prevention and treatment of colon cancer in the United States [31].

2.5. 2″-Oxovoruscharin and UNBS1450

From *Calotropis procera* (Aiton) W.T. Aiton (Asclepiadaceae) is isolated the cardenolide, 2″-oxovoruscharin with a demonstrated *in vitro* antitumor and Na+/K+-ATPase inhibitory activities [32]. *Calotropis procera* is native to North Africa, Tropical Africa, Western Asia, South Asia, and Indochina [33]. Reduction of the formyl group in the 2″-oxovoruscharin molecule into a hydroxymethyl group yields UNBS1450 with an improved *in vitro* cytotoxicity profile when compared with the parent compound [34]. UNBS1450 has been established to induce the disruption of the actin cytoskeleton to affect multiple signaling pathways by binding to the sodium pump, and that leads to nonapoptotic cell death [35]. UNBS1450 has entered Phase I clinical studies in Europe for patients with solid tumors and lymphomas [36]. *Calotropis procera* is widely distributed in Africa and also employed in folkloric medicine as an abortifacient, hepatoprotective agent, anti-inflammatory agent as well as treating leprosy, syphilis, and cutaneous infections [37].

2.6. Combretastatin A1 and combretastatin A4

Combretastatins isolated from the South African tree, *Combretum caffrum* Kuntze (Combretaceae) are simple stilbenoid compounds with a number of activities including anticancer activity. The A series combretastatin are cis-stilbenes with potent *in vitro* antiproliferative activity against the leukemic P388 and L1210 cell lines. Combretastatin A4, the most potent member of the group, in sodium phosphate prodrug form, has not long ago completed phase I clinical trials as an anti-angiogenic tubulin-binding agent and in nonsmall cell lung cancer and cervix carcinoma, and is presently being assessed in a phase II trial with regards to ovarian, anaplastic thyroid, gastric, and other solid tumors [19, 38]. A propanamide derivative of combretastatin A4 exhibits even more potent antitumor effect than the phosphate by inducing an irreversible blockage of tumor blood flow and is now in phase I clinical studies in Europe and the United States [39, 40]. Again, a bisphosphate prodrug of combretastatin A1 has also been reported to be more potent than combretastatin A4 phosphate and is undergoing phase I anticancer clinical trials in the United Kingdom [40].

2.7. Perillyl alcohol

The essential oils of *Lavandula X intermedia* (Lamiaceae) and *Prunus avium* L. (Rosaceae) are rich in perillyl alcohol, a monoterpenoid with a monocyclic carbon skeleton [41]. *Lavandula*

X intermedia and *Prunus avium* are plants which are widely distributed in South and North Africa, respectively. *In vitro* studies have established the cytotoxicity of perillyl alcohol to cell lines derived from lung cancer, pancreatic cancer, prostate cancer, breast cancer, and leukemia. *In vivo* studies also revealed the inhibitory effects of perillyl alcohol against UVB-induced skin carcinogenesis and DMBA-induced murine melanoma models [42, 43]. Its antiproliferative activity was shown to be due to its arrest of the G0/G1 phase, by modulating the protein levels of cyclin-dependent kinases and cyclin-dependent kinase inhibitors [44]. Currently, perillyl alcohol is undergoing phase I/II clinical trials in patients with breast cancer, ovarian cancer, and glioblastoma multiform [45].

2.8. Alvocidib (Flavopiridol)

Alvocidib, a semisynthetic rohitukine, is an N-methylpiperidine alkaloid first isolated from *Aphanamixis polystachya* (Roxb.) Wight & Arn. (Meliaceae) and later from the African plant *Schumanniophyton magnificum* (K.Schum.) Harms. (Rubiaceae) [46]. It is also present in the stem bark of *Dysoxylum binectariferum* Hiern (Meliaceae) from India and documented to have immunomodulatory and anti-inflammatory activity [46, 47]. Alvocidib has been established to exhibit cytotoxicity for a wide range of cancer cell lines and has demonstrated *in vivo* activity against prostate cancer, head and neck cancer, hematopoietic neoplasia, leukemia, and lymphoma xenograft murine models [48, 49]. Its mechanism has been established to involve inhibition of cyclin-dependent kinases (CDKs) by competing with adenosine triphosphate (ATP) at their nucleotide binding sites and causes cell cycle arrest at either the G1 or G1/M phases. Also, it exhibits apoptosis induction, and antiangiogenic and antiproliferative effects, by interacting at other target sites besides CDK [50, 51]. Alvocidib is the first cyclin-dependent kinase inhibitor in clinical trials for the treatment of patients with non-Hodgkin's lymphoma, renal, prostate, colon, and gastric cancers [50–53].

2.9. Maytansinoids

The parent nitrogen-containing macrocylic substance, maytansine, was first isolated by Kupchan and colleagues from the Ethiopian shrub *Maytenus serrata* (Hochst. ex A. Rich.) R. Wilczek (Celastraceae) [54]. Maytansinoids exhibits antimitotic activity due to tubulin binding hence resulting in inhibition of microtubule assembly [55, 56]. However, there is an overlap of maytansinoids with vincristine in their binding site activity [57, 58]. Maytansinoids has exhibited antiproliferative activity against Lewis lung carcinoma, B-16 melanocarcinoma, murine solid tumor test system, and antileukemic activity against P-388 lymphocytic leukemia, significantly over a 50–100 fold dosage range at the μg/kg level [54, 59]. Clinical trials with maytansine, both alone and as a monoclonal antibody conjugate, however, showed toxicity as well as low response rates in adults with advanced cancer [12, 31, 60]. This informed further metabolic studies involving maytansine to be undertaken to produce analogs with better clinical potential [61]. The extremely high *in vitro* potency of the maytansinoids has sustained interest in structure-activity relationship studies, analog development, total synthesis, and preclinical studies [62].

2.10. Indirubin and 1-methylisoindigo

These are indole alkaloids isolated from the leaves and/or stems of several plants which include the African plant, *Indigofera tinctoria* L. (Fabaceae), as well as *Baphicacanthus cusia* (Nees) Bremek. (Acanthaceae), *Indigofera suffruticosa* Mill. (Fabaceae), *Isatis tinctoria* L. (Brassicaceae), and *Polygonum tinctorium* Ait. (Polygonaceae) [63, 64]. Indirubin has been demonstrated to exert its antileukemic effect by competing with ATP for binding to the catalytic subunit of cyclin-dependent kinase (CDK), via hydrogen bonding, leading to the inhibition of this enzyme [65]. 1-Methylisoindigo is a derivative developed to improve water solubility and other pharmaceutical properties of indirubin. 1-methylisoindigo exhibited significant anticancer activity through a multitargeting profile including inhibition of DNA biosynthesis and assembly of microtubules, induction of cell differentiation, and down-regulation of c-myb gene expression [65, 66]. 1-Methylisoindigo is under clinical trial in the People's Republic of China for chronic myelogenous leukemia (CML) [67].

3. Plant-derived compounds with potential anticancer activity but not yet in clinical trials

3.1. Fagaronine

Fagaronine is a benzophenanthridine alkaloid isolated from *Fagara zanthoxyloides* Lam. (syn. *Zanthoxylum zanthoxyloides*) (Rutaceae), which is widely distributed in Uganda and some other African countries. The root bark extract of the plant is used in the treatment of elephantiasis, malaria, dysmenorrhoea, impotence, and abdominal pain. Fagaronine exhibits antitumor activity against P388 and L1210 murine leukemic cell lines. Its mechanism of action is via inhibition of DNA and RNA polymerase activities as well as inhibition of protein synthesis. This results in disruption of replication in rapidly dividing neoplastic cells. Again, there has been observed inhibition of reverse transcriptase by fagaronine (**Tables 1** and **2**) [68, 69].

3.2. Isofuranonaphthoquinone

Isofuranonaphthoquinone is a phytochemical constituent that occurs in *Bulbine* species (Asphodelaceae) such as *Bulbine abyssinica* A. Rich., *Bulbine capitata* Poelln., and *Bulbine frutescens* (L.) Willd., which are found in Australia and southern Africa. Traditionally, *Bulbine frutescens* is used for a wide range of skin conditions including acne, burns, blisters, cold sores, cracked lips, fingers, nails and heels, insect bites, fever blisters, mouth sores, sunburn, and ringworm among others. It is used internally for coughs, cold, and arthritis. Cell viability assay was used to investigate the action of isofuranonaphthoquinone found in *Bulbine frutescens* on Jurkat T cells [70]. In this study, it was concluded that the effect of isofuranonaphthoquinone was comparable to 1,3-bis(2-chloroethyl)-1-nitrosourea (BCNU), an anticancer agent, and its effects were irreversible. The study showed that isofuranonaphthoquinone could be exerting its activity by generating reactive oxygen species which result in cell death and that it inhibits drug efflux pumps which have been implicated in drug resistance in cancer cells. A combination with BCNU

http://dx.doi.org/10.5772/intechopen.68568

Class of compounds	Structure	References
1. Terpenoids		
– **Monoterpenes**	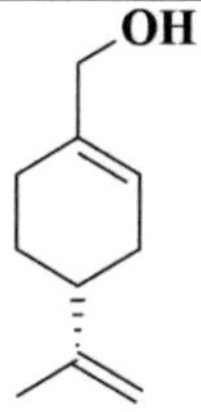 **Perillyl alcohol**	[41–45]
– **Triterpenes**	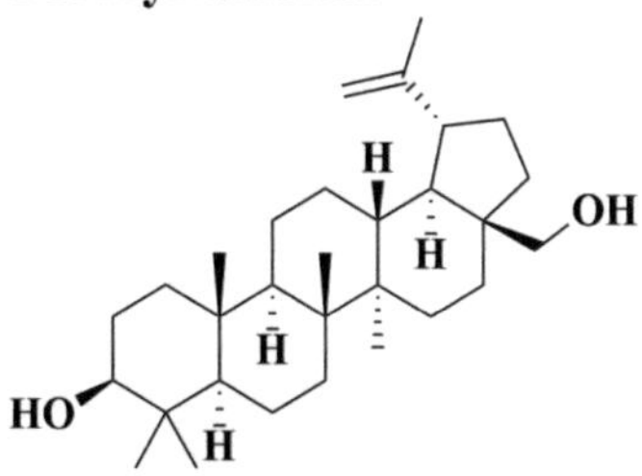 **Betulin**	[18]
		[18]
– **Tetraterpene**	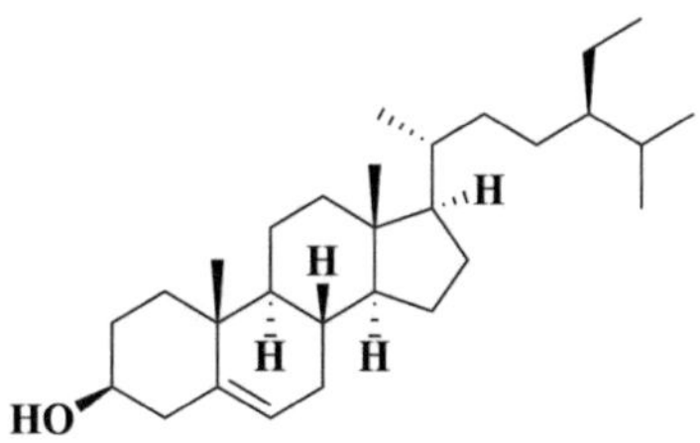 **β-sitosterol**	[14–18]
	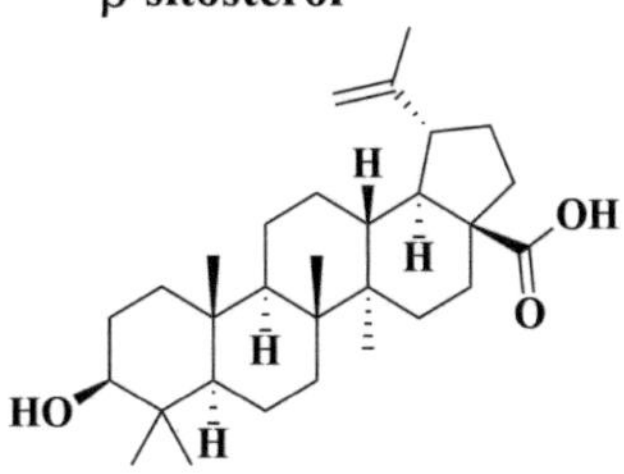 **Betulinic acid**	[24–26]
	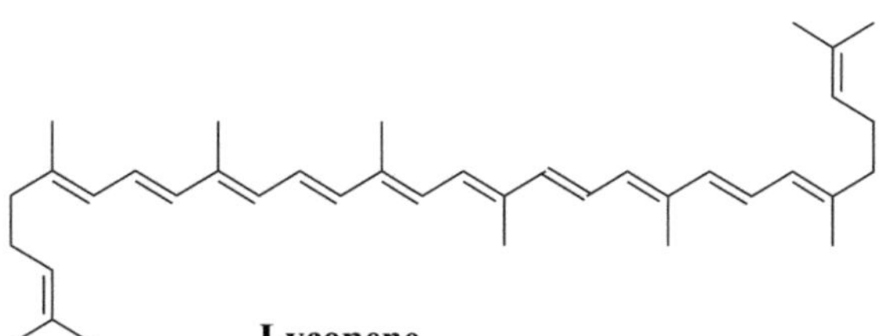 **Lycopene**	

Class of compounds	Structure	References
2. Alkaloids – **Indole**	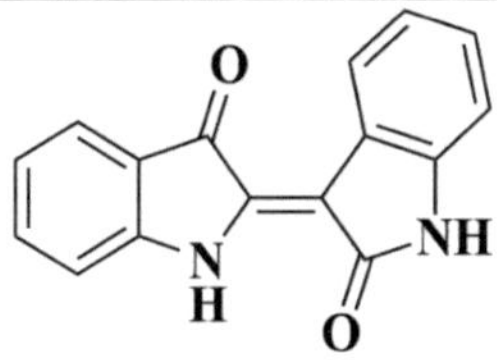 **Indirubin**	[63–65]
	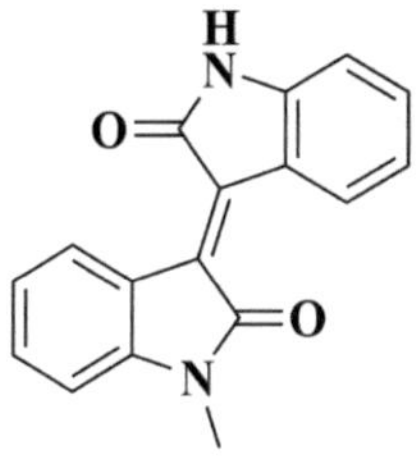 **1-methylisoindigo**	[63–67]
3. Polyphenols – **Diarylheptanoid**	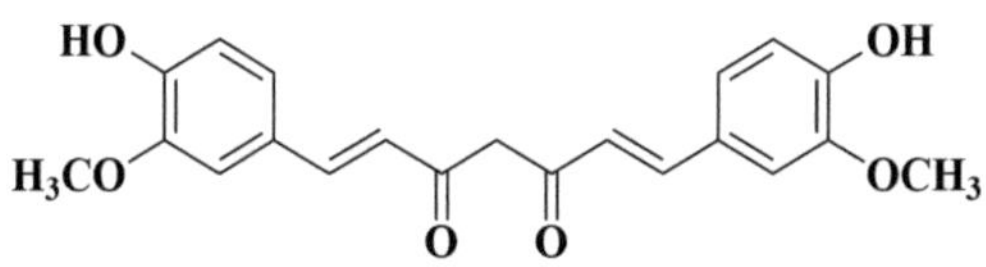 **Curcumin**	[22]
– **Stilbenoid**	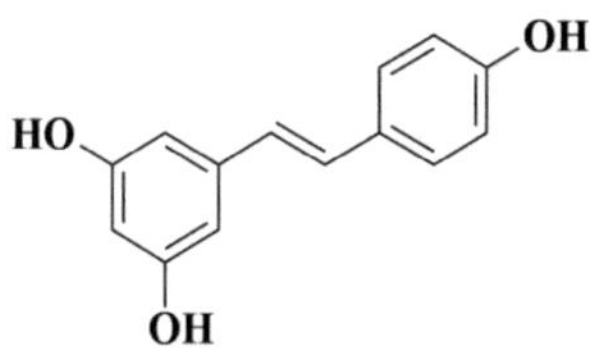 **Resveratrol**	[27–31]
	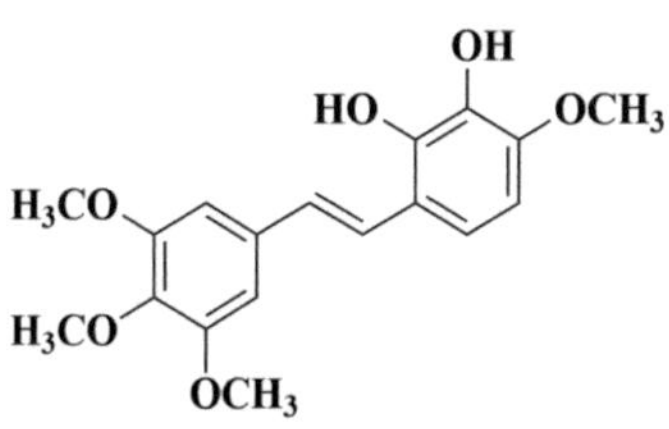 **Combretastatin A1**	[40]
	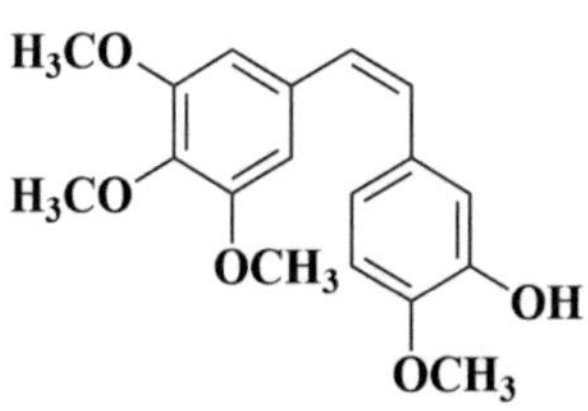 **Combretastatin A4**	[19, 38–40]

http://dx.doi.org/10.5772/intechopen.68568

Class of compounds	Structure	References
4. Steroids – Cardenolides	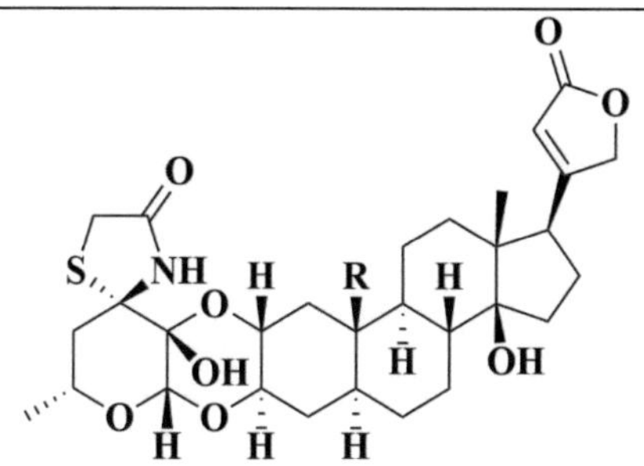 2''-oxovoruscharin R = CHO UNBS1450 R = CH_2OH	[32–37]
5. Flavoalkaloid	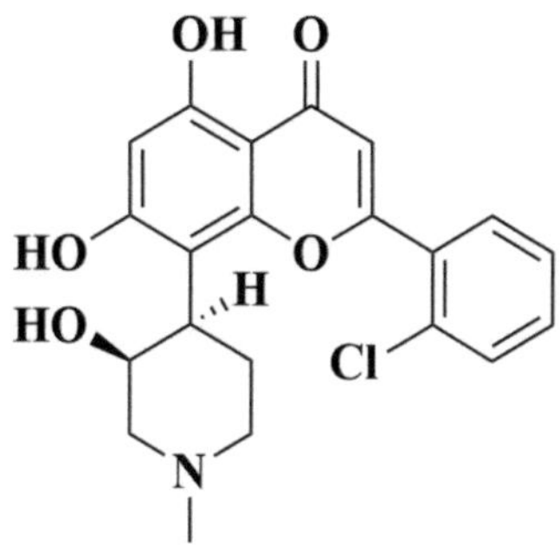 Alvocidib	[46–53]
6. Maytansinoids	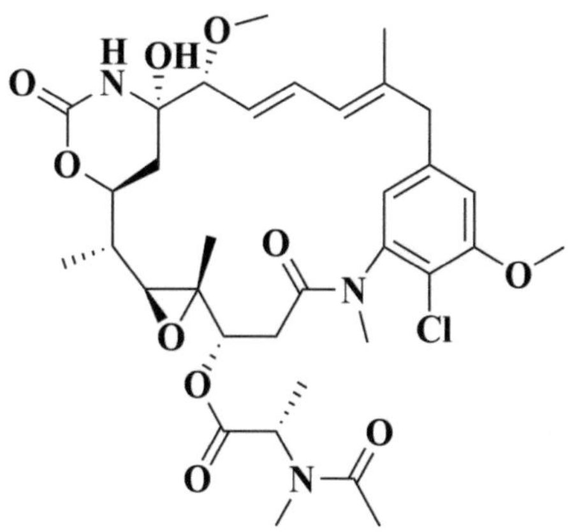 Maytansine	[12, 31, 54–62]

Table 1. Plant-derived compounds currently under clinical trial as anti-cancer drugs.

showed greater toxicity effects on the Jurkat T cells than the individual compounds. Thus, this compound is a potential lead candidate for anticancer drug development and an adjunct compound in combination treatment regimens [70].

Class of compounds	Structure	References
1. Terpenoids		
– Monoterpenes		
• Iridoid lactone	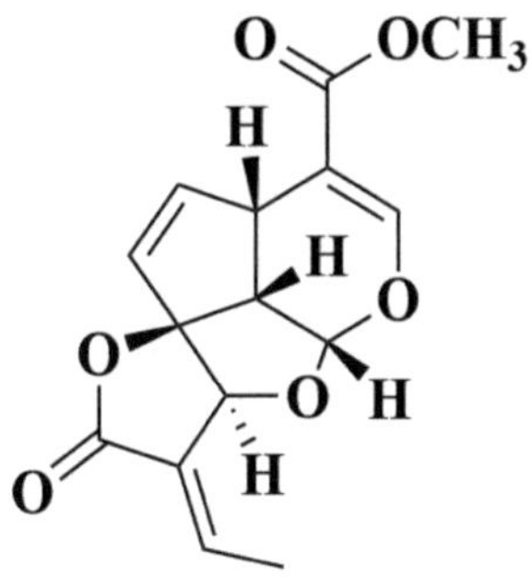 Plumericin	[72]
– Diterpenes • Kaurane	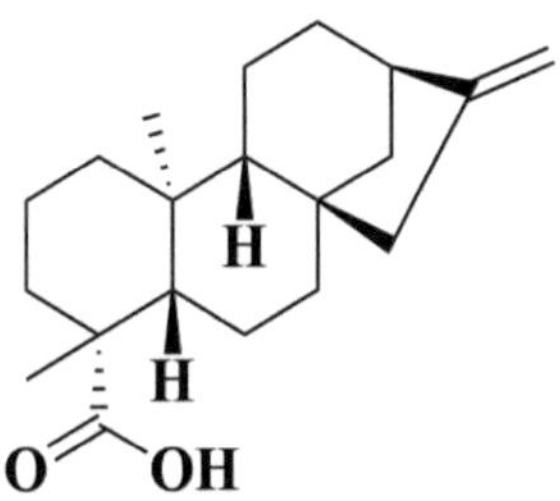 Kaurenoic acid	[76]
2. Alkaloids		
– Benzophen-anthridine	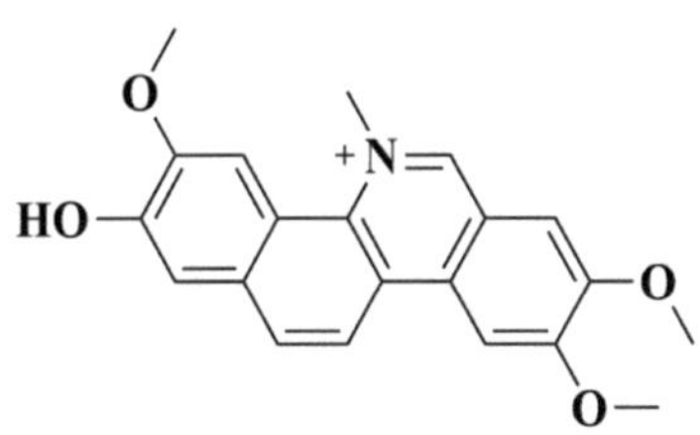 Fagaronine	[68, 69]
3. Quinones	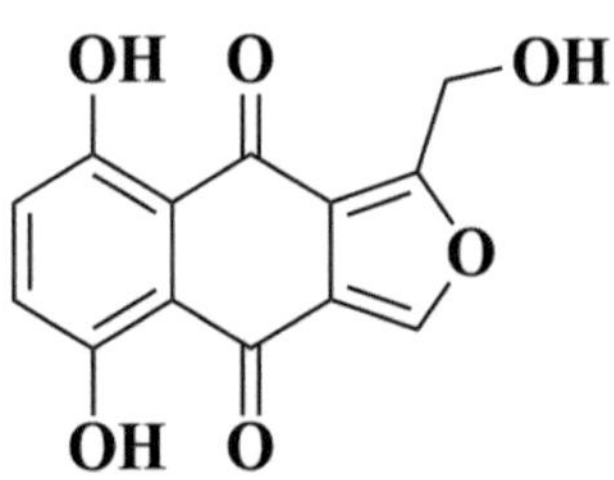 Isofuranonaphthoquinone	[70]

http://dx.doi.org/10.5772/intechopen.68568

Class of compounds	Structure	References
4. Saponins	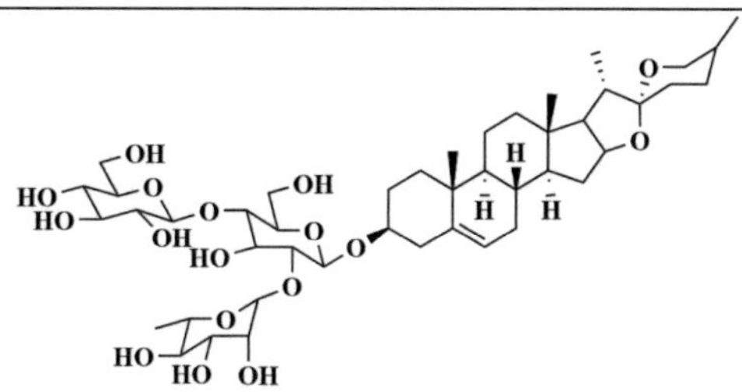 Balanitin-6	[74]
	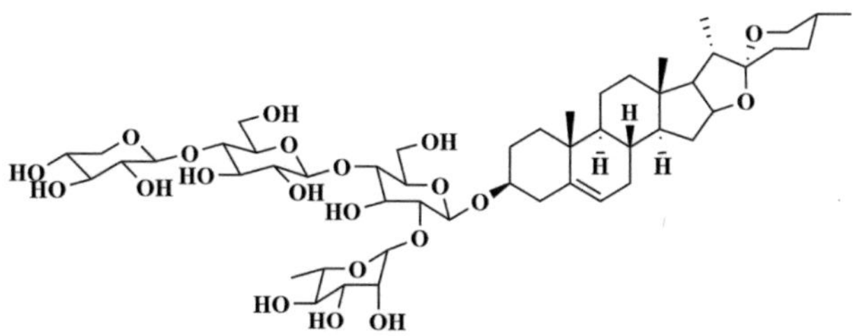 Balanitin-7	[74]
5. Steroids	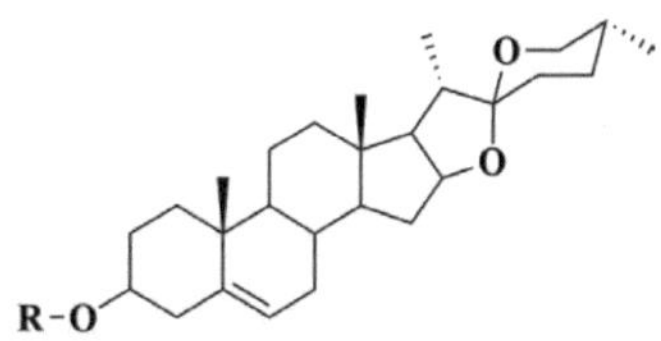 SAP-1016 R = Glu(Rha)—Glu—Xyl SAP-884 R = Glu(Rha)—Glu Spirostanes	[73]
	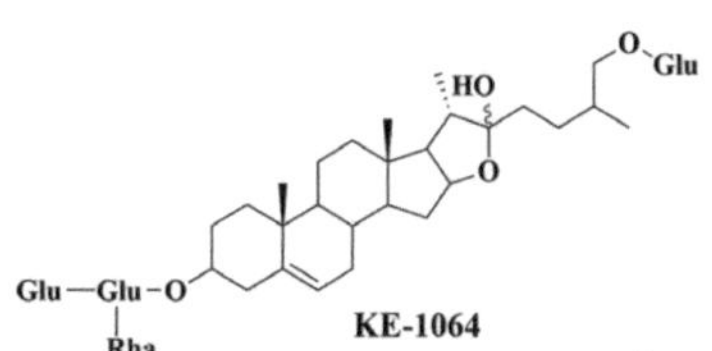 KE-1064 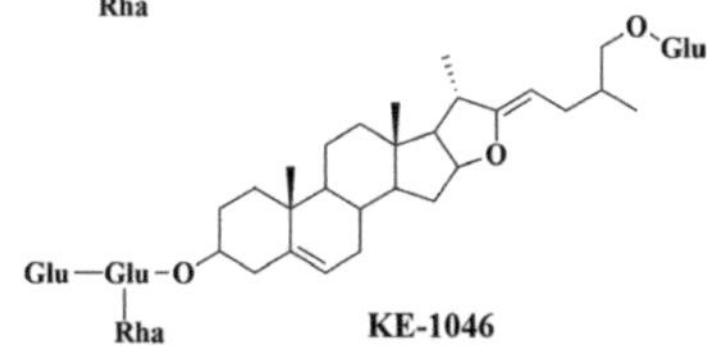 KE-1046 Furostanes	[73]

Class of compounds	Structure	References
6. Crotophorbolanes	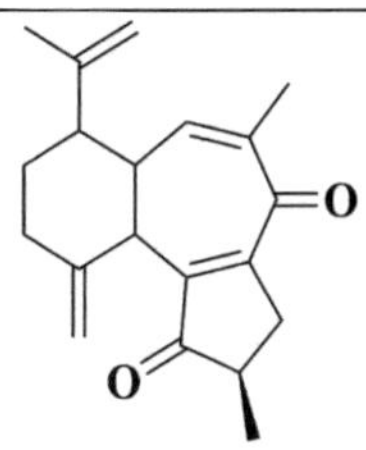 Curcusone A	[75]
	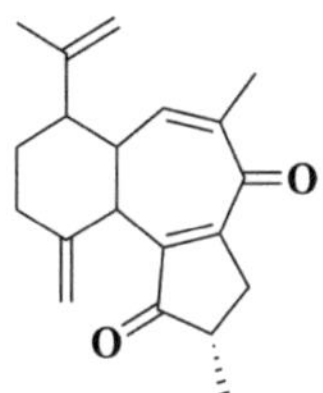 Curcusone B	[75]
	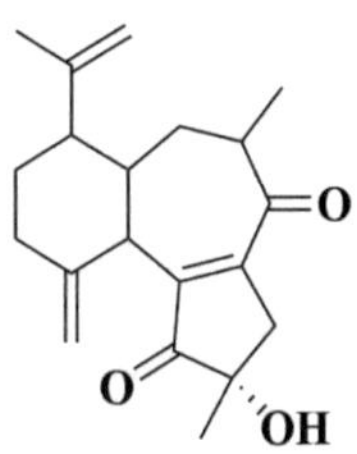 Curcusone C	[75]
	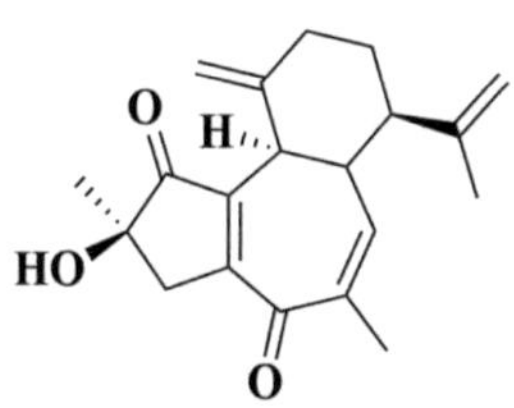 Curcusone D	[75]
	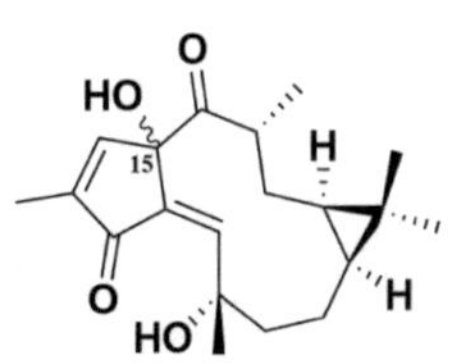 4Z-jatrogrossidentadion 15β- OH 15-epi-4Z-jatrogrossidentadion 15α- OH	[75]

Class of compounds	Structure	References
	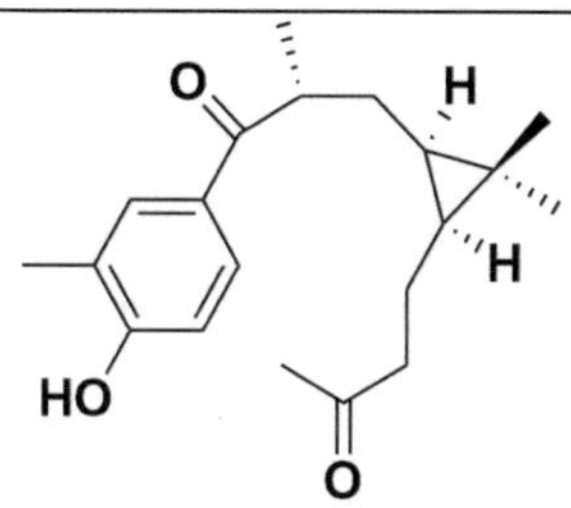 **Multidione**	[75]
	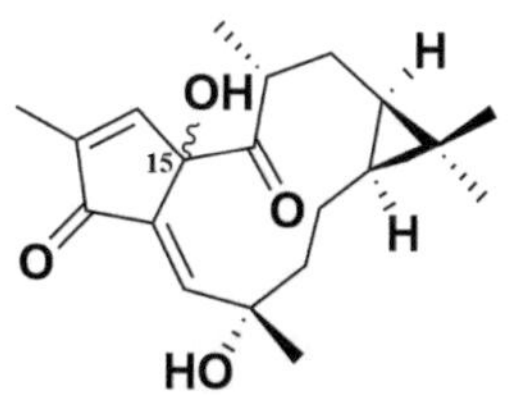 **4E-jatrogrossidentadion 15β- OH**	[75]
	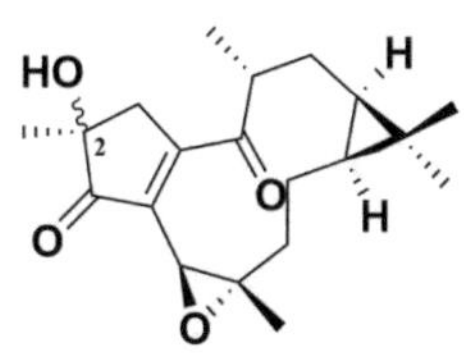 **12-epi-hydroxyisojatrogrossidion 2β- OH** **2-hydroxyisojatrogrossidion 2α- OH**	[75]
7. Anthraquinone	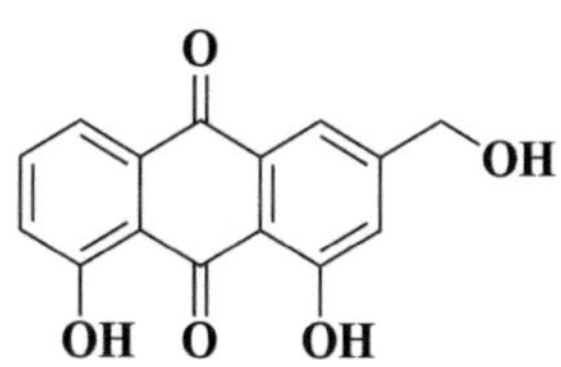 **Aloe-emodin**	[77–79]

Table 2. Plant-derived compounds with potential anti-cancer activity but not yet in clinical trials.

3.3. Plumericin

Momordica charantia L., (Cucurbitaceae) is a plant commonly known as bitter gourd or bitter melon which is widely distributed in Asia and tropical Africa. Bitter gourd extracts have been shown to have antioxidant, antimicrobial, antiviral, antihepatotoxic, hypoglycemic, and antiulcerogenic properties [71]. It has also been shown to have anticancer properties. MTT (3-(4,5-dimethylthiazol-2-yl)-2,5-diphenyltetrazoliumbromide) assay was used in this experiment to investigate the antiproliferative activity of plumericin, isolated from this plant. The results indicated it to have high antiproliferative effect against leukemia (NB4 and K562), breast cancer (T47D) cell lines, and a moderate activity against liver cancer cell line (C3A) [72].

3.4. Balanitin-6 and balanitin-7

Balanites aegyptiaca Del (Balanitaceae) is a spiny evergreen tree found in the dry regions of the Middle East, Africa, and Southern Asia. [73]. Traditionally in Egypt, the fruits are used as antidiabetic agents. In Sudan, it is used in the treatment of jaundice and as an anthelminthic. Additionally, the extracts have been shown to show abortive and antiseptic characteristics [74]. A study was conducted to further characterize the anticancer activity of the steroidal saponins of *B. aegyptiaca* kernels, which contain a mixture of Balanitin-6 (28%) and balanitin-7 (72%). The mixture was found to display greater antiproliferative activity than oxaliplatin as well as etoposide against human cancer cell lines U373 glioblastoma and A549 nonsmall cell lung cancer, though it was less active compared to taxol. The results also showed that the balanitin-6, balanitin-7 mixture is more cytotoxic than it is cytostatic. Its antiproliferative activity does not appear to be by inducing apoptotic cell death and it does not appear to induce detergent-like effects on the cells tested in the study. Rather, its *in vitro* activities are indicated to be at least partially as a result of ATP depletion, the result of which is considerable disorganization of the actin cytoskeleton, finally leading to impaired cancer cell proliferation and migration. Additionally, the study showed that the mixture does not cause intracellular reactive oxygen species levels to increase, unlike a number of anticancer agents of natural origin. In *in vivo* studies, the extent of increase of survival time reported for vincristine was found to be the same for the mixture when tested on mice bearing murine L1210 leukemia grafts. The preliminary *in vivo* results obtained showed that new hemi synthetic derivatives of balanitin-6 and -7 which have enhanced *in vivo* and *in vitro* anticancer activity coupled with decreased toxicity could possibly be produced, which would markedly improve the therapeutic ratio of these compounds [74].

3.5. Spirostanes and furostanes

Another study used the MTT assay to evaluate the antiproliferative activity of furostane (KE-1046 and KE-1064) as well as spirostane (SAP-1016 and SAP-884) saponins isolated from *Balanites aegyptiaca* Del. Potent antiproliferative activity was observed for SAP-1016 against HT-29 human colon and MCF-7 human breast cancer cells. Additionally, for furostane saponins, there was considerable selectivity in growth inhibition between HFF normal cells and MCF-7 breast cancer cells. It was shown that SAP-1016 works by generation of reactive oxygen species in a time-dependent manner in both MCF-7 and HT-29 cancer cells. It also induced apoptosis through the activation of caspase-3 in HT-29 cells [73].

3.6. Curcusones

Found in Africa and Asia, *Jatropha curcas* L. (Euphorbiaceae) is a large drought-resistant shrub, which is used for multiple purposes. The seeds and the oil obtained from them are used for biodiesel production, as a cure for syphilis, and also as a purgative. Different forms of this plant are used in West Africa to treat ailments such as jaundice, mouth sores as well as sores due to guinea worm infestation, fever, and joint rheumatism. The crushed leaves and the latex show antiparasitic activity as well as antibacterial activity against Staphylococcus aureus. Extracts of the stem have been suggested to have anti-insect, anti-inflammatory, cytotoxic, and molluscicidal activities. The MTT method was used to determine the anticancer activity of curcusone A, B, C, and D, pure compounds obtained from the stem of this plant. Curcusone A and B were revealed to possess antiproliferative activity with curcusone B, additionally, suppressing the metastatic process effectively at nontoxic doses. Curcusone C and D were shown to be active against L5178y mouse lymphoma cells. 2-Epi-hydroxyisojatrogrossidion, 4Z-jatrogrossidentadion, 2-hydroxyisojatrogrossidion, 4E-jatrogrossidentadion, and Multidione, 15-epi-4Z-jatrogrossidentadion have also been reported to exhibit potent cytotoxic activity against HeLa human cervix carcinoma cells and L5178y mouse lymphoma cells but exhibited no or low activities against the neuronal cell, PC12 [75].

3.7. Kaurenoic acid

Annona senegalensis Pers. (Annonaceae), (popular names: African custard apple or wild custard apple) has been reported to possess cytotoxic and anticancer effects. Kaurenoic acid, a diterpenoid, has been shown to have anticonvulsant, anti-inflammatory as well as antimicrobial properties. A cytotoxicity assay on Kaurenoic acid was performed using the MTT assay method against Henrietta Lack's cervical (HeLa) and pancreatic tumor (PANC-1) cell lines. Okoye et al. reported that kaurenoic acid exhibited better cytotoxic and antiproliferative activity against HeLa cells, than PANC-1 cells [76]. The anticancer effect of kaurenoic acid on breast, leukemia, and colon cancer cells has been documented, as well as activity on human glioblastoma, murine, and human melanoma cell lines. Terpenoids have been shown to exhibit antitumor activities by inducing apoptosis in various cancer cells by activating various pro-apoptotic signaling cascades and by the inhibition of metastatic progression and tumor-induced angiogenesis. Thus, kaurenoic acid, a terpenoid can potentially be further studied for its potential anticancer activity [76].

3.8. Aloe emodin

Aloe emodin is an anthraquinone compound found in many medicinal plants including the widely grown *Aloe vera* L. and *Rheum palmatum* L. (Rhei rhizome), used in traditional medicine in China and Africa. Previous studies report that aloe emodin has laxative, antibacterial, antiviral, antifungal, and hepatoprotective properties [77]. A recent study has shown that it possesses *in vivo* and *in vitro* antineuroectodermal tumor activity [78]. Another study indicated that aloe emodin showed inhibition of cell proliferation as well as induction of apoptosis in both Hep 3B and Hep G2 human liver cancer cell lines but through different antiproliferative mechanisms. p53 expression was induced in Hep G2 cells, along with a cell cycle arrest in the G1 phase. Added to this, there was a considerable increase in Bax and FAS/APO1 receptor expression. In the Hep 3B cells, the antiproliferative activity was in a p21-dependent manner which did not lead to cell cycle arrest or rise in Fas/APO1 receptor level. Rather, aloe emodin induced apoptosis was promoted through enhanced Bax expression. As a result, aloe emodin may be instrumental in preventing liver cancer [79].

4. Conclusion

A sizeable number of plant-derived compounds are currently under clinical trial for the management of cancers though much needs to be identified. This goes a long way to affirm the therapeutic benefits plants hold. It is therefore prudent that scientist and researchers in Africa and the world as a whole to continue to work on identifying newer compounds of natural origin that would hold potential in the management of cancers.

Author details

Newman Osafo[1]*, Yaw Duah Boakye[2], Christian Agyare[2], Samuel Obeng[3], Judith Edem Foli[2] and Prince Amankwaah Baffour Minkah[2]

*Address all correspondence to: nosafo.pharm@knust.edu.gh

1 Department of Pharmacology, Faculty of Pharmacy and Pharmaceutical Sciences, College of Health Sciences, Kwame Nkrumah University of Science and Technology, Kumasi, Ghana

2 Department of Pharmaceutics, Faculty of Pharmacy and Pharmaceutical Sciences, College of Health Sciences, Kwame Nkrumah University of Science and Technology, Kumasi, Ghana

3 Department of Medicinal Chemistry, Virginia Commonwealth University, Richmond, Virginia, USA

References

[1] Kuipers SE, Farnsworth NR, Fong HMS, Segelman AB. Herbal medicines—A continuing world trend. Presentation at the 1st World Federation of Proprietary Medicine Manufacturers Asia Pacific Regional Meeting; Jakarta. 2010. Unpublished

[2] Agyare C, Obiri DD, Boakye YD, Osafo N. Analgesic Activities of African Medicinal Plants. In: Medicinal Plant Research in Africa. USA: Elsevier Inc; 2013. pp. 726

[3] Bindseil KU, Jakupovica J, Wolf D, Lavayre J, Leboul J, van der Pyl D. Pure compound libraries: A new perspective for natural product based drug discovery. Drug Discovery Today. 2001;**6**:840-847

[4] Firn RD, Jones CG. Natural products—A simple model to explain chemical diversity. Natural Product Reports. 2003;**20**:382-391

[5] Vuorela P, Leinonen M, Saikku P, Tammela P, Rauha J-P, Wennberg T, Vuorela H. Natural products in the process of finding new drug candidates. Current Medicinal Chemistry. 2004;**11**:1375-1389

[6] Newman DJ, Cragg GM. Natural products as sources of new drugs over the last 25 years. Journal of Natural Products. 2007;**70**:461-477

[7] Koehn FE, Carter GT. The evolving role of natural products in drug discovery. Nature Reviews Drug Discovery. 2005;**4**:206-220

[8] Lam KS. New aspects of natural products in drug discovery. Trends in Microbiology. 2007;**15**:279-289

[9] Li JW-H, Vederas JC. Drug discovery and natural products: End of an era or an endless frontier? Science. 2009;**325**:161-165

[10] Saklani A, Kutty SK. Plant-derived compounds in clinical trials. Drug Discovery Today. 2008;**13**:161-171

[11] Harvey AL. Natural products in drug discovery. Drug Discovery Today. 2009;**13**:894-901

[12] Butler MS. Natural products to drugs: Natural product-derived compounds in clinical trials. Natural Product Reports. 2008;**25**:475-516

[13] Orwa C. *Parinari curatellifolia* Planch. ex Benth. *Parinari curatellifolia* Planch. ex Benth. Agroforestry database 4.0 [Internet]. 2009. Available from: www.worldagroforestry.org/treedb/AFTPDFS/Parinari_curatellifolia.PDF

[14] Zuco V, Supino R, Righetti SC, Cleris L, Marchesi E, Gambacorti-Passerini C, Formelli F. Selective cytotoxicity of betulinic acid on tumor cell lines, but not on normal cells. Cancer Letters. 2002;**175**:17-25

[15] Laszczyk MN. Pentacyclic triterpenes of the lupane, oleanane and ursane group as tools in cancer therapy. Planta Medica. 2009;**75**:1549-1560

[16] Sami A, Tarua Mk, Salmea K, Jari Y-K. Pharmacological properties of the ubiquitous natural product betulin. European Journal of Pharmaceutical Sciences. 2006;**29**:1-13

[17] U.S. National Institutes of Health. Evaluation of 20% Betulinic Acid Ointment for Treatment of Dysplastic Nevi (Moderate to Severe Dysplasia) [Internet]. 2010. Available from: http://www.cancer.gov/search/ViewClinicalTrials.aspx?cdrid=494341&version=HealthProfessional&protocolsearchid=3664931 [Accessed: August 2010]

[18] Halilu ME, October N, Balogun M, Lall N, Abubakar MS. Studies of *in vitro* antioxidant and cytotoxic activities of extracts and isolated compounds from *Parinari curatellifolia* (Chrysobalanaceae). Journal of Natural Sciences Research. 2013;**3**(13):149-155

[19] Pan L, Chai H, Kinghorn AD. The continuing search for antitumor agents from higher plants. Phytochemistry Letters. 2010;**3**(1):1-8

[20] Fagbemi JF, Ugoji, Esther AT, Adelowotan O. Evaluation of the antimicrobial properties of unripe banana (*Musa sapientum* L.), lemon grass (*Cymbopogon citratus* S.) and turmeric (*Curcuma longa* L.) on pathogens. African Journal of Biotechnology. 2009;**8**(7):1176-1182

[21] Bhowmik DC, Kumar KS, Chandira M, Jayakar B. Turmeric: A herbal and traditional medicine. Archives of Applied Science Research. 2009;**1**(2):86-108

[22] Dhillon N, Aggarwal BB, Newman RA, Wolff RA, Kunnumakkara AB, Abbruzzese JL, Ng CS, Badmaev V, Kurzrock R. Phase II trial of curcumin in patients with advanced pancreatic cancer. Clinical Cancer Research. 2008;**14**:4491-4499

[23] Kong K-W, Khoo H-E, Nagendra PK, Ismail A, Tan C-P, Rajab NF. Revealing the power of the natural red pigment lycopene. Molecules. 2010;**15**:959-987

[24] Nahum A, Hirsch K, Danilenko M, Watts CK, Prall OW, Levy J, Sharoni Y. Lycopene inhibition of cell cycle progression in breast and endometrial cancer cells is associated with reduction in cyclin D levels and retention of p27 (Kip1) in the cyclin E-cdk2 complexes. Oncogene. 2001;**20**(26): 3428-3436

[25] Bhuvaneswari V, Nagini S. Lycopene: A review of its potential as an anticancer agent. Current Medicinal Chemistry—Anti-Cancer Agents. 2005;**5**:627-635

[26] U.S. National Institutes of Health. Lycopene in Treating Patients with Metastatic Prostate Cancer [Internet]. 2009. Available from http://clinicaltrials.gov/ct2/show/NCT00068731 [Accessed: January 2017]

[27] Aggarwal BB, Bhardwaj A, Aggarwal RS. Seeram, NP, Shishodia S, Takada Y. Role of resveratrol in prevention and therapy of cancer: Preclinical and clinical studies. Anticancer Research.. 2004;**24**:2783-2840

[28] Bishayee A, Politis T, Darvesh AS. Resveratrol in the chemoprevention and treatment of hepatocellular carcinoma. Cancer Treatment Reviews. 2010;**36**:43-53

[29] Athar M, Back JH, Tang X, Kim KH, Kopelovich L, Bickers DR, Kim AL. Resveratrol: A review of preclinical studies for human cancer prevention. Toxicology and Applied Pharmacology. 2007;**224**:274-283

[30] Fulda S, Debatin K-M. Sensitization for anticancer drug-induced apoptosis by the chemopreventive agent resveratrol. Oncogene. 2004;**23**:6702-6711

[31] ClinicalTrials.gov. Resveratrol for Patients with Colon Cancer. [Internet]. 2009. Available from: http://clinicaltrials.gov/ct2/show/NCT00256334. [Accessed: December 2016]

[32] Van Quaquebeke E, Simon G, Andre A, Dewelle J, El Yazidi M, Bruyneel F, Tuti J, Nacoulma O, Guissou P, Decaestecker C, Braekman J-C, Kiss R, Darro F. Identification of a novel cardenolide (2″-oxovoruscharin) from *Calotropis procera* and the hemisynthesis of novel derivatives displaying potent *in vitro* antitumor activities and high *in vivo* tolerance: structure-activity relationship analyses. Journal of Medicinal Chemistry. 2005;**48**:849-856

[33] United States Department of Agriculture (USDA). *Calotropis procera* (Aiton) W. T. Aiton. Germplasm Resources Information Network. 2001. [Accessed: January 2017]

[34] Mijatovic T, Lefranc F, Van Quaquebeke E, Van Vynckt F, Darro F, Kiss R. UNBS1450: A new hemi-synthetic cardenolide with promising anti-cancer activity. Drug Development Research. 2007;**68**:164-173

[35] Juncker T, Schumacher M, Dicato M, Diederich M. UNBS1450 from *Calotropis proceraas* a regulator of signaling pathways involved in proliferation and cell death. Biochemical Pharmacology. 2009;**78**:1-10

[36] Unibioscreen. The piperline—UNBS 1450 [Internet]. 2009. Available from http://www.unibioscreen.com/randd/pipeline_unbs1450.html [Accessed: August 2010]

[37] Sharma P, Sharma JD. *In-vitro* schizonticidal screening of *Calotropis procera*. Fitoterapia. 2000;**71**:77-79

[38] Tsopmo A, Awah FM, Kuete V. Lignans and Stilbenes from African Medicinal Plants. Medicinal Plant Research in Africa. Elsevier Inc. Jamestown Road, London UK. 2013;435-478pp. https://doi.org/10.1016/B978-0-12-405927-6.00012-6

[39] Lippert JW, III. Vascular disrupting agents. Bioorganic & Medicinal Chemistry. 2007;**5**:605-615

[40] Delmonte A, Sessa C. AVE8062: A new combretastatin derivative vascular disrupting agent. Expert Opinion on Investigational Drugs. 2009;**18**:1541-1548

[41] Belanger JT. Perillyl alcohol: Applications in oncology. Alternative Medicine Review. 1998;**3**:448-457

[42] Barthelman M, Chen W, Gensler HL, Huang C, Dong Z, Tim BG. Inhibitory effects of perillyl alcohol on UVB-induced murine skin cancer and AP-1 transactivation. Cancer Research. 1998;**58**:11-716

[43] Lluria-Prevatt M, Morreale J, Gregus J, Alberts DS, Kaper F, Giaccia A, Powell MB. Effects of perillyl alcohol on melanoma in the TPras mouse model. Cancer Epidemiology, Biomarkers & Prevention. 2002;**11**:573-579

[44] Wiseman DA, Werner SR, Crowell PL. Cell cycle arrest by the isoprenoids perillyl alcohol, geraniol, and farnesol is mediated by p21Cip1 and p27Kip1 in human pancreatic adenocarcinoma cells. Journal of Pharmacology and Experimental Therapeutics. 2007;**320**:1163-1170

[45] da Gama Fischer JdS, Carvalho PC, da Costa Neves-Ferreira AG, da Fonseca CO, Perales J, da Costa Carvalho MdG, Domont GB. Anti-thrombin as a prognostic biomarker candidate for patients with recurrent glioblastoma multiform under treatment with perillyl alcohol. Journal of Experimental Therapeutics & Oncology. 2008;**7**:285-290

[46] Lakdawala AD, Shirole MV, Mandrekar SS, Dohadwalla AN. Immunopharmacological potential of rohitukine: A novel compound isolated from the plant *Dysoxylum binectariferum*. Asia Pacific Journal of Pharmacology. 1988;**3**:91-98

[47] Harmon AD, Weiss U, Silverton JV. The structure of rohitukine, the main alkaloid of *Amoora rohituka* (syn. *Aphanamixis polystachya*) (Meliaceae). Tetrahedron Letters. 1979;**20**:721-724

[48] Bible KC, Kaufmann SH. Flavopiridol: A cytotoxic flavone that induces cell death in noncycling A549 human lung carcinoma cells. Cancer Research. 1996;**56**:4856-4861

[49] Arguello F, Alexander M, Sterry JA, Tudor G, Smith EM, Kalavar NT, Greene JFJr, Koss W, David MC, Stinson SF, Siford TJ, Gregory AW, Klabansky RL, Sausville EA. Flavopiridol induces apoptosis of normal lymphoid cells, causes immunosuppression, and has potent antitumor activity *in vivo* against human leukemia and lymphoma xenografts. Blood. 1998;**91**:2482-2490

[50] Senderowicz AM. Flavopiridol: The first cyclin-dependent kinase inhibitor in human clinical trials. Investigational New Drugs. 1999;**17**:313-320

[51] Krystof V, Uldrijan S. Cyclin-dependent kinase inhibitors as anticancer drugs. Current Drug Targets. 2010;**11**:291-302

[52] Schwartz GK, Ilson D, Saltz L, O'Reilly E, Tong W, Maslak P, Werner J, Perkins P, Stoltz M, Kelsen D. Phase II study of the cyclin-dependent kinase inhibitor flavopiridol administered to patients with advanced gastric carcinoma. Journal of Clinical Oncology. 2001;**19**:1985-1992

[53] Karp JE, Blackford A, Douglas SB, Alino K, Seung AH, Bolanos-Meade J, Greer JM, Carraway HE, Gore SD, Jones RJ, Levis MJ, McDevitt MA, Austin DL, Wright JJ. Clinical activity of sequential flavopiridol, cytosine arabinoside, and mitoxantrone for adults with newly diagnosed, poor-risk acute myelogenous leukemia. Leukemia Research. 2010;**34**:877-882

[54] Kupchan SM, Komoda Y, Court WA, et al. Maytansine, a novel antileukemic ansa macrolide from *Maytenus ovatus*. Journal of the American Chemical Society. 1972;**94**:1354-1356

[55] Remillard S, Rebhun LI, Howie GA, Kupchan SM. Antimitotic activity of the potent tumor inhibitor maytansine. Science. 1975;**189**:1002-1005

[56] Wolpert-Defilippes MK, Adamson RH, Cysyk RL, Johns DG. Initial studies on the cytotoxic action of maytansine, a novel ansa macrolide. Biochemical Pharmacology. 1975;**24**:751-754

[57] Hamel E. Natural products which interact with tubulin in the vinca domain: maytansine, rhizoxin, phomopsin A, dolastatins 10 and 15 and halichondrin B. Pharmacology & Therapeutics. 1992;**55**:31-51

[58] Rai SS, Wolff J. Localization of the vinblastine-binding site on beta-tubulin. The Journal of Biological Chemistry. 1996;**271**:14707-14711

[59] Kupchan SM, Komoda Y, Branfman AR, Dailey RG Jr. Tumor inhibitors. 96. Novel maytansinoids. Structural interrelationships and requirements for antitumor activity. Journal of the American Chemical Society. 1974;**96**:3706-3708

[60] Ravry MJ, Omura GA, Birch R. Phase II evaluation of maytansine (NSC 153858) in advanced cancer. A Southeastern Cancer Study Group trial. American Journal of Clinical Oncology. 1985;**8**:148-150

[61] Liu Z, Floss HG, Cassady JM, Chan KK. Metabolism studies of the anti-tumor agent maytansine and its analog ansamitocin P-3 using liquid chromatography/tandem mass spectrometry. Journal of Mass Spectrometry. 2005;**40**:389-399

[62] Cassady JM, Chan KK, Floss HG, Leistner E. Recent developments in the maytansinoid antitumor agents. Chemical and Pharmaceutical Bulletin. 2004;**52**:1-26

[63] Deng B. Direct colorimetric method for determination of indigo and indirubin in Qingdai. Zhong Cao Yao. 1986;**17**:163-164

[64] Hoessel R, Leclerc S, Endicott JA, Nobel MEM, Lawrie A, Tunnah P, Leost M, Damiens E, Marie D, Marko D, Niederberger E, Tang W, Eisenbrand G, Meijer L. Indirubin, the active constituent of a Chinese antileukaemia medicine, inhibits cyclin-dependent kinases. Nature Cell Biology. 1999;**1**:60-67

[65] Xiao Z, Hao Y, Liu B, Qian L. Indirubin and meisoindigo in the treatment of chronic myelogenous leukemia in China. Leukemia & Lymphoma. 2002;**43**:1763-1768

[66] Zuo M, Li Y, Wang H, Zhou J, Li H, Liu H, Xin H, Zhang S, Chen X. The antitumor activity of meisoindigo against human colorectal cancer HT-29 cells *in vitro* and *in vivo*. Journal of Chemotherapy. 2008;**20**:728-733

[67] Cooperative Study Group of Phase III Clinical Trial on Meisoindigo (CSGPCTM). Phase II clinical trial on meisoindigo in the treatment of chronic myelogenous leukemia. Zhonghua Xueyexue Zazhi. 1997;**18**:69-72

[68] Fleury F, Sukhanova A, Ianoul A, Devy J, Kudelina I, Duval O, Alix AJ, Jardillier JC, Nabiev I. Molecular determinants of site-specific inhibition of human DNA topoisomerase I by fagaronine and ethoxidine. Relation to DNA binding. The Journal of Biological Chemistry. 2000;**275**:3501-3509

[69] Raina H, Soni G, Jauhari N, Sharma N, Bharadvaja N. Phytochemical importance of medicinal plants as potential sources of anticancer agents. Turkish Journal of Botany. 2014;**38**:1027-1035

[70] Tambama P, Abegaz B, Mukanganyama S. Antiproliferative activity of the isofuranonaphthoquinone isolated from *Bulbine frutescens* against Jurkat T cells. BioMed Research International. 2014;1-14 pp. Article ID 752941, 14 pages. DOI: 10.1155/2014/752941

[71] Behera TJ, Behera S, Bharathi LK. Bitter Gourd: Botany, Horticulture, and Breeding. Horticultural Reviews. 2010;**37**:101-141

[72] Saengsai J, Kongtunjanphuk S, Yoswatthana N, Kummalue T, Jiratchariyakul W. Antibacterial and antiproliferative activities of plumericin, an iridoid isolated from *Momordica charantia* vine. Evidence-Based Complementary and Alternative Medicine. 2015;**2015**:1-11

[73] Beit-Yannai E, Ben-Shabat S, Goldschmidt N, Chapagain BP, Liu RH, Wiesman Z. Antiproliferative activity of steroidal saponins from *Balanites aegyptiaca*—An *in vitro* study'. Phytochemistry Letters. 2011;**4**(1):43-47

[74] Gnoula C, Mégalizzi V, De Nève N, Sauvage S, Ribaucour F, Guissou P, Duez P, Dubois J, Ingrassia L, Lefranc F, Kiss R, Mijatovic T. Balanitin-6 and -7: Diosgenyl saponins isolated from *Balanites aegyptiaca* Del. display significant anti-tumor activity *in vitro* and *in vivo*. International Journal of Oncology. 2008;**32**(1):5-15

[75] Aiyelaagbe OO, Hamid AA, Fattorusso E, Taglialatela-Scafati O, Schröder HC, Müller WEG. Cytotoxic activity of crude extracts as well as of pure components from jatropha species, plants used extensively in African traditional medicine. Evidence-Based Complementary and Alternative Medicine. 2011;1-7pp. ArticleID 134954,7 pages. DOI: http://dx.doi.org/10.1155/2011/134954

[76] Okoye TC, Akah PA, Nworu CS, Ezike AC. Kaurenoic acid isolated from the root bark of *Annona senegalensis* induces cytotoxic and antiproliferative effects against PANC-1 and HeLa cells. European Journal of Medicinal Plants. 2014;**4**(5):579-589

[77] Yordanova A, Koprinarova M. Is aloe-emodin a novel anticancer drug? Trakia Journal of Sciences. 2014;**12**(1):92-95

[78] Pecere T, Gazzola MV, Mucignat C, Parolin C, Vecchia FD, Cavaggioni A, Basso G, Diaspro A, Salvato B, Carli M, Palu G. Aloe-emodin is a new type of anticancer agent with selective activity against neuroectodermal tumors. Cancer Research. 2000;**60**(11):2800-2804

[79] Kuo P-L, Lin T-C, Lin C-C. The antiproliferative activity of aloe-emodin is through p53-dependent and p21-dependent apoptotic pathway in human hepatoma cell lines. Life Sciences. 2002;**71**(16):1879-1892

Chapter 2

Anticancer Effects of Some Medicinal Thai Plants

Pongtip Sithisarn and Piyanuch Rojsanga

Additional information is available at the end of the chapter

http://dx.doi.org/10.5772/67648

Abstract

Ethanolic extracts from thirty Thai edible plants collected from Sa Keao province, Thailand, were screened for *in vitro* antiproliferative effect on HCT-116 human colon cancer cell line using cell titer 96 aqueous one solution cell proliferation assay. It was found that leaf extract of *Crateva adansnii*, fruit and leaf extracts of *Ardisia elliptica*, shoot extract of *Colocasia esculenta*, leaf extract of *Cratoxylum fomosum*, and leaf extract of *Millettia leucantha* exhibited antiproliferative activities. The fruit extract of *Ardisia elliptica* showed the highest antiproliferative activity. Ethanolic extract of the stems from *C. fenestratum* and its dichloromethane and aqueous fractions showed antiproliferative activity to human colorectal cancer cells (HCT-116) determined by cell growth assay. Berberine, one of the major alkaloid in the stems of *C. fenestratum*, also promoted antiproliferative effect. Extracts from the leaves of three *Azadirachta* species in Thailand, *A. indica*, *A. indica* var. *siamensis*, and *A. excelsa*, were reported to promote *in vitro* antioxidant effects determined by various methods. Ten *Russula* mushroom collected from northeastern part of Thailand were tested for *in vitro* antioxidant activities using photochemiluminescence assay for both lipid-soluble and water-soluble antioxidant capacities. *R. medullata* extract exhibited the highest antioxidant effects in both lipid-soluble and water-soluble models.

Keywords: anticancer, *Coscinium fenestratum*, berberine, *Azadirachta*, *Russula*

1. Introduction

Cancer cells uncontrollably divide to form masses of tissue, which are called tumors. Tumors can grow and interfere with the functions of many bodily systems including the digestive, nervous, and cardiovascular systems. Cancer has been reported to be the first in the rank of causes of the death in the Thai population. Liver, colon, and lung cancers are the most prevalent cancers in Thai males, while breast, cervical, and colon cancers are the most prevalent cancers in Thai females [1].

The development of cancer or carcinogenesis occurs through a multistep process involving the mutation, selection of cells with a progressive increasing capacity for proliferation, survival, invasion, and metastasis [2]. The first step in the process, tumor initiation, relates to the genetic alteration leading to the changes in normal cells. Then, in the promotion or development stage, the cells abnormally proliferate leading to the outgrowth of a population of clonally derived tumor cells [2]. This stage can be stimulated by carcinogens, which are a group of substances such as tobacco, asbestos, arsenic, radiation such as gamma and X-rays, sun light, polycyclic hydrocarbons, nitrosamines, and aflatoxins: these substances do not directly cause cancers but promote or aid the development of cancers [2, 3]. After that, tumor progression continues as additional mutations occur within the cells of the tumor population to further advantage the cancer cells, such as more rapid growth, which will allow them to become dominant within the late tumor population. The process is called clonal selection, since a new clone of tumor cells evolves on the basis of its increased growth rate or other properties such as survival, invasion, or metastasis. Clonal selection continues throughout tumor development, so tumors continuously become more rapid-growing and increasingly malignant [2].

2. Cancer therapy

The modern treatments for cancers mainly are surgery, radiation, and chemotherapy. However, most of chemotherapeutic drugs are not specific to only cancer cells, but also cause damage to normal cells, especially bone marrow, mucous glands, mucous membranes, hair, and nails and can lead to the suppression of the immune system [3]. The success of chemotherapy depends on the number of cancer cells, the proliferation rate, the duration of the drug administration, and the therapeutic interval. To avoid drug resistance, polychemotherapy is always used instead of monochemothearpy [3]. The anticancer drugs can also cause some other side effects including nausea, vomiting, agranulocytosis, inhibition of spermatogenesis and ovulation, alopecia, inflammation of mucous membranes, and terratogenesis [3].

Some compounds separated from natural products are now being developed as modern medicines for the treatments of cancers including paclitaxel, catharanthus alkaloids, and derivatives of podophyllotoxin.

Paclitaxel was separated from the bark of *Taxus brevifolia* Nutt. (Pacific Yew), which is a tree in Taxaceae. Paclitaxel will bind with b-tubulin and stimulate the aggregation of a tubulin subunit to become a nonphysiological microtubule composed of 12 proto-filaments, which cause the inhibition of cell cycles in mitosis and interphase (G_2-phase) and lead to cell apoptosis. This compound is normally used in an injection formulation as the adjuvant chemotherapy for the treatments of ovarian, breast, and bronchial cancers [3].

Some alkaloids are separated from the leaves of *Catharanthus roseus* (L.) G. Don., such as vincristine and vinblastine. Vincristine is used for the treatment of lymphatic leukemia, neuroblastoma, and Wilms tumor, while vinblastine is used to treat lymphogranuloma (Morbus Hodgin), lymphosarcoma, testicular carcinoma, and chorionic carcinoma [3].

Podophyllotoxin was separated from the rhizome of *Podophyllum peltatum* L. or American mandrake. Two derivatives of podophyllotoxin, etoposide and teniposide, are now being developed and used as anticancer drugs. Etoposide is used for the treatment of bronchial cancer, testicular carcinoma, and chorionic carcinoma, while tenoposide is used to treat brain or bladder cancers [3]. The chemical structures of some anticancer compounds from natural products are shown in **Figure 1**.

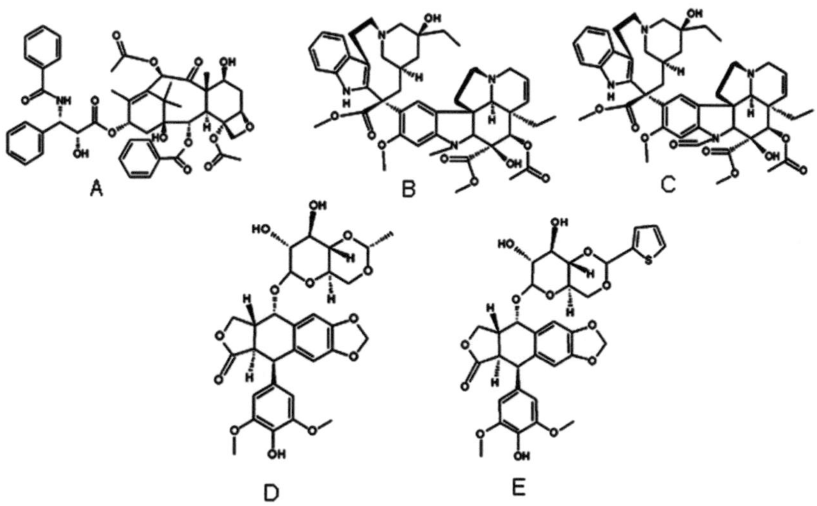

Figure 1. Chemical structures of some anticancer compounds from natural products. A = paclitaxel, B = vinblastine, C = vincristine, D = etoposide, E = teniposide.

3. Anticancer effects of medicinal plants and natural products

Natural products from plants, animals, marine sources, and minerals have been used for the treatments of ailments and diseases for a long time. In Thai traditional medicine, the word "cancer" could refer to the symptom of chronic wound, abscess, emaciation, and weak [4]. Active phytochemicals in plants can be classified into two main groups of primary metabolites, which are the compounds necessary for plant growth and development such as carbohydrates, proteins, and fats. Another group is secondary metabolites, which promote the defense mechanisms or support the lives of the plants; they include polyphenolic compounds, flavonoids, terpenoids, and alkaloids [5]. Ethanolic extracts from thirty Thai local edible plants collected from Wang Nam Yen district, Sa Keao province, Thailand were screened for the *in vitro* anti-proliferative effect on HCT-116 human colon cancer cell lines using a cell titer 96 aqueous one solution cell proliferation assay. It was found that six ethanolic plant extracts, including a leaf extract of *Crateva adansnii*, fruit and leaf extracts of *Ardisia elliptica*, a shoot extract of *Colocasia esculenta*, a leaf extract of *Cratoxylum fomosum*, and a leaf extract of *Millettia leucantha* exhibited antiproliferative activities on the HCT-116 cell line. The fruit extract of *Ardisia elliptica* showed the highest antiproliferative activities with an IC_{50} value of 5.12 ± 0.54 μg/ml [6]. The mechanisms of the action of medicinal plants for anticancer effects have been reported as following [4]:

3.1. Inhibition of cell division in the cancer cell cycle

Alpha-mangostin from mangosteen (*Garcinia mangostana*) fruit rind promoted inhibitory effects to breast cancer cell line (MDA-MB-231) by inhibition of cell division in G1 and S phases [7]. Methanol extract of *Morus alba* L. leaves inhibited liver cancer cell line Hep G2 by inhibition of cell division in G2/M phase [8]. Cucurbitacin B, a triterpenoid from *Trichosanthes cucumerina* L., also inhibited breast cancer cell division in G2/M phase [9].

3.2. Induction of cancer cell apoptosis

This mechanism includes some minor mechanisms which stimulate anticancer genes, induction of caspase enzymes, induction of free radical formation, inhibition or induction of enzymes relating to histone protein, and the formation of spingosine or ceramide [4]. Dehydrocostus lactone from the root of *Saussurea lappa* induced the apoptosis of liver cancer cells Hep G2 and PLC/PRF/5 via p53 protein [10]. Water extract of the seed from *Sapindus rarak* Candolle. induced lung cancer cells A549 apoptosis through the induction of the caspase enzyme [11], while methanol extract of *Derris scandens* Benth. induced apoptosis of colon cancer cells SE480 by increased caspase-3 activity and down-regulated Bcl-2 and up-regulated Bax protein of SW480 cells; it also significantly induced cell necrosis determined by the release of LDH [12]. Alpha-mangostin separated from the fruit rind of mangosteen also upregulated Bax and down-regulated Bcl-2 proteins in rat liver tissue [13]. Methanol extract from stem bark of *Myristica fragrans* Houtt. promoted the apoptosis of lymphoblast Jurkat by controlling the SIRT1 gene [14]. G1 b, a glycospingolipid from *Murdannia loriformis* (Hassk.) R.S.Rao & Kammathy, inhibited breast, lung, colon, and liver cell lines [15].

3.3. Immune stimulation

Methanol extract from the leaves of *Moringa oleifera* Lam. exhibited immune stimulation effect both cell-mediated immunity and humoral immunity by induction of neutrophile production and stimulation of macrophages in animals damaged by the toxicity of anticancer drugs [16].

In Thai traditional medicine, there are some medicinal formulas compose of several plants in different ratios. These formulas are traditionally used for a long time usually for the treatments of cancers in patient with the late stage cancers, patients who cannot improve after treatment with chemotherapy, radiation or surgery, patients with cancers in several organs or patients with incurrent diseases [4]. The sources of anticancer herbal formulas usually come from local traditional doctors or priests in the temples (in Thai, temple is called as "Wat"), with the normal method of preparation being the decoction of plant materials with water [4]. A herbal remedy from Wat Tha-it (Tha-it temple), Ang Thong province, Thailand, composed of several plant materials including *Gelonium multiflorum* A. Juss., *Erycibe elliptilimba* Merrill & Chun, *Balanophora abbreviate* Blume, *Smilax china* L., *Smilax glabra* Wall. ex Roxb., and *Millingtonia hortensis* Linn. was reported to significantly promote synergistic effects on doxorubicin in the treatment of A549 cancer cells by the inhibition of cell divisions in the G2/M phase [4, 17]. Another herbal remedy is from a Thai herbal nursing home, Wat Khampramong, Sakon Nakhon province comprises of several plant materials such as *Rhinacanthus nasutus* (L.) Kurz, *Acanthus ebrateatus* Wall., *Smilax glabra* Wall. ex Roxb.,

Artemisia annua L., *Angelica sinensis* (Oliv.) Diels, *Salacia chinensis* L., and *Orthosiphon aristatus* Miq [18]. This herbal remedy can inhibit the growth of some cancer cell lines such as breast adenocarcinoma MDA-MB 231, synovial sarcoma SW982, hepatocellular carcinoma HepG2, cervical adenocarcinoma HeLa, and lung carcinoma A549 [18].

4. Some potential Thai medicinal plants with anticancer effects

4.1. *Coscinium fenestratum* (Gaertn.) Colebr

NAG-1 or nonsteroidal anti-inflammatory drug (NSAID)-activated gene was identified in COX-negative cells by PCR-based subtractive hybridization from an NSAID-induced library as a divergent member of the TGF-β superfamily [19]. The overexpression of NAG-1 in cancer cells results in growth arrest and an increase in apoptosis, suggesting that NAG-1 has antitumorigenic activity [20]. NAG-1 expression is also upregulated by a number of dietary compounds, medicinal plants, and anticancer drugs [21–25]. *Coscinium fenestratum* is one of the medicinal plants that promoted antiproliferative effects on colon cancer cell lines with mechanisms related to NAG-1 [20].

Coscinium fenestratum (Gaertn.) Colebr. is a large climber with yellow wood and sap, known in the Thai language as Hamm or Khamin khruea. The genus *Coscinium* belongs to the tribe Coscinieae of the family Menispermaceae. This genus comprises two species, which are *Coscinium blumeanum* Miers. and *C. fenestratum* (Gaertn.) Colebr. Both of them are stout woody climbers growing in the tropical rain forest regions of Asia [26]. *Coscinium* species are characterized by the axillary flowers, extra-axillary or cauliflorous in racemiform, or peduncled subumbellate aggregate, of 20–50 cm in length. The inflorescences are axillary or cauliflorous with 6–12 florets. Male flowers are sessile or with pedicels, up to 1 mm. Sepals are broadly elliptic to obovate with the inner 3–6 spreading, yellow, and 1.5–2 mm long. Stamens are 6 with 1 mm long. The Sepals of female flower are as in male flowers. Staminodes are 6 and claviform with 1 mm long. Drupes are subglobose, tomentellous, brown to orange or yellowish, 2.8–3 cm diameter. Pericarp is drying woody. Seeds are whitish and subglobose with the enveloping condyle. The leaves are subpeltate or ovate, large, hard-coriaceous, palmately nerved, reticulate, and densely hairy beneath [26]. Physical characteristic of the *Coscinium fenestratum* stem (cross section) is shown in **Figure 2**.

The stem decoction and maceration extracts of *Coscinium fenestratum* have been traditionally used in the Northeastern part of Thailand for the treatment of various diseases such as cancer, diabetes mellitus, and arthritis [27]. The ethanolic extract of the stems from *C. fenestratum* and its dichloromethane and aqueous fractions showed antiproliferative activity on human colorectal cancer cells (HCT-116) determined by a cell growth assay. Berberine, one of the major alkaloids in the stems of *C. fenestratum*, also promoted an antiproliferative effect [20]. The mechanisms of action of the extracts from *C. fenestratum* were reported as the activation of proapoptotic proteins and pparγ [20]. It was also reported that berberine facilitated the apoptosis of cancer cells, and the molecular targets for its activity are NAG-1 and AFT3 [24]. The chemical structure of Berberine is shown in **Figure 3**.

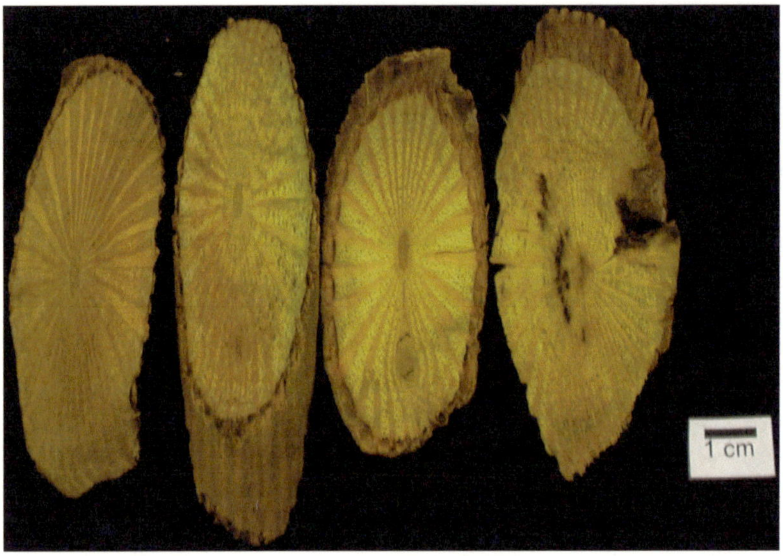

Figure 2. Physical characteristic of *Coscinium fenestratum* stem purchased from Nongkhai province, Thailand (cross section ×1).

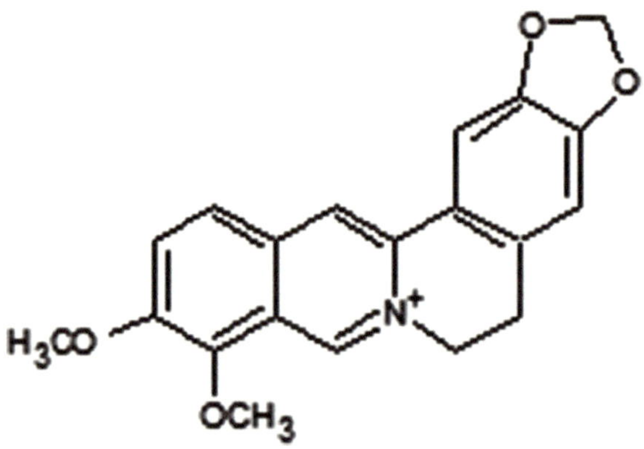

Figure 3. Chemical structure of Berberine.

4.2. *Azadirachta* plants

Oxidative stress is considered to be of some importance for many ailments and pathologies; including cardiovascular diseases, cancers, rheumatoid arthritis, and Alzheimer's disease [28]. Polyphenolic compounds have been reported to have important anticancer and chemopreventive effects [29]. Phenolic acids such as gallic acid, ellagic acid, and ferulic acid induce apoptosis in cancer cells, activated caspase, prevented cancer formation, and suppress the angiogenesis of cancer [29–32]. Flavonoids such as quercertin and kaempferol also promote apoptosis, inhibit oncogenes, and generated cell cycle arrest [29, 33–35].

Suttajit et al. [36] studied the antioxidant activities of extracts from many Thai medicinal plants using a ABTS-metmyoglobin assay and reported some plants with high antioxidant activities; including *Uncaria gambier* Roxb., *Piper betle* Linn., *Camellia sinensis* (L.) Kuntze., *Azadirachta indica* A. Juss. var. *siamensis* Valeton., *Curcuma zedoaria* Roxb., *Syzygium aromaticum* (L.) Merr. & Perry and *Tamarindus indica* Linn. When focusing on Thai medicinal plants, the Siamese neem tree (*Azadirachta indica* A. Juss. var. *siamensis* Valeton.) is an interesting plant that showed high antioxidant activity in the screening test [36, 37]. Moreover, there are reports about its antioxidant potential based on the antioxidant content as the butylated hydroxyanisole (BHA) equivalent of Thai indigenous vegetable extracts. From this report, the Siamese neem tree leaf extract appeared to be a high potency antioxidant, containing more than 100 mg BHA equivalent in 100 g fresh weight.

Azadirachta plants comprise of three different plant species; *Azadirachta indica* A. Juss or *A. indica* A. Juss var. *indica* (neem), *Azadirachta indica* A. Juss. var. *siamensis* Valeton (Siamese neem tree), and *Azadirachta excela* (Jack) Jacobs. (marrango tree). The Siamese neem tree leaves are wider, longer, and thicker than the leaves of neem, while the marrango tree has the widest, longest, and thickest leaves. The margin of the leaflet of Siamese neem tree is crenate to entire, while the margin of neem is serrate and that of marrango tree is entire to undulate. The colors of the leaflet blade of the Siamese neem tree, neem, and marrango tree are green, light green, and dark shiny green, respectively [38, 39]. The physical characteristics of Siamese neem tree, neem, and marrango tree leaves are shown in **Figure 4**.

The leaves and flowers of Siamese neem tree and neem have been traditionally used as element tonics and antipyretic and gastric secretion stimulating agents, while the stem bark of all *Azadirachta* plants is used to treat amoebic dysentery and diarrhea [40, 41]. There also reports suggesting that polysaccharides and limonoids found in neem bark, leaves, and seed oil reduce tumors and cancers and showed effectiveness against lymphocytic leukemia [42–44]. Moreover, the young leaves and flowers of the Siamese neem tree are popularly consumed as vegetables [39].

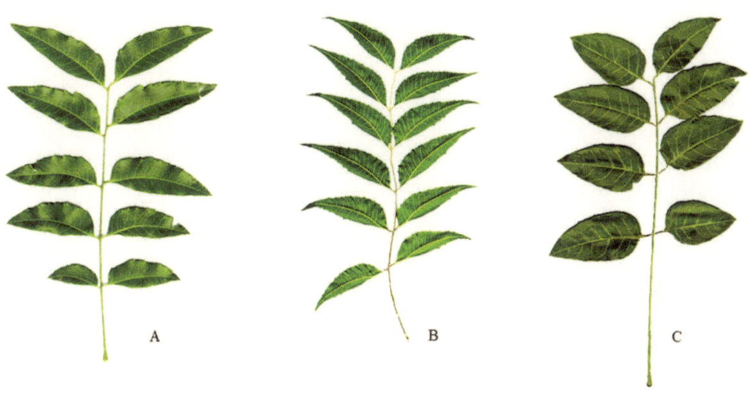

Figure 4. Physical characteristics of *Azadirachta* plants; A = Siamese neem tree (*Azadirachta indica* var. *siamensis*), B = neem (*Azadirachta indica*), C = marrango tree (*Azadirachta excela*).

For the antioxidant effect, *Azadirachta* plants were reported to promote *in vitro* activities tested by various methods. Extracts from the leaves of *A. indica, A. indica* var. *siamensis,* and *A. excelsa* were reported to promote *in vitro* antioxidant effects determined by a DPPH scavenging assay, Fremy's salt assay, ESR detection of POBN spin adducts, and an oxygen consumption assay [45, 46]. The leaf's aqueous and flower ethanol extracts from the Siamese neem tree provide antioxidant activity on lipid peroxidation formation induced by UV-irradiation of a Chago K-1 bronchogenic cell culture at a concentration of 100 μg/ml determined by the thiobarbituric acid reactive substances (TBARS) method [47].

Cloning and expression analysis of genes involving flavonoid biosynthesis showed that Siamese neem tree leaves total RNA contained nucleotide sequences related to enzymes F3′H, FLS, DFR, and F3′5′H, which could be responsible for the biosynthesis of the antioxidant flavonoids [48]. Some flavonoids that were separated from Siamese neem tree and neem leaves and flowers are kaempferol, myricetin, quercetin, and rutin [39, 49–51]. The chemical structures of some flavonoids found in *Azadirachta* plants are shown in **Figure 5**.

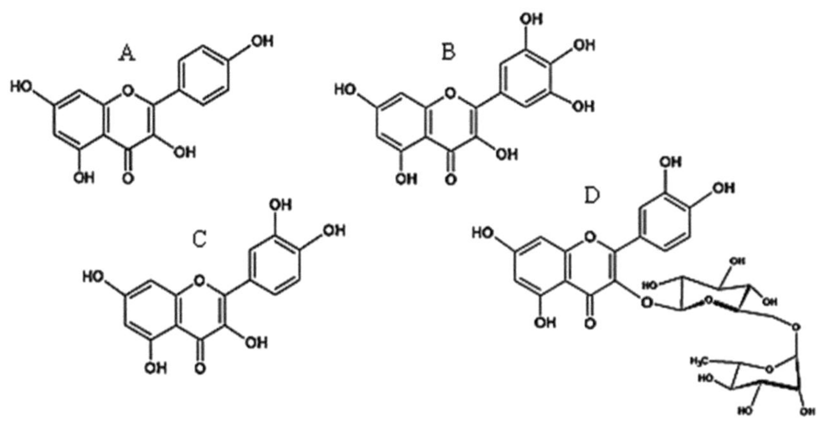

Figure 5. Chemical structures of some flavonoids found in *Azadirachta* plants. A = kaempferol, B = myricetin, C = quercetin, D = rutin.

4.3. *Russula* mushrooms

It is well established that many compounds separated from mushrooms can be used as immuno-modulators or as biological response modifiers [52]. Several mushroom species in Basidiomycetes have been reported to possess anti-tumor activity [53, 54].

Many phytochemical compounds have been reported in various mushrooms, and they can be classified into two main groups: high molecular weight compounds such as beta-glucan and other polysaccharides [55] and low molecular weight compounds including polyphenolics, flavonoids, and terpenoids [52]. Polyphenolics such as caffeic acid, chlorogenic acid, ferulic acid, and gallic acid and flavonoids such as myricetin and catechin were found in *Agaricusbisporus, Boletus edulis, Calocybe gambosa,* and *Cantharellus cibarius* [56]. Triterpeniods were found in *Agaricus bisporus, Ganoderma lucidum,* and *Russula lepida*. Moreover, aristolane sesquiterpenoids were also found in *Russula lepida* [57]. Polysaccharides were found in *Agaricus bisporus, Agaricus brasiliensis, Ganoderma lucidum,* and *Phellinus linteus* [58]. Some polysaccharides such as beta-glucan are reported to promote immunomodulatory effects via CR3, the leukocytemembrane receptor for β-glucans [59]. The mechanisms of the action of the mushrooms to promote anticancer effects have been reported as NF-κB inhibitors, protein kinase inhibitors, protein and DNA alkylating agents, modulators of G1/S and G2/M phases, inhibitors of MAPK protein kinase signaling pathways, aromatase and sulfatase inhibitors, matrix metalloproteinases inhibitors, cyclooxygenase inhibitors, DNA topoisomerases, and DNA polymerase inhibitors and anti-angiogenic substances [52].

A previous study reported the presence of 1147 mushroom species in the Northeast part of Thailand. They are composed of 647 consumed mushroom species, 222 trade mushroom species, and 400 poisonous mushroom species [60]. Thirty-seven species of these mushrooms are used in traditional medicine [60]. However, there are still some mushrooms in Thailand, especially in the Northeastern part of the country, that have never been studied for their biological properties and phytochemical compounds.

The Russula mushroom's shape resembles an umbrella. There have a clear cap and stem, with the gills underneath the cap. The cap is thin and has an underlying radius arranged around the center. The mushroom has no ring and no latex in the cap. The mushroom is fresh, soft, fragile, and perishable [61]. There are around 750 worldwide species of *Russula* [62, 63]. The distribution of the *Russula* species shows that they are present in several countries, including the United States of America, Sweden, France, Norway, Madagascar, Italy, Belgium, Taiwan, China, Japan, and Thailand [64]. In Thailand, *Russula* mushrooms have been found in 17 provinces in the Northeastern region of Thailand [65]. Numerous *Russula* mushrooms have been consumed as food such as *R. monspeliensis, R. virescens, R. alboareolata, R. medullata,* and *R. helios* [65, 66]. Various *Russula* mushrooms have been traditionally used for the treatments of various diseases such as *R. cyanoantha* and *R. nobilis,* which are used for the treatment of fever; *R. luteotacta,* which is used for wound healing; and *R. delica* and *R. parazurea,* which are used for the treatment of gastritis and high blood pressure, while *R. acrifolia* is used for treatments of skin cancer [36]. Moreover, some *Russula* mushrooms have also been traditionally used for tonic purposes such as *R. cyanoxantha, R. nobilis, R. delica, R. parazurea, R. acrifolia,* and *R. luteotacta* [67]. In addition, *Russula luteotacta* has been used as a sleep promoting agent [67]. Physical characteristics of some *Russula* mushrooms found in Thailand are shown in **Figure 6**.

Ten *Russula* mushroom collected from northeastern part of Thailand: *R. crustosa, R. delica, R. monspeliensis, R. velenovskyi, R. virescens, R. lepida, R. alboareolata, R. paludosa, R. medullata,* and *R. helios* were tested for their *in vitro* antioxidant activities using a photochemiluminescence assay for both lipid-soluble and water-soluble antioxidant capacities. *R. medullata* extract exhibited the highest antioxidant effects in both lipid-soluble and water-soluble models with antioxidant capacities of 1.1658 nmol of trolox equivalence and 1.323 nmol of ascorbic acid equivalence, respectively [68].

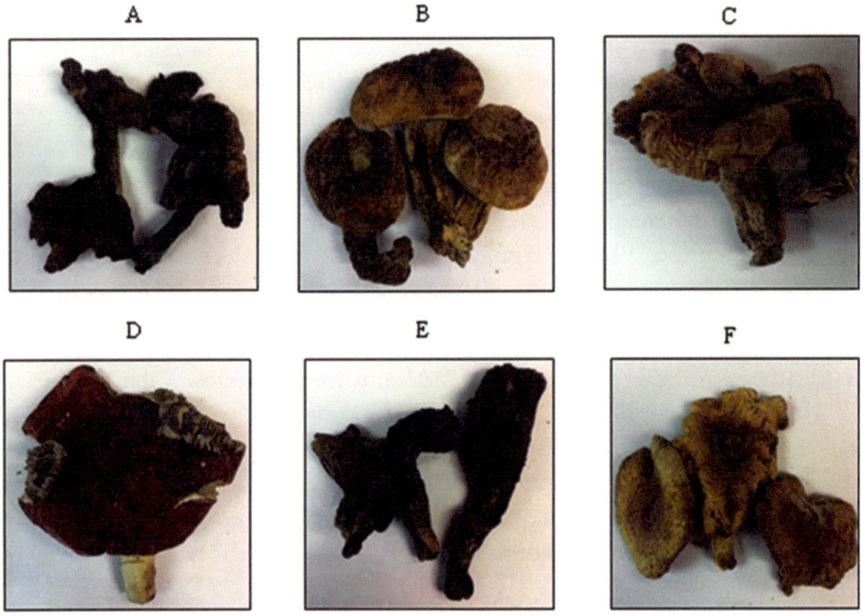

Figure 6. Physical characteristics of some Russula mushrooms found in Thailand; A = *Russula crustosa* Peck, B = *Russula delica* Fries, C = *Russula monspeliensis* Sarnari, D = *Russula velenovskyi* Melzer & Zvára, E = *Russula virescens* (Schaeff) Fries, F = *Russula alboareolata* Hongo.

Some chemical constituents have been reported from *Russula* mushrooms including phenolic acids such as ϱ-hydroxy-benzoic acid, chlorogenic acid, ferulic acid, caffeic acid, protocatechuic acid, and coumaric acid and flavonoids such as quercetin, chrysin, and catechin [69–71]. Some terpeniods were also found in *Russula* mushrooms including aristolane and marasmane [57, 72]. The chemical structures of the constituents found in *Russula* mushrooms are shown in **Figure 7**.

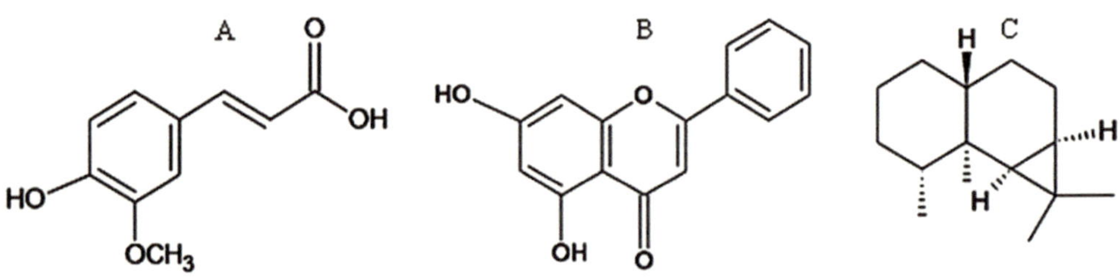

Figure 7. Chemical structures of some flavonoids found in *Russula* mushrooms. A = ferulic acid, B = chrysin, C = aristolane.

5. Conclusion

Natural products have been main sources of drug discoveries including the development of active compounds or formulas for the treatment of cancers. Even though it has become difficult to discover or synthesize new active components, with the knowledge and intelligence regarding traditional medicine, there are still several ethnomedical herbal formulas and regional plants that could be studied and developed for further medicinal utilizations. Herbal remedies from Wat Tha-it and Wat Khampramong, Thailand, are examples of the efforts to develop anticancer therapies from traditional knowledge. Both remedies can inhibit the growth of various cancer cell lines. The stem extract and active compound, Berberine from the Thai medicinal plant *Coscinium fenestratum*, significantly promoted anti-proliferative activity on human colorectal cancer cells with the mechanism of action via NAG-1 and AFT3. Plants in the genus *Azadirachta* have been traditionally used as a tonic. They promote significant antioxidant activities, which could support the body's systems and prevent oxidative stress, which is one of the causes of carcinogenesis. *Russula* is the local mushroom species in the Northeastern part of Thailand. They promote significant antioxidant effects in both lipid-soluble and water-soluble models. These plants and natural products have the potential to be sources of anticancer compounds or active extracts for the treatments of cancer. However, standardization and quality control of the extract or active compounds should be performed before studying the toxicity, *in vivo* biological activity tests, and further clinical studies in the future.

Acknowledgements

The authors acknowledge the Thailand Institute of Scientific and Technological Research for the support in supplying the photos of *Russula* mushrooms. The authors would like to thank Dr. Prapaipat Klungsupya for her valuable guidance and support about photochemiluminescence assays. The authors also thank Ms. Charinan Jaengklang for her assistance in the *Russula* mushrooms work.

Author details

Pongtip Sithisarn[1]* and Piyanuch Rojsanga[2]

*Address all correspondence to: pongtip.sit@mahidol.ac.th

1 Department of Pharmacognosy, Faculty of Pharmacy, Mahidol University, Bangkok, Thailand

2 Department of Pharmaceutical Chemistry, Faculty of Pharmacy, Mahidol University, Bangkok, Thailand

References

[1] Attasara P, Buasom R (2009). Hospital-based cancer registry. National Cancer Institute. Department of Medical Services. Ministry of Public Health. [Access on January 10, 2017] http://www.nci.go.th/th/File_download/Nci%20Cancer%20Registry/hospital%20based%20cancer%20registry.pdf

[2] Cooper GM, Sunderland MA (2000). The development and causes of cancer. The cell: a molecular approach. 2nd edition. Sinauer Associates.

[3] Jiratchariyakul W (2015). Anticancer substances in medicinal plants. M and M Laser Printing Co. Ltd. Bangkok (book in Thai).

[4] Kummalue T (2012). Anticancer mechanisms of medicinal plants, a medical research. Faculty of Medicine Siriraj Hospital, Mahidol University. Bangkok (book in Thai).

[5] Evans WC (2009). Trease and Evans Pharmacognosy. 16th edition. Elsevier. London.

[6] Ondee S, Sithisarn P, Ruangwises N, Rojsanga P (2015). Anti-proliferative activity on colorectal cancer cells of thirty Thai edible plants. Proceeding in the 1st international conference on pharmacy education and research network of ASEAN, Bangkok, Thailand, December, 2-4.

[7] Shibata MA, Iinuma M, Morimoto J, Kurose H, Akamatsu K, Okuno Y, Akao Y, Otsuki Y (2011). α-Mangostin extracted from the pericarp of the mangosteen (*Garcinia mangostana* Linn) reduces tumor growth and lymph node metastasis in an immunocompetent xenograft model of metastatic mammary cancer carrying a p53 mutation. BMC Med. 9(69):1-18.

[8] Naowaratwattana W, De-eknamkul W, De Mejia EG (2010). Phenolic containing organic extracts of mulberry (Morusalba L.) leaves inhibit Hep G2 hepatoma cell through G2/M phase arrest, induction of apoptosis, and inhibition of topoisomerase II alpha activity. J Med Food. 13(5):1045-56.

[9] Dakeng S, Duangmano S, Jiratchariyakul W, U-pratya Y, Bogler O, Patmasiriwat P (2012). Inhibition of Wnt signaling by cucurbitacin B in breast cancer cells: reduction of Wnt-associated proteins and reduced translocation of galectin-3-mediated β-catenin to the nucleus. J Cell Biochem. 113(1):49-60.

[10] Hsu YL, Wu LY, Kuo PL (2009). Dehydrocostus lactone, a medicinal plant-derived sesquiterpene lactone, induces apoptosis coupled to endoplasmic reticulum stress in liver cancer cells. J Pharmacol Exp Ther. 329(2):808-19.

[11] Kummalue T, Sujiwattanarat P, Jiratchariyakul W (2011). Apoptosis inducibility of Sapindusrorak water extract on A549 human lung cancer cell line. J Med Plant Res. 5(7):1087-94.

[12] Kaewkon W, Khamprasert N, Limpeanchob N (2011). Derris scandens Benth extract induced necrosis rather than apoptosis of SW480 colon cancer cell. Thai J Pharmacol. 33(2):118-21.

[13] Moongkarndi P, Jaisupa N, Kosem N, Konlata J, Samer J, Pattanapanyasat K, Rodpai E (2015). Effect of purified α-mangostin from mangosteen pericarp on cytotoxicity, cell cycle arrest and apoptotic gene expression in human cancer cells. World J Pharm Sci. 3(8):1473-84.

[14] Chirathaworn C, Kongcharoensuntorn W, Dechdoungchan T, Lowanitchapat A, Sa-nguanmoo P, Poovorawan Y (2007). Myristica fragrans Houtt. methanolic extract

induces apoptosis in a human leukemia cell line through SIRT1 mRNA downregulation. J Med Assoc Thai. 90(11):2422-8.

[15] Jiratcgariyakul W, Okabe H, Moongkarndi P, Frahm AW (1998). Cytotoxic glycosphingolipid from Murdannia loriformis (Hassk.) Rolla Rao et Kammathy. Thai J Phytopharm. 5(1):10-20.

[16] Sudha P, Syed M, Sunil D, Gowda C (2010). Immunomodulatory activity of methanolic leaf extract of Moringa oleifera in animals. Indian J Physiol Pharmacol. 54(2):133-40.

[17] Srisapoomi T, Jiratchariyakul W, O-partkiattikul N, Kummalue T (2008). Effects of two Thai herbal remedies on the sensitivity of chemotherapeutic agents in human cancer cells. Asian J Trad Med. 3(4):144-52.

[18] Soonthornchareonnon N, Sireeratawong S, Wiwat C, Ruangwises N, Wongnopphavich A, Jaijoy K (2011). Research and development of anti-cancer formula from Wat Khampramong. National Research Council of Thailand. Faculty of Pharmacy, Mahidol University, Bangkok.

[19] Baek SJ, Kim KS, Nixon JB, Wilson LC, Eling TE (2001). Cyclooxygenase inhibitors regulate the expression of a TGF-beta superfamily member that has proapoptotic and antitumorigenic activities. Mol Pharmacol 59:901-8.

[20] Rojsanga P, Sukhthankar M, Krisanapan C, Gritsanapun W, Lawson DB, Baek SJ (2010). In vitro anti-proliferative activity of alcoholic stem extract of *Coscinium fenestratum* in human colorectal cancer cells. Exp Ther Med. 1:181-6.

[21] Baek SJ, Kim JS, Jackson FR, Eling TE, McEntee MF, Lee SH (2004). Epicatechin gallate induced expression of NA G-1 is associated with growth inhibition and apoptosis in colon cancer cells. Carcinogenesis. 25:2425-32.

[22] Baek SJ, Wilson LC, Eling TE (2002). Resveratrol enhances the expression of non-steroidal anti-inflammatory drug-activated gene (NA G-1) by increasing the expression of p53. Carcinogenesis. 23: 425-34.

[23] Martinez JM, Sali T, Okazaki R, Anna C, Hollingshead M, Hose C, Monks A, Walker NJ, Baek SJ, Eling TE (2006). Drug-induced expression of nonsteroidal anti-inflammatory drug-activated gene/macrophage inhibitory cytokine-1/prostate-derived factor, a putative tumor suppressor, inhibits tumor growth. J Pharmacol Exp Ther. 318:899-906.

[24] Rojsanga P, Sukhthankar M, Baek SJ (2007). Berberine, a natural isoquinoline alkaloid, induces NAG-1 and AFT3 expression in human colorectal cancer cells. Cancer Lett. 258(2): 230-40.

[25] Lee SH, Cekanova M, Baek SJ (2008). Multiple mechanisms are involved in 6-gingerol-induced cell growth arrest and apoptosis in human colorectal cancer cells. Mol Carcinog. 47:197-208.

[26] Forman LL (1991). Menispermaceae. Bangkok: The Forest Herbarium.300-65.

[27] Wattanathorn J, Uabundit N, Itarat W, Mucimapura S, Laopatarakasem P, Sripanidkulchai B (2006). Neurotoxicity of Coscinium fenestratum stem, a medicinal plant used in traditional medicine. Food Chem Toxicol. 44:1327-33.

[28] Cross EC (1987). Oxygen radicals and human disease. Ann Intern Med. 107: 526-45.

[29] Carocho M, Ferreira ICFR (2013). The role of phenolic compounds in the fight against cancer-a review. Anticancer Agents Medicinal Chem. 13:1236-58.

[30] Ji B, Hsu W, Yang J, Hsia T, Lu C, Chiang J, Yang J, Lin C, Lin J, Suen L, Wood WG, Chung J (2009). Gallic acid inducesapoptosisviacaspase-3 and mitochondrion-dependent pathways in vitro and suppresses lung xenograft tumor growth in vivo. J Agric Food Chem. 57:7596-7604.

[31] Kim S, Gaber MW, Zawaski JA, Zhang F, Richardson M, Zhang XA, Yang Y (2009). The inhibition of glioma growth in vitro and in vivo by a chitosan/ellagic acid composite biomaterial. Biomaterials. 30:4743-51.

[32] Baskaran N, Manoharan S, BalakrishnanS, Pugalendhi P (2010). Chemopreventive potential of ferulic acid in 7,12-dimethylbenz[a]anthracene-induced mammary carcinogenesis in Sprague-Dawley rats. Eur J Pharmacol. 637:22-9.

[33] Nair H, Rao KVK, Aalinkeel R, Mahajan S, Chawda R, Schwartz SA (2004). Inhibition of prostate cancer cell colony formation by the flavonoid quercetin correlates with modulation of specific regulatory genes. Clin Diagn Lab Immunol. 11:63-9.

[34] Yuan Z, Chen L, Fan L, Tang M, Yang G, Yang H, Du X, Wang G, Yao W, Zhao Q, Ye B, Wang R, Diao P, Zhang W, Wu H, Zhao X, Wei Y (2006). Liposomal quercetin efficiently suppresses growth of solid tumors in murine models. Clin Cancer Res. 12:3193-9.

[35] Zhang H, Zhang M, Yu L, Zhao Y, HeN, Yang, X (2012).Antitumor activitiesofquercetin and quercetin-50,8-disulfonate in human colon and breast cancer cell lines. Food Chem Toxicol. 50:1589-99.

[36] Suttajit S, Khansuwan U, Suttajit M (2002). Antioxidative activity of Thai medicinal herbs. Thai J Pharm Sci. 26(suppl.):32.

[37] Trakoontivakorn G, Saksitpitak J (2000). Antioxidative potential of Thai indigenous vegetable extracts. Journal of Food Research and Product Development. Kasetsart University. 30(3):164-76.

[38] Sombatsiri K, Ermel K, Schmutterer H (1995). Other Meliaceous plants containing ingredients for integrated pest management and further purpose. In: Schmutter H. The neem tree Azadirachtaindica A. Juss. and other meliaceous plants. Germany: VCH.

[39] Sithisarn P, Gritsanapan W (2008). Siamese neem tree: A plant from kitchen to antioxidative health supplement. Advances in Phytotherapy Research. Research Signpost. Kerala. India.

[40] Clayton T, Soralump P, Chaukul W, Temsiririrkkul R (1996). Medicinal plants in Thailand volume 1. Bangkok: Amarin Printing.

[41] Te-Chato S, Rungnoi O (2000). Induction of somatic embryogenesis from leaves of Sadao Chang (Azadirachta excelsa (Jack) Jacobs). Sci Horticult. 86:311-21.

[42] Arivazhagan S, Balasenthil S, Nagini S (2000). Garlic and neem extracts enhance hepatic glutathione-dependent enzymes during N-methyl-N-nitro-N-nitrosoguanidine (MNNG)-induced gastric carcinogenesis in rats. Phytother Res. 14:291-3.

[43] Akudugu J, Gade G, Bohm L (2001). Cytotoxicity of axadirachtin A inhuman glioblastoma cell lines. Life Sci. 68:1153-60.

[44] Subapriya R, Nagini S (2003). Ethanolicneem leaf extracts protects againstN-methyl-N-nitro-N-nitrosoguanidine-induced gastric carcinogenesis inWistar rats. Asian Pac J Cancer Prev. 4:215-23.

[45] Sithisarn P, Gritsanapan W, Supabphol R (2004). Free radical scavenging activity of three Azadirachta plants. Proceeding in the 21st Annual Research meeting in Pharmaceutical Sciences, Bangkok, Thailand, December, 23-24, 2004.

[46] Sithisarn P, Carlsen CU, Andersen ML, Gritsanapan W, Skibsted LH (2007). Antioxidative effects of leaves from Azadirachta species of different provenience. Food Chem. 104: 1539-49.

[47] Sithisarn P, Supabphol R, Gritsanapan W (2005). Antioxidant activity of Siamese neem tree. J Ethophamacol. 99: 109-12.

[48] Sithisarn P, Suksangpanomrung M, Gritsanapan W (2007). Gene expression of enzymes related to biosynthesis of antioxidative flavonoids in Siamese neem tree leaves. Planta Med. 73: 222.

[49] Pankadamani KS, Seshadri TR (1952). Survey of anthoxanthins. Proc Indian Acad Sci Ser A 36: 157-69.

[50] Nakov N, Labode O, Akahtaedzhiev K (1982). Study of the flavonoid composition of *Azadirachta indica*. Farmatsiya (Sofia). 32:24-8.

[51] Siddiqui S, Mahmood T, Siddiqui BS, Faizi S (1985). Studies in the nonterpenoial constituents of Azadirachtaindica. Pak J Sci Ind Res. 28(1):1-4.

[52] Zaidman BZ, Yassin M, Mahajna J, Wasser SP (2005). Medicinal mushroom modulators of molecular targets as cancer therapeutics. Appl Microbiol Biotechnol. 67: 453-68.

[53] Mizuno T (1995). Bioactive biomolecules of mushrooms: food function and medicinal effect of mushroom fungi. Food Rev Int. 11:7-21.

[54] Wasser SP (2002). Medicinal mushrooms as a source of antitumor and immunomodulating polysaccharides. Appl Microbiol Biotechnol. 60:258-274.

[55] Jaruntorn B, Chanida H (2010). Spatial distribution of Beta glucan containing wild mushroom communities in subtropical dry forest, Thailand. Fungal Divers. 46(1): 29-42.

[56] Palacios I, Lozano M, Moro C, D'Arrigo M, Rostagno MA, Martínez JA, García-Lafuente A, Guillamón E, Villares A (2011). Antioxidant properties of phenolic compounds occurring in edible mushrooms. Food Chem. 128:674-8.

[57] Jian-Wen T, Ze-Jun D, Ji-Kai L (2000). New terpenoids from Basidiomycetes Russula lepida. Helv Chim Acta. 83:3191-7.

[58] Kozarski M, Klaus A, Niksic M, Jakovljevic D, Helsper JPFG, Van Griensven LJLD (2011). Antioxidative and immunomodulating activities of polysaccharide extracts of the medicinal mushrooms Agaricusbisporus, Agaricusbrasiliensis, Ganodermalucidum and Phellinuslinteus. Food Chem. 129(4):1667-75.

[59] Xia Y, Vetvicka V, Yan J, Hanikyrova M, Mayadas T, Ross GD (1999). The beta-glucan-binding lectin site of mouse CR3 (CD11b/CD18) and its function in generating a primed state of the receptor that mediates cytotoxic activation in response to iC3b-opsonized target cells. J Immunol. 162:2281-90.

[60] The Bureau of Thai Indigenous Medicine, Department for Development of Thai Traditional and Alternative Medicine. Ministry of Public Health (2011). Mushrooms are health food from folk medicine. The Bureau of Thai Indigenous Medicine, Department for Development of Thai Traditional and Alternative Medicine. Ministry of Public Health. Nonthaburi. (book in Thai).

[61] Sonoamuang N (2010). Wild mushrooms of Thailand: biodiversity and utilization. Department of Plant Science and Natural Resources. Faculty of Agriculture, Khon Kaen University.

[62] Joshi S, Bhatt RP, Stephenson SL (2012). The current status of the family Russulaceae in the Uttarakhand Himalaya, India. Mycosphere. 3(4):486-501.

[63] Jain N, Pande V (2013). Diversity analysis of ectomycorrhizal genus Russula using RAPD markers. Octa Jour Env Res. 1(4):332-5.

[64] Buyck B, Hofstetter V, Eberhardt U, Verbeken A, Kauff F (2008). Walking the thin line between *Russula* and *Lactarius*: the dilemma of Russula subsect. Ochricompactae. Fungal Divers. 28:15-40.

[65] Manassila M, Sooksa-Nguan T, Boonkerd N, Rodtongb S, Teaumroonga N (2005). Phylogenetic diversity of wild edible Russula from Northeastern Thailand on the basis of internal transcribed spacer sequence. Science Asia. 31:323-8.

[66] Quiñónez-Martínez M, Ruan-Soto F, AguilarMoreno IE, Garza-Ocañas F, LebgueKeleng T, Lavín-Murcio PA, Enríquez-Anchondo ID (2014). Knowledge and use of edible mushrooms in two municipalities of the Sierra Tarahumara, Chihuahua, Mexico. J Ethnobiol Ethnomed. 10(67):1-13.

[67] Sanmeea R, Dellb B, Lumyongc P, Izumorid K, Lumyong S (2003). Nutritive value of popular wild edible mushrooms from northern Thailand. Food Chem. 82: 527-32.

[68] Jaengklang C, Jarikasem S, Sithisarn P, Klungsupya P (2015). Determination on antioxidant capacity and TLC analysis of ten Thai Russula mushroom extracts. Isan J Pharm Sci. 10:241-50.

[69] Yaltirak T, Aslim B, Ozturk S, Alli H (2009). Antimicrobial and antioxidant activities of Russula delica Fr. Food Chem Toxicol. 47:2052-6.

[70] Chen XH, Xia LX, Zhou HB, Qiu GZ (2010). Chemical composition and antioxidant activities of Russula griseocarnosa sp. nov. J Agric Food Chem. 58:6966-71.

[71] Kalogeropoulos N, Yanni AE, Koutrotsios G, Aloupi M (2013). Bioactive microconstituents and antioxidant properties of wild edible mushrooms from the island of Lesvos, Greece. Food Chem Toxicol. 55:378-85.

[72] Clericuzio M, Cassino C, Corana F, Vidari G (2012). Terpenoids from Russula lepida and Russula amarissima (Basidiomycota, Russulaceae). Phytochemistry. 84:154-9.

Section 2

Nutrients and Herbal Anticancer Agents

Phytocompounds Targeting Cancer Angiogenesis Using the Chorioallantoic Membrane Assay

Stefana Avram, Roxana Ghiulai, Ioana Zinuca Pavel,
Marius Mioc, Roxana Babuta, Mirela Voicu,
Dorina Coricovac, Corina Danciu,
Cristina Dehelean and Codruta Soica

Additional information is available at the end of the chapter

http://dx.doi.org/10.5772/intechopen.68506

Abstract

Cancer is the second cause of mortality worldwide. Angiogenesis is an important process involved in the growth of primary tumors and metastasis. New approaches for controlling the cancer progression and invasiveness can be addressed by limiting the angiogenesis process. An increasingly large number of natural compounds are evaluated as angiogenesis inhibitors. The chorioallantoic membrane (CAM) assay represents an *in vivo* attractive experimental model for cancer and angiogenesis studies as prescreening to the murine models. Since the discovery of tumor angiogenesis, the CAM has been intensively used in cancer research. The advantages of this *in vivo* technique are in terms of low time-consuming, costs, and a lower number of sacrificed animals. Currently, a great number of natural compounds are being investigated for their effectiveness in controlling tumor angiogenesis. Potential reducing of angiogenesis has been investigated by our group for pentacyclic triterpenes, in various formulations, and differences in their mechanism were registered. This chapter aims to give an overview on a number of phytocompounds investigated using *in vitro*, murine models and the chorioallantoic membrane assay as well as to emphasize the use of CAM assay in the study of natural compounds with potential effects in malignancies.

Keywords: phytocompounds, tumor angiogenesis, chorioallantoic membrane assay

1. Introduction

Angiogenesis represents the process by which new vessels are formed from preexisting vessels [1] and has important implications associated with tumor growth and metastasis [2]. Studies have shown that neovascularization is essential for tumor survival and growth, whereas in angiogenic absent conditions, tumor may display necrosis or even apoptosis [3, 4]. The angiogenic switch represents the process in which endothelial cells are led to a rapid growth state induced by stimuli secreted by the tumor microenvironment, comprising tumor and stromal cells, extracellular matrix components, immunologic cells, fibroblasts, adipocytes, muscle cells, and pericytes [5]. The switch may also involve downregulation of endogenous inhibitors of angiogenesis such as endostatin, angiostatin, or thrombospondin.

The undergoing of tumor angiogenesis represents a four-step process [6]: (i) tissue basement membrane injury; (ii) migration of endothelial cells, activated by angiogenic factors; (iii) endothelial cell proliferation and stabilization; (iv) continuous angiogenesis induced by angiogenic factors. Therefore, key elements in the angiogenesis process are the endogenous angiogenic factors. The most relevant angiogenic activators, signal mediators, and signaling effects are represented in **Figure 1**.

A class of proteins that is widely responsible for tumor angiogenesis is represented by growth factors, such as the vascular endothelial growth factor (VEGF), fibroblast growth factor (FGF), platelet-derived endothelial growth factor (PDGF), tumor necrosis factor-α (TNF-α), epidermal growth factor (EGF), placental growth factor (PGF), transforming growth factor (TGF), granulocyte colony stimulating factor (GCSF), hepatocyte growth factor (HGF), angiostatin, and angiogenin [7]. However, VEGF is thought to be the main proangiogenic growth factor, because it induces all four phases of angiogenesis by augmenting vascular permeability, endothelial cell proliferation, endothelial cell migration, and capillary like tube formation [8]. Angiogenic cytokines or other growth factors such as VEGF are expressed under hypoxia conditions or by various oncogenes (e.g., mutant ras, erbB-2/HER2) [9].

As shown in **Figure 1**, after binding the tyrosine kinase specific domain of the receptors, multiple ways of signaling are possible for the angiogenic factors. Important molecular mechanisms involve activation of RAS/RAF1/kinase through the extracellular signal (ERK-1 și-2), inducing proliferation and differentiation; RAS/p38 mitogen-activated kinase (MAPK) and JUN/kinase 1-3 N-terminal, modulating inflammation, apoptosis, and differentiation; phosfatidyl-3-inositol kinase-1 (PI3K) and AKT dependent, regulating cell survival, mammalian receptor for rapamycin (mTOR), highly involved in proliferation and cell growth. Other inductor factors of the signaling pathways of angiogenesis are found in the cytoplasm (e.g., GAB1, SHC, SRC, PI3K, and phosfolipase γ C) [10].

VEGF and its receptors, the VEGFR family, remain intensively researched for targeting angiogenesis in different tumors. At the same time, other angiogenesis suppressing-related targets are being studied for the development of anticancer therapies for tumors resistant to anti-VEGF therapy. A number of therapeutic agents are currently in use for several malignancies: monoclonal antibodies against angiogenic growth factors (e.g., antibody against VEGF, Bevacizumab), inhibitors of angiogenic factors synthesis (e.g., mTOR inhibitor Rapamycin), and inhibitors of angiogenic factor receptors (tyrosine-kinase inhibitors, e.g., imatinib and sorafenib) [11]. Unfortunately, clinical response to the new molecular advances in cancer therapy by targeting angiogenesis is unsatisfactory. Resistance and low survival rates are signaled. New therapeutic approaches with minimal side effects are desired to act by targeting the multiple factors that are activated during tumor progression.

http://dx.doi.org/10.5772/intechopen.68506

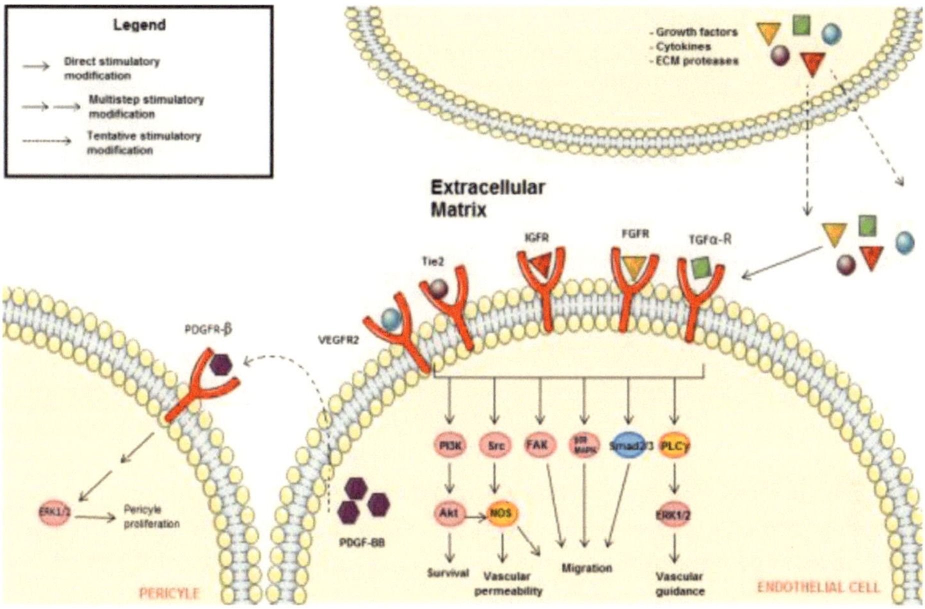

Figure 1. Angiogenic factors and signaling pathways involved in angiogenesis mediation. Abbreviations: Akt, RAC-alpha serine/threonine-protein kinase, ERK1/2, mitogen-activated protein kinase 1/2, FAK, focal adhesion kinase; FGFR, fibroblast growth factor receptor; IGFR, insulin growth factor receptor; MAPK, mitogen-activated protein kinases; NOS, nitric oxide synthase; p38, mitogen-activated protein kinase 11; PDGFR, olated-delivered endothelial growth factor receptor; PI3K, phosphatidylinositol 4,5-bisphosphate 3-kinase; PLCγ, phospholipase C gamma; Smad, Smad protein; Src, proto-oncogene tyrosine-protein kinase; TGFα-R, transforming growth factor α receptor; Tie, angiopoietin receptor; VEGFR, vascular endothelial growth factor receptor.

Based on the preventive effect that healthy diets have on the epidemiology of cancer, medicinal plants, spices, fruits, and vegetables represent an interesting source of phytochemicals. Natural compounds or even plant extracts are now considered important and accessible therapeutic or chemopreventive agents in cancer. In the search of the suitable phytocompounds to test for specific effects, virtual screening methods can be successfully applied in the selection of selective compounds for specific targets [12]. To avoid lack of selectivity, computational filtering schemes can be used [13]. Extensive studies demonstrate the high potential of plant-derived chemicals in controlling tumor angiogenesis with minimal secondary effects and drug resistance, by targeting multiple key pathways in a synergistic manner.

2. Experimental models for tumor angiogenesis: focus on the CAM assay

An important issue in angiogenesis studies is the appropriate choice of the assays. To evaluate the efficacy of potential phytocompounds and to identify potential targets within the angiogenic process, several methods both *in vitro* and *in vivo* can be applied. Each of them having one or more drawbacks, ideally more techniques are to be applied. *In vitro* techniques are used by co-culturing endothelial cell and other tumor microenvironment factors with tumor cells in 2D or even 3D models which facilitate the identification of the involved molecular mechanisms. Despite the advances made in the direction of designing *in vitro* assays, the *in vivo* environment can be difficultly reproduced with such protocols [14]. To better assess the key aspects of tumor angiogenesis and therapeutic approaches, *in vivo* assays can be applied, such as the chick chorioallantoic membrane (CAM), the zebrafish, the sponge implantation, the corneal, or dorsal air sac and tumor angiogenesis models in rodents or rabbits [15]. Several drawbacks can still be cited, especially for the murine models, including high costs, complex technical and surgical abilities, and important quantities of test compounds.

2.1. Chorioallantoic membrane assay

The chorioallantoic membrane (CAM) assay represents an attractive *in vivo* experimental model for angiogenesis and cancer studies. The advantages of this *in vivo* technique in terms of costs, time, simplicity, reproducibility, and ease of the approval by the ethic committee make it a good prescreening assay to murine models in the research of biological systems and new therapeutic targets. Especially tumor angiogenesis and metastasis protocols benefit for a much shorter time for the tumor to grow and metastasize than the classical animal models.

The limitations of the model include a restricted number of reagents to work with due to low compatibility, nonspecific inflammatory reactions, keratinization of the membrane, and a vascular reaction that interferes with the visualization of vascular modifications. Technical skills may be significant to counteract these limitations [16, 17].

The chorioallantoic membrane is the vascularized respiratory extraembryonic tissue of avian species. First, this biologic system has been used for embryologic, immunological, and tumor grafting studies [18], and more recently, since the discovery of tumor angiogenesis [19], it is intensively applied in cancer research [20]. During the stages of embryo development, the immunologic, nervous, and nociceptive systems are not fully developed [21]. Several types of CAM assay protocols have been developed.

2.2. Uses in biological studies

The method can be applied for bioengineering development, morphology, biochemistry, transplant biology, cancer research, and drug development, but also in immunology, wound healing, tissue repair, or drug toxicity [22, 23]. The possibilities of imaging and evaluation have attracted many research studies. Nutritional therapeutics is an example of products approved by the U.S. Food and Drug Administration (FDA) that were preclinically evaluated in the CAM model [16].

Phytocompounds can be tested in order to evaluate their potential bioavailability, tolerability, and lack of irritation effects. For this purpose, the variations of the HET-CAM protocol can be applied, according the Interagency Coordinating Committee on the Validation of Alternative Methods (ICCVAM) recommendations published in November 2006 in Appendix G of reference [24]. Our previous evaluations proved its applicability in testing different sets of compounds, i.e., surfactants and aflatoxins [25].

In the attempt of finding new means for cancer chemoprevention, the chorioallantoic membrane assay can be used to test natural compounds that could reduce or inhibit several pathways involved in malignancies, especially pro-inflammatory cytokine activation and excessive angiogenesis. Tumor microenvironment, including inflammation and angiogenesis next to the development of new therapeutic targets for these pathological conditions, is intensively researched on murine models [26]. Previously, we have evaluated mast cell involvement in the angiogenesis process implementing a mastocytoma model on the CAM assay [27], which can be further developed for the evaluation of natural compounds on mast cells as key participants in the tumor microenvironment.

2.3. General *in ovo* method

Ex ovo or *in ovo* techniques are applicable. The *ex ovo* protocol involves the transfer of the egg content on day 3 of incubation into a Petri dish. It facilitates the visualization of the experiment, but the unnatural milieu of development of the embryo is detrimental to the survival rate of the specimens. Therefore, we prefer the *in ovo* protocol and is the type of method described here.

Fertilized eggs are horizontally incubated 7 days prior to use, at 37°C, in a controlled wet atmosphere. On the third day of incubation, in order to detach the chorioallantoic membrane, a volume of 2–3 ml of albumen is aspired through a perforation at the more pointed end of the eggs. The hole is resealed and returned to the incubator. The next day, a window is cut and resealed on the superior side of the shell. The eggs are returned to incubation until the day of the experiment [28]. Generally, 5–10 eggs are used for each test sample. Samples are applied inside a sterile plastic ring on the surface of the membrane. Samples are applied in triplicate. *In ovo* investigation by means of a stereomicroscope is performed throughout the experiment. Photographs are recorded for further analysis (**Figure 2**).

Starting with day 11 of incubation, samples can be considered active on excessive angiogenesis. The rapid growth of the vessels occurs during days 7–11; therefore, applying substances during this interval can be evaluated in terms of antiangiogenic effects. Morphometric evaluation of the angiogenic reaction can be conducted using a 0–5 arbitrary scale, the mean values expressing the vascular density around the site of application [20]. Finally, specimens are sacrificed and membranes are submitted to histological and immunohistological evaluation. On slides with immunohistochemical marked vessels, the mean microvascular density can be determined using the hotspot method, and counting the blood vessels, to calculate an antiangiogenic index, with the aid of the formula: $AAI = 1 - No_{BVtest}/No_{BVcontrol,}$ AAI = antiangiogenic index, BV = blood vessels [29].

2.4. Tumor angiogenesis model on CAM

Tumor cells are used on the CAM in order to obtain tumors, to study their microenvironment and the effects that phytochemicals might have. Tumor grafts can be used as well. Usually, cultured cancer cells are inoculated on the surface of the CAM, on day 10 of incubation, after being trypsinized and resuspended in culture medium to final concentrations in the range of 10^5–10^6 ml^{-1}. Cells can be applied directly on the CAM using a plastic ring for localizing the cells or using Matrigel impregnated with cells. Further, test compound solutions diluted with minimal DMSO (dimethyl sulfoxide) concentration in phosphate buffer can be applied on the

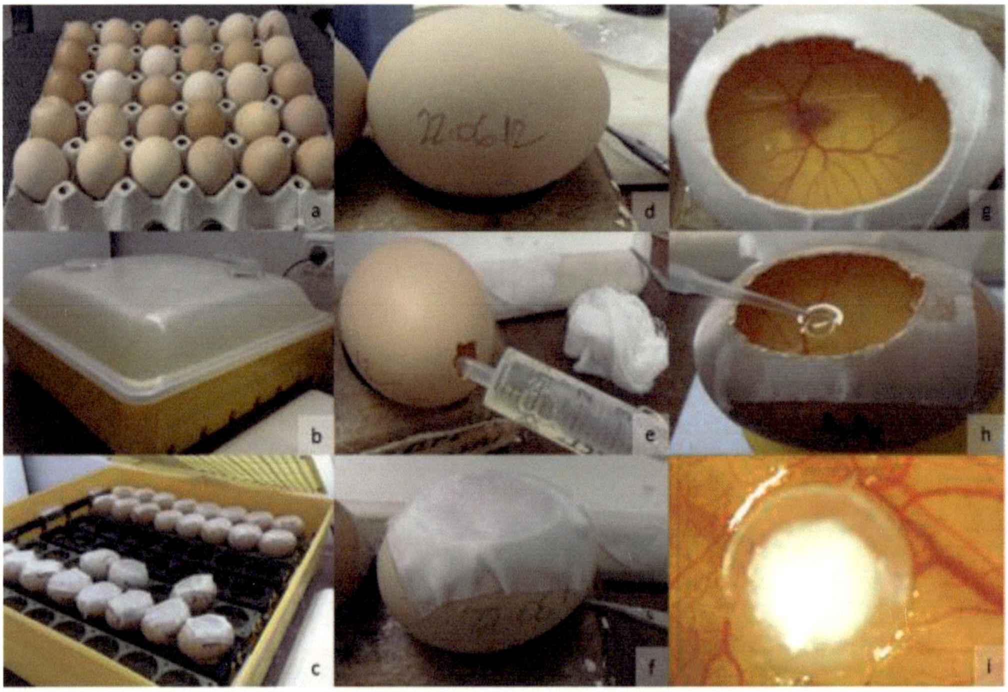

Figure 2. Chorioallantoic membrane assay—*in ovo* practical approach: incubation of the eggs (a–c); albumen removal, shell opening, and resealing (d–f); visualization of the CAM, sample application, and sample application inside a plastic ring (g–i) [30].

same spot as the cancer cell samples. *In ovo* stereomicroscopic follow-up is performed daily to register the changes in the vascular response around the tumor developing area that will be used for the morphometric analysis. On the final day of the experiment, after sacrificing the embryos, tumor masses are measured; the chorioallantoic membrane, the formed tumors, and some organs suspected to have metastasis are harvested and histologically processed.

In order to observe morphologic changes in the chorioallantoic membrane, hematoxylin eosin staining is analyzed. Different panels of immunohistochemical markers can be further applied: tumor cell markers and specific antibodies for different key proteins involved in the tumor microenvironment (e.g., endothelial cell marker-factor VIII, smooth muscle actin (SMA) marker, vascular endothelial growth factors, and its receptors, mast cells marker—Tryptase, the proliferation marker—Ki67). Results can reveal molecular modifications and serve to vascular density quantification.

Our experience is related to testing phytocompounds and plant extracts for the effect on angiogenesis. Using the angiogenesis method in the rapid stage of CAM development, we found that pentacyclic triterpenes, betulinic (BA) acid, and betulin (Bet) in various formulations with cyclodextrin and in nanoemulsion are potential antiangiogenic compounds, acting differently, both through direct and indirect mechanisms [31, 32]. Immunohistochemical staining for smooth muscle actin (SMA) on the specimens treated with betulin in nanoemulsion, next to blank and control samples, are shown in **Figure 3**. The low expression of the marker in the betulin-treated specimen indicates a minimal implication of pericytes in the angiogenesis process [32]. On the contrary, we found that betulinic acid determined rapid maturation of the vessels and high levels of SMA [31]. We also evaluated triterpenes and other types of natural compounds in melanoma models on CAM, which confirms the inhibitory effect on tumor angiogenesis (data not published).

Most studies that use the CAM assay are evaluated through stereomicroscopy that allows a series of quantitative measurements, and by histologic an immunohistological interpretation. Advances in the evaluation techniques include fluorescence microscopy, confocal microscopy, microCT scanning, and imaging, *in situ* hybridization (ISH), quantitative PCR (qPCR) determination of specific targets [16, 33].

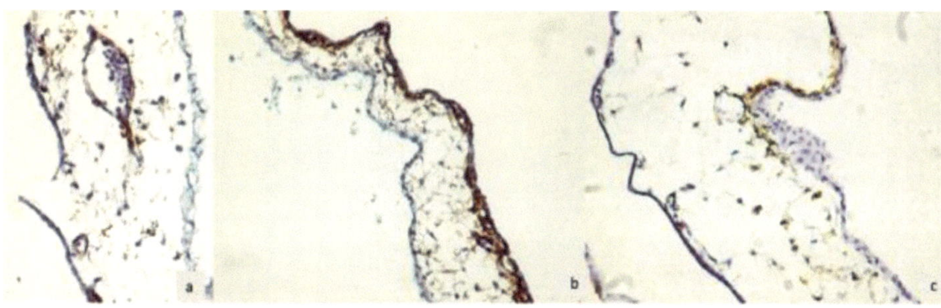

Figure 3. Light microscopic evaluation of CAM sections from ID 11 smooth muscle actin marker: (a) blank specimen, ×40, (b) control specimen treated with nanoemulsion, ×40, (c) specimen treated with betulin in nanoemulsion, ×40 [32].

3. Phytocompounds targeting cancer angiogenesis: *in vitro*, on the chorioallantoic membrane assay, in animal model

Chemicals derived from plant sources as well as various types of extracts have been already investigated for their effects on angiogenesis and on cancer. Currently, based on the failure of the approved therapeutics and also by crediting the traditional medicine philosophy that pathologies are imbalances that have to be rebalanced, the idea of multiple targeting through synergetic phytocompounds mixtures is gaining more attention. Extensive research is being dedicated to the understanding of their mechanism and their efficacy using *in vitro* and *in vivo* methods. The most in depth evidence comes from the results on cell cultures. *In vivo* methods also offer other accurate data on their effects. The chorioallantoic membrane assay is being used by more and more researchers for the evaluation of plant-derived chemicals or extracts. Correlations can be made using the results obtained for *in vitro*, animal and CAM assays, which will improve the knowledge and the future analysis to perform for the active compounds. We reviewed here some of the most investigated phytocompounds concerning the results obtained on all the three experimental models (**Table 1**).

Phytochemical class	Compound	Chemical structure	Plant source	*In vitro* effects	Effects on CAM	*In vivo* effects
Polyphenols	Curcumin	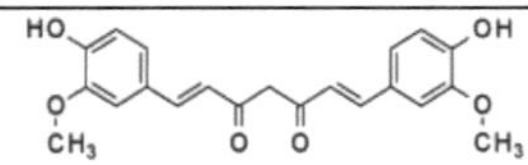	*Curcuma longa* L.	MiaPaCa-2; BxPC-3; Panc-1; MPanc-96 prostate cancer cell lines Reduced expression of NF-κB [34]	Angiogenesis inhibitor on small capillaries [35]	Athymic nude mice xenograft with prostate cancer cells Reduced expression of NFκB-p65, STAT3 and SRC; Reduced expression of ANXA2 and VEGFR2 [36]
	Epigallocatechin-gallate	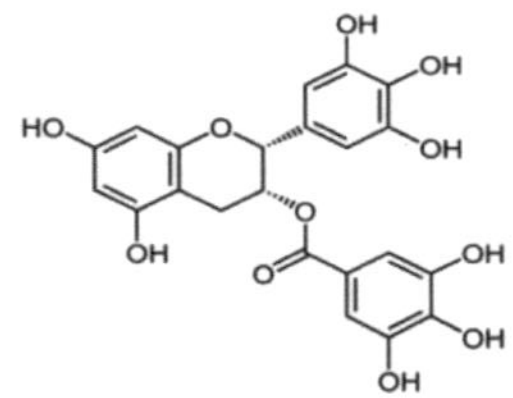	*Camellia sinensis* L.	Hepatocellular carcinoma Inhibition of the VEGF-VEGFR axis [37]	Inhibition of fibroblast growth factor (FGF) and inhibition of mean branch formation and tumor weight of neuroblastoma-induced angiogenesis [38]	BGC-823 human gastric cancer xenograft mice model Reduction of VEGF [39]
Phloroglucinol derivative	Hyperforin	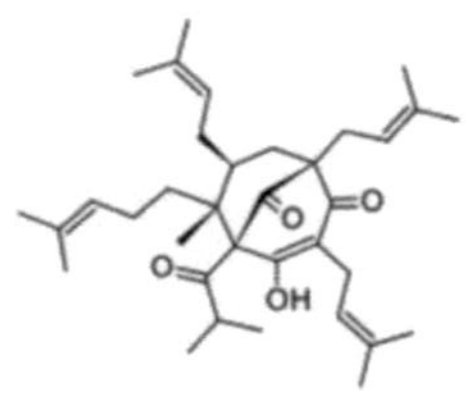	*Hypericum perforatum* L.	BAE—bovine aortic endothelial cell MDA-MB231 human breast cancer and NIH-3T3 mouse fibroblast cell Inhibition of capillary tube formation; Inhibition of urokinase and MMP2 [40]	Multiple target angiogenesis inhibitor [40]	Wistar rats inoculated with MT-450 at mammary tumor cells Suppression tumor-induced lymphangiogenesis [41]
Stilbene phytoalexin derivative	Resveratrol	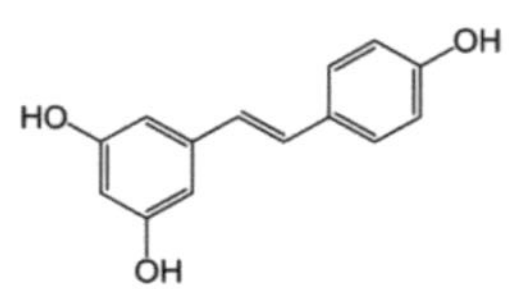	*Vitis vinifera* L., *Polygonum cuspidatum* L.	YUZAZ6, M14, A375 melanoma cell lines Downregulation of VEGF and upregulation of TSP1 [42]	Significant reduction in angiogenesis in higher doses [43]	C57BL/6 Mice inoculated with Lewis lung carcinoma cells Inhibition of neovascularization [44]

Phytochemical class	Compound	Chemical structure	Plant source	*In vitro* effects	Effects on CAM	*In vivo* effects
Phenols	Carnosic acid	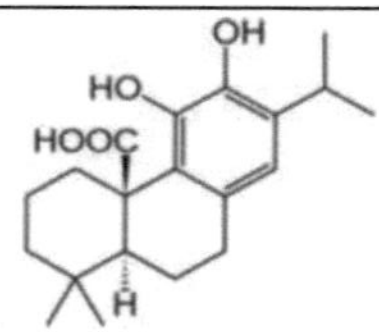	*Rosmarinus officinalis* L	HT-1080 Human fibrosarcoma cells, HL60 Human promyelocytic leukemia cells, HUVECs cells Inhibition of capillary tube formation; Decrease in the endothelial cells MMP-2 activity [45]	Antiangiogenic effect; emphasized activity for carnosic acid [45]	DMBA-induced hamster buccal Pouch carcinogenesis Suppressed expression of Cyclin D1 and NFκB; modulation of VEGF [46]
	Carnosol	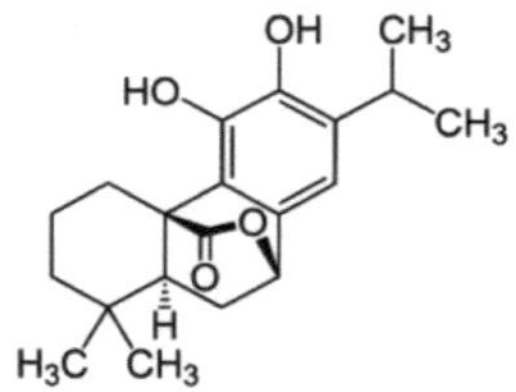	*Rosmarinus officinalis* L	HT-1080 Human fibrosarcoma cells, HL60 Human promyelocytic leukemia cells, HUVECs cells capillary tube formation; Decrease in the endothelial cells MMP-2 activity [45]	Antiangiogenic effect; emphasized activity for carnosic acid [45]	n/a
	Capsaicin	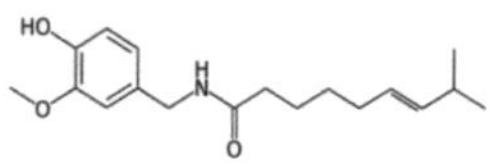	*Capsicum* sp.	Hy-A549CoCl2-stimulated A549 lung cancer cells Inhibition of VEGF by downmodulation of HIF-1α; Increased p53 level [47]	Potent inhibitor of tumor-induced angiogenesis [48]	C57BL/6 mice Inhibition of VEGF and hemoglobin [48]
Isoflavones	Daidzein	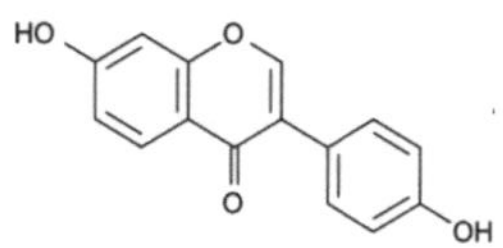	*Trifolium pratense* L., *Glycine maxima* L.	LNCaP, PC-3, and DU-145 PCa cells - Down-regulation of ECGF1, FGF1, IGF1, FGFR3, IL-1β, IL-6, IL-8, PECAM1[49]	Antiangiogenic effect, anti-inflammatory effect with no membrane-irritating and toxic side effects[50]	n/a
	Genistein	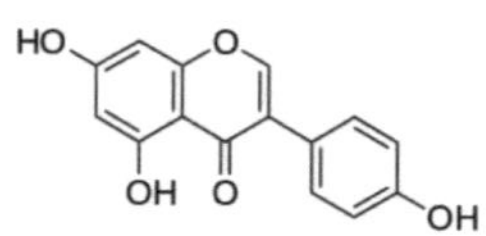	*Trifolium pratense* L., *Glycine maxima* L.	BME cloned bovine microvascular endothelial cells Inhibition of bFGF [51]	Antiangiogenic effect, anti-inflammatory effect with no membrane-irritating and toxic side effects[50]	BALB/C nu/nu mice inoculated with Bel 7402 hepatocellular carcinoma Significant decrease of positive unit (PU) of the microvessels[52]

Phytochemical class	Compound	Chemical structure	Plant source	*In vitro* effects	Effects on CAM	*In vivo* effects
Flavonoids	Quercetin	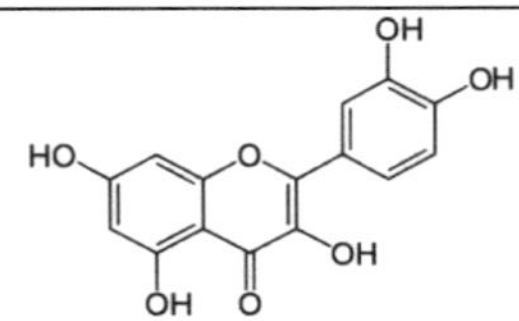	*Camelia sinensis* L., *Angelica keiskei* *Momordica cochinchinensis*,	PC-3 prostate cells Inhibition of VEGF [53]	Potent angiogenesis inhibitor [53]	DMBA-induced experimental mammary carcinoma in rats Inhibition of H-ras protein; inhibition of VEGF and bFGF [54]
	Naringenin	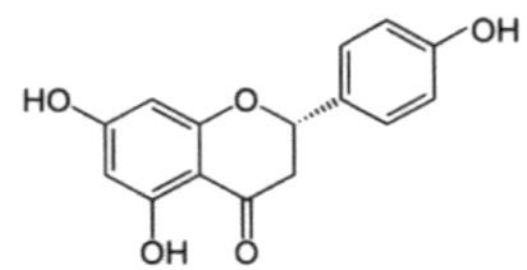	*Citrus* sp.	Aspc-1 and panc-1 prostate cancer cells Inhibition of TGF-β1-induced migration; Decreased expression of MMP2 and MMP9 proteins [55]	Potent angiogenesis inhibitor [56]	n/a
	Apigenin	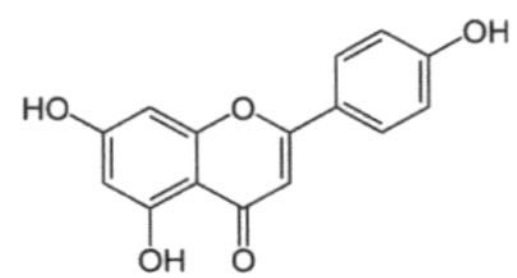	*Entada africana*, *Matricaria chamomilla* L	PC-3 and DU145 prostate cancer cells Inhibition of HIF-1α and VEGF LNCaP prostate cancer cells, HCT-8 colon cancer cells, and MCF-7breast cancer cells Inhibition of hypoxia-induced HIF-1α and VEGF[57]	Promising antiangiogenic effect [58]	BALB/cA-nu nude mice injected with PC-3 prostate cancer cells and OVCAR-3 ovarian cancer cells Inhibition of blood vessels formation; Inhibition of hemoglobin levels [57]
	Isoliquiritigenin	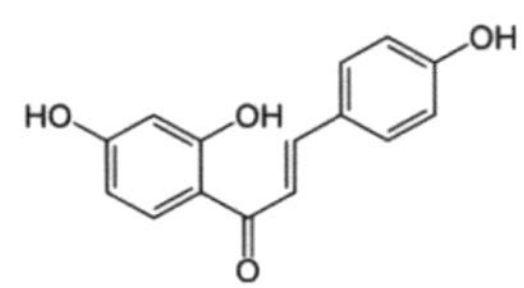	*Glycyrrhiza glabra* L	ACC-M, ACC-2 adenoid cystic carcinoma cells and EAhy926 endothelial hybridoma cell line Prevention of tube formation; Downregulation of VEGF [59]	Angiogenesis suppressor [60]	BALB/c nude mice injected with ACC-M cells Reduction in S6 phosphorylation; Decreased VEGF; Inhibition of the mTOR signaling pathway[59]
	Silibinin	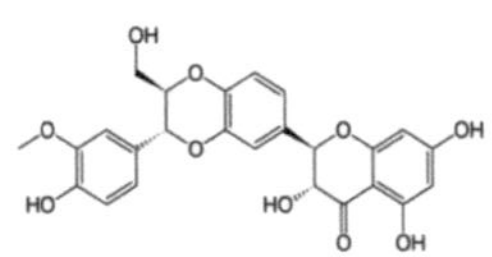	*Silybum marianum* L	SW480, HT-29 and LoVo colorectal cancer cells Inhibition of NF-κB; Reduction of MMP9, COX-2 and VEGF[61]	dose-dependent suppressive on angiogenesis [62]	A/J mice with Urethane-induced lung tumors Inhibition of new microvessels formation; Decreased levels of IL-1α,-6, -9, -13, -16, IFN-γ and TNF-α[63]

http://dx.doi.org/10.5772/intechopen.68506

Phytochemical class	Compound	Chemical structure	Plant source	*In vitro* effects	Effects on CAM	*In vivo* effects
Alkaloids	Vinblastine	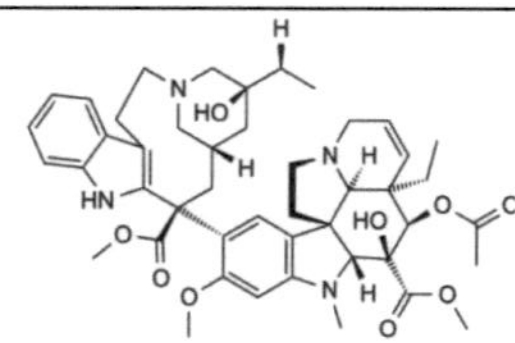	*Vinca* sp.	Human neuroblastoma cell lines Downmodulation of VEGF and VEGF-R2 [64]	Angiostatic activity [64]	Athymic (Nude-nu) mice injected with GI-LI-N cells Decrease of CD31-positive blood vessels; Downmodulation of VEGF and VEGF-R2[64]
	Vincristine	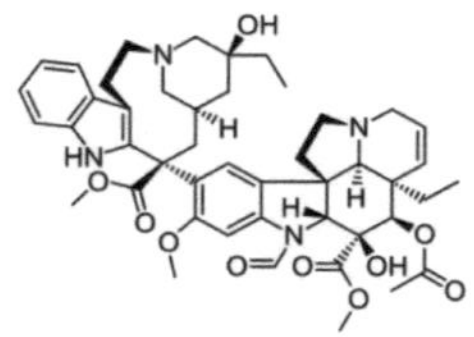	*Vinca* sp.	Glioblastoma cells—decreased expression of VEGF mRNA and the level of HIF-1α protein [65]	Antiangiogenic effects in neuroblastoma tumors in high doses [66]	Swiss nu/nu mice injected with Caki-l and Caki-2 renal carcinoma cells Inhibition of angiogenesis [67]
Pentacyclic triterpenes	Betulin	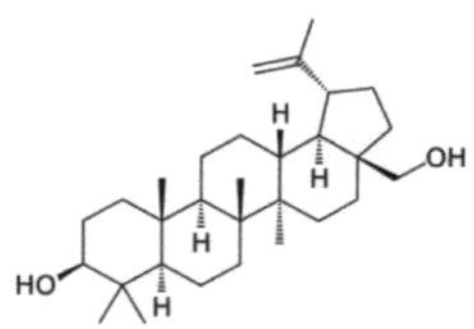	*Betula pendula, Prunus dulcis*	Apoptotic induction in MCF-7, A431 [68]	Strong direct antiangiogenic effects [32]	Balb/C mice DMBA/TPA skin carcinoma model Decreased expression of VEGF [32]
	Betulinic acid	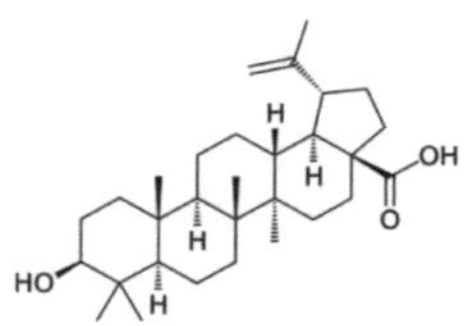	*Betula pendula, Prunus dulcis*	SK-MEL2 melanoma and LNCaP prostate cancer cells - Decreased expression of Sp1, Sp3, Sp4, and VEGF [69]	Strong antiangiogenic effects [31]	Athymic nude mice with LNCaP cells as xenografts Tumor tissue less vascular; Decreased expression of Sp1, Sp3, Sp4, AR, and VEGF [69]
Tetracyclic Triterpenoid saponins	Ginsenoside Rg3	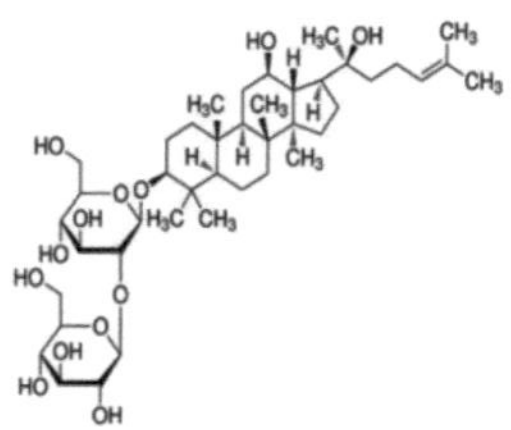	*Panax ginseng*	Eca-109—human esophageal carcinoma cell line and 786-0 renal cell carcinoma cell line Downregulation of VEGF expression via COX-2 pathway; Reduction of STAT3 phosphorylation; Decreased HIF-1α protein expression in Eca-109 cells[70]	Strong, multi-target inhibition of neovascularization, without affecting endothelial cell proliferation; lack of cytotoxicity [71]	C57BL/6 mice injected with LLC Lewis lung carcinoma cells Decreased tube formation of circulating progenitor cells; Suppression of VEGF dependent p38 and ERK signal pathways [72]

Phytochemical class	Compound	Chemical structure	Plant source	*In vitro* effects	Effects on CAM	*In vivo* effects
Flavones	Baicalein	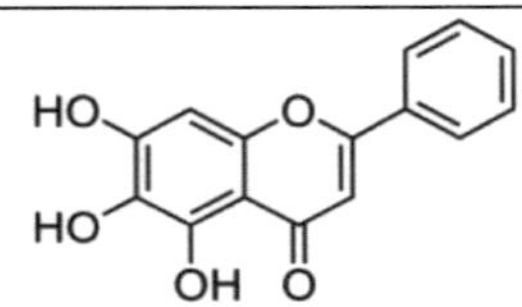	*Scutellaria baicalensis* Georgi	H-460 cells assessed using BrdU assay Significant antiproliferative and pro apoptotic; inhibit bFGF-induced HUVEC tube formation in Matrigel stronger than baicalin [74, 75]	Dose-dependent antiangiogenic activity [74]	H-460 athymic nude mice, tumor growth and survival *low expression of* 12-LOX, *VEGF* and *FGFR-2 gene* [73]
	Baicalin	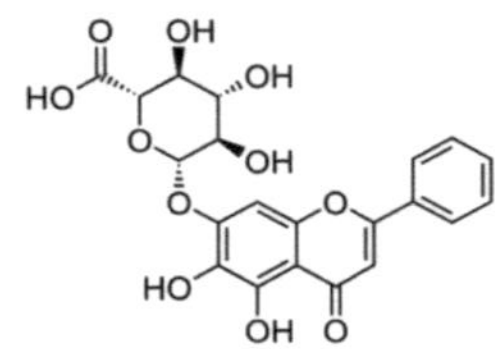	*Scutellaria baicalensis* Georgi	Growth and survival, MMP-2 expression, inhibit bFGF-induced HUVEC tube formation in Matrigel [74]; increases VEGF expression by activating the ERRα/PGC-1α pathway [75]	Dose-dependent antiangiogenic activity [74]	Inhibit growth of S180 solid tumor in mice [76]
Steroids	Withaferin A	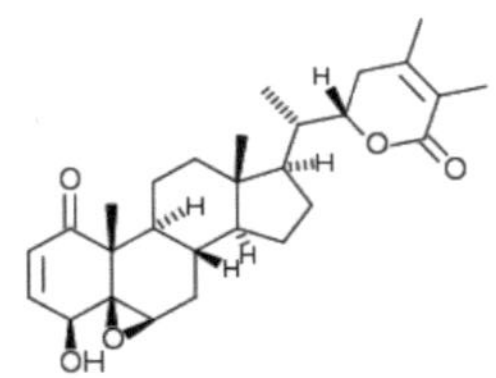	*Withania somnifera* Dunal	Antiangiogenic activity in primary endothelial cells HUVEC [77]	Significant antiangiogenic activity [78]	Inhibits FGF-2 Induced angiogenesis in C57BL/6J mice [77]

Table 1. Common phytocompounds with *in vitro* and *in vivo* antiangiogenic activity.

4. Clinical trials correlation

Implementation of clinical trials is vital for the validation and future use of the active phytocompounds as additional therapies to the oncologic protocols or as chemopreventive strategies. These types of experiments are difficult to implement and therefore not many trials are finalized for the evaluation of antiangiogenic effect in cancer. Two of the above-listed phytochemicals (**Table 1**) benefit from large investigations among which some are clinical trials, but the modulation of the angiogenic process does not appear as a distinct evaluation, cancer effects being the first ones to be described.

Most of the controlled clinical trials of curcumin supplementation in cancer patients aimed to determine its feasibility, tolerability, safety, and to provide early evidence of efficacy [79]. For patients with advanced colorectal cancer, oral doses up to 3.6 g/day for 4 months were well tolerated, although the systemic bioavailability of oral curcumin was low [80]. For this dose, trace levels of curcumin metabolites were measured in liver tissue, but curcumin itself was not detected [81]. These findings suggested that oral curcumin is effective as a therapeutic agent in cancers of the gastrointestinal tract. Other trials found that combining curcumin with anticancer drugs like gemcitabine in pancreatic cancer [82], docetaxel in breast cancer [83], and imatinib in chronic myeloid leukemia may confer additional benefits to conventional drugs against different types of cancer.

Green tea made from *Camellia sinensis* L. leaves, originated in China, is one of the most extensively consumed beverages and achieved significant attention due to health benefits against cancer. Representative compounds are polyphenols and catechins with therapeutic potential against cancer [84]. Recent clinical trials proved that green tea extract and epigallocatechin gallate (EGCG) can be active in several forms of cancer. There is an increasing trend to employ green tea extract and EGCG as conservative management for patients diagnosed with less advanced prostate cancer. Combinations of chemopreventive agents should be carefully investigated because mechanisms of action may be additive or synergistic [85]. Several clinical examinations reported different molecular mechanisms regarding green tea beneficial effects against oral cancer chemoprevention [86–88]. Lung cancer induction may also be inhibited by tea polyphenols. Some studies suggest that individuals who never drank green tea have an elevated lung cancer risk compared to those who drank green tea at least one cup per day, and the effect is more pronounced in smokers [88]. Hepatocellular carcinoma (HCC) usually develops in a cirrhotic liver due to hepatitis virus infection. Green tea catechins (GTCs) may possess potent anticancer and chemopreventive properties for a number of different malignancies, including liver cancer. Antioxidant and anti-inflammatory activities are key mechanisms through which GTCs prevent the development of neoplasms, and they also exert cancer chemopreventive effects by modulating several signaling transduction and metabolic pathways where angiogenesis is exacerbated. Several interventional trials in humans have shown that GTCs may ameliorate metabolic abnormalities and prevent the development of precancerous lesions [89].

5. Conclusion

Currently, a great number of natural compounds are being investigated for their potential effectiveness in controlling tumor angiogenesis and therefore the reduction of tumor growth and metastasis. Observing the high number of molecular pathways that are deregulated in tumor angiogenesis and that many phytocompounds are active on several key factors, it is recommendable that more *in vivo* studies should investigate mixture of compounds for broader targeting, having eventually lower secondary effects and resistance. The optimal experimental technique is an important factor in order to get a useful output. More types of assays are always a good choice, including *in vivo* assays. The chorioallantoic membrane protocol is a good candidate for one type of "golden standardized method" in tumor angiogenesis, being a versatile, rapid, easy, and cheap method to apply in the research of phytocompounds. A great number of plant-derived chemicals, alone or in combination, are studied using this method, but standardization, next to applying new analysis techniques will outcome useful data that will be easier translated to clinical trials.

Acknowledgements

This work was supported by a grant of the Romanian National Authority for Scientific Research and Innovation, CNCS—UEFISCDI, project number PN-II-RU-TE-2014-4-2842 to S.A., R.G., I.Z.P. and D.C. Special thanks to the Histology and Angiogenesis Department, University of Medicine and Pharmacy Victor Babes Timisoara, for the technical support and help in setting up the CAM assay.

Author details

Stefana Avram[1], Roxana Ghiulai[2*], Ioana Zinuca Pavel[1], Marius Mioc[2], Roxana Babuta[2], Mirela Voicu[3], Dorina Coricovac[4], Corina Danciu[1], Cristina Dehelean[4] and Codruta Soica[2]

*Address all correspondence to: roxana.ghiulai@umft.ro

1 Department of Phamacognosy, Faculty of Pharmacy, Victor Babeş University of Medicine and Pharmacy, Timisoara, Romania

2 Department of Pharmaceutical Chemistry, Faculty of Pharmacy, Victor Babeş University of Medicine and Pharmacy, Timisoara, Romania

3 Department of Phamacology, Faculty of Pharmacy, Victor Babeş University of Medicine and Pharmacy, Timisoara, Romania

4 Department of Toxicology, Faculty of Pharmacy, Victor Babeş University of Medicine and Pharmacy, Timisoara, Romania

References

[1] Ribatti D, Djonov V. Intussusceptive microvascular growth in tumors. Cancer Letters. 2012;**316**(2):126-131

[2] Folkman J. Tumor angiogenesis: Therapeutic implications. The New England Journal of Medicine. 1971;**285**(21):1182-1186

[3] Holmgren L, O'Reilly MS, Folkman J. Dormancy of micrometastases: Balanced proliferation and apoptosis in the presence of angiogenesis suppression. Nature Medicine. 1995;**1**:149-153

[4] Parangi S, O'Reilly M, Christofori G, Holmgren L, Grosfeld J, Folkman J, Hanahan D. Antiangiogenic therapy of transgenic mice impairs de novo tumor growth. Proceedings of the National Academy of Sciences of the United States of America. 1996;**93**(5):2002-2007

[5] Ziyad S, Iruela-Arispe ML. Molecular mechanisms of tumor angiogenesis. Genes Cancer. 2011;**2**(12):1085-1096

[6] Denekamp J. Angiogenesis, neovascular proliferation and vascular pathophysiology as targets for cancer therapy. The British Journal of Radiology. 1993;**66**(783):181-196

[7] Nishida N, Yano H, Nishida T, Kamura T, Kojiro M. Angiogenesis in cancer. Vascular Health and Risk Management. 2006;**2**(3):213-219

[8] Prager GW, Poettler M, Unseld M, Zielinski CC. Angiogenesis in cancer: Anti-VEGF escape mechanisms. Translational Lung Cancer Research. 2012;**1**(1):14-25

[9] Ferrara N, Kerbel RS. Angiogenesis as a therapeutic target. Nature. 2005;**438**(7070):967-974

[10] Oklu R, Walker TG, Wicky S, Hesketh R. Angiogenesis and current antiangiogenic strategies for the treatment of cancer. Journal of Vascular Interventional Radiology. 2010;**21**(12):1791-805; quiz 1806

[11] Wang Z, Dabrosin C, Yin X, Fuster MM, Arreola A, Rathmell WK, Generali D, Nagaraju GP, El-Rayes B, Ribatti D, Chen YC, Honoki K, Fujii H, Georgakilas AG, Nowsheen S, Amedei A, Niccolai E, Amin A, Ashraf SS, Helferich B, Yang X, Guha G, Bhakta D, Ciriolo MR, Aquilano K, Chen S, Halicka D, Mohammed SI, Azmi AS, Bilsland A, Keith WN, Jensen LD. Broad targeting of angiogenesis for cancer prevention and therapy. Seminars in Cancer Biology. 2015;**35**:S224–S243

[12] Bora A, Avram S, Ciucanu I, Raica M, Avram S. Predictive models for fast and effective profiling of kinase inhibitors. Journal of Chemical Information and Modeling. 2016;**56**(5):895-905

[13] Avram SI, Pacureanu LM, Bora A, Crisan L, Avram S, Kurunczi L. ColBioS-FlavRC: A collection of bioselective flavonoids and related compounds filtered from high-throughput screening outcomes. Journal of Chemical Information and Modeling. 2014;**54**(8):2360-2370

[14] Roudsari LC, West JL. Studying the influence of angiogenesis in in vitro cancer model systems. Advanced Drug Delivery Reviews. 2016;**97**:250-259

[15] Staton CA, Reed MWR, Brown NJ. A critical analysis of current in vitro and in vivo angiogenesis assays. International Journal of Experimental Pathology. 2009;**90**(3):195-221

[16] Dupertuis YM, Delie F, Cohen M, Pichard C. In ovo method for evaluating the effect of nutritional therapies on tumor development, growth and vascularization. Clinical Nutrition Experimental. 2015;**2**:9-17

[17] Nowak-Sliwinska P, Segura T, Iruela-Arispe ML. The chicken chorioallantoic membrane model in biology, medicine and bioengineering. Angiogenesis. 2016;**17**(4):779-804

[18] Harris RJ. Multiplication of Rous No. 1 sarcoma agent in the chorioallantoic membrane of the embryonated egg. British Journal of Cancer. 1954;**8**(4):731-736

[19] Folkman J, Cotran R. Relation of vascular proliferation to tumor growth. International Review of Experimental Pathology. 1976;**16**:207-248

[20] Ribatti D. The Chick Embryo Chorioallantoic Membrane in the Study of Angiogenesis and Metastasis. Springer Netherlands; 2010

[21] Friend JV, Crevel RW, Williams TC, Parish WE. Immaturity of the inflammatory response of the chick chorioallantoic membrane. Toxicology In Vitro. 1990;**4**(4-5):324-326

[22] Rashidi H, Sottile V. The chick embryo: Hatching a model for contemporary biomedical research. Bioessays. 2009;**31**(4):459-465

[23] Vargas A, Zeisser-Labouèbe M, Lange N, Gurny R, Delie F. The chick embryo and its chorioallantoic membrane (CAM) for the in vivo evaluation of drug delivery systems. Advanced Drug Delivery Reviews. 2007;**59**(11):1162-1176

[24] Scheel J, Kleber M, Kreutz J, Lehringer E, Mehling A, Reisinger K, Steiling W. Eye irritation potential: Usefulness of the HET-CAM under the globally harmonized system of classification and labeling of chemicals (GHS). Regulatory Toxicology and Pharmacology. 2011;**59**(3):471-492

[25] Ardelean S, Feflea S, Ionescu D, Năstase V, Dehelean CA. Toxicologic screening of some surfactants using modern in vivo bioassays. Revista Medico-Chirurgicala a Societatii De Medici Si Naturalisti Din Iasi Nat. din Iaşi. 2011;**115**(1):251-258

[26] Lokman NA, Elder ASF, Ricciardelli C, Oehler MK. Chick chorioallantoic membrane (CAM) assay as an in vivo model to study the effect of newly identified molecules on ovarian cancer invasion and metastasis. International Journal of Molecular Sciences. 2012;**13**(8):9959-9970

[27] (Feflea) Avram S, Cimpean AM, Raica M. Behavior of the P1.HTR mastocytoma cell line implanted in the chorioallantoic membrane of chick embryos. Brazilian Journal of Medical and Biological Research. 2013;**46**(1):52-57.

[28] Ribatti D. The chick embryo chorioallantoic membrane in the study of tumor angiogenesis. Romanian Journal of Morphology and Embryology. 2008;**49**(2):131-135

[29] Demir R, Peros G, Hohenberger W. Definition of the 'Drug-Angiogenic-Activity-Index' that allows the quantification of the positive and negative angiogenic active drugs: A study based on the chorioallantoic membrane model. Pathology and Oncology Research. 2011;**17**(2):309-313

[30] Feflea S. Stimulators and Inhibitors Of Angiogenesis in Experimental Model. (Doctoral Dissertation). University of Medicine and Pharmacy Victor Babes Timisoara; Timisoara;2013

[31] Dehelean CA, Feflea S, Ganta S, Amiji M. Anti-angiogenic effects of betulinic acid administered in nanoemulsion formulation using chorioallantoic membrane assay. Journal of Biomedical Nanotechnology. 2011;**7**(2):317-324

[32] Dehelean CA, Feflea S, Gheorgheosu D, Ganta S, Cimpean AM, Muntean D, Amiji MM. Anti-angiogenic and anti-cancer evaluation of betulin nanoemulsion in chicken chorioallantoic membrane and skin carcinoma in Balb/c mice. Journal of Biomedical Nanotechnology. 2013;**9**(4):577-589

[33] Xue X, Xiaoying Z, Huixin M, Zhang J, Huang G, Zhang Z, Li P. Chick chorioallantoic membrane assay: A 3D animal model for study of human nasopharyngeal carcinoma. PLoS One. 2015;**10**(6):e0130935

[34] Kunnumakkara AB, Guha S, Krishnan S, Diagaradjane P, Gelovani J, Aggarwal BB. Curcumin potentiates antitumor activity of gemcitabine in an orthotopic model of pancreatic cancer through suppression of proliferation, angiogenesis, and inhibition of nuclear factor-kappa B-regulated gene products. Cancer Research. 2007;**67**(8):3853-3861

[35] Gururaj AE, Belakavadi M, Venkatesh DA, Marmé D, Salimath BP. Molecular mechanisms of anti-angiogenic effect of curcumin. Biochemical and Biophysical Research Communications. 2002;**297**(4):934-942

[36] Ranjan AP, Mukerjee A, Helson L, Gupta R, Vishwanatha JK. Efficacy of liposomal curcumin in a human pancreatic tumor xenograft model: Inhibition of tumor growth and angiogenesis. Anticancer Research. 2013;**33**(9):3603-3609.

[37] Shirakami Y, Shimizu M, Adachi S, Sakai H, Nakagawa T, Yasuda Y, Tsurumi H, Hara Y, Moriwaki H. (-)-Epigallocatechin gallate suppresses the growth of human hepatocellular carcinoma cells by inhibiting activation of the vascular endothelial growth factor-vascular endothelial growth factor receptor axis. Cancer Science. 2009;**100**(10):1957-1962

[38] Siddiqui IA, Adhami VM, Bharali DJ, Hafeez BB, Asim M, Khwaja SI, Ahmad N, Cui H, Mousa SA, Mukhtar H. Introducing nanochemoprevention as a novel approach for cancer control: Proof of principle with green tea polyphenol epigallocatechin-3-gallate. Cancer Research. 2009;**69**(5):1712-1716

[39] Wu H, Xin Y, Xu C, Xiao Y. Capecitabine combined with (-)-epigallocatechin-3-gallate inhibits angiogenesis and tumor growth in nude mice with gastric cancer xenografts. Experimental and Therapeutic Medicine. 2012;**3**(4):650-654

[40] Martínez-Poveda B, Quesada AR, Medina MÁ. Hyperforin, a bio-active compound of St. John's Wort, is a new inhibitor of angiogenesis targeting several key steps of the process. International Journal of Cancer. 2005;**117**(5):775-780

[41] Rothley M, Schmid A, Thiele W, Schacht V, Plaumann D, Gartner M, Yektaoglu A, Bruyère F, Noël A, Giannis A, Sleeman JP. Hyperforin and aristoforin inhibit lymphatic endothelial cell proliferation in vitro and suppress tumor-induced lymphangiogenesis in vivo. International Journal of Cancer. 2009;**125**(1):34-42

[42] Trapp V, Basmina P, Papazian V, Lyndsay W, Fruehauf JP. Anti-angiogenic effects of resveratrol mediated by decreased VEGF and increased TSP1 expression in melanoma-endothelial cell co-culture. Angiogenesis. 2010;**13**:305-315

[43] Wang H, Zhou H, Zou Y, Liu Q, Guo C, Gao G, Shao C, Gong Y. Resveratrol modulates angiogenesis through the GSK3β/β-catenin/TCF-dependent pathway in human endothelial cells. Biochemical Pharmacology. 2010;**80**(9):1386-1395

[44] Kimura Y, Okuda H. Resveratrol isolated from Polygonum cuspidatum root prevents tumor growth and metastasis to lung and tumor-induced neovascularization in Lewis lung carcinoma-bearing mice. The Journal of Nutrition. 2001;**131**(6):1844-1849

[45] López-Jiménez A, García-Caballero M, Medina MÁ, Quesada AR. Anti-angiogenic properties of carnosol and carnosic acid, two major dietary compounds from rosemary. European Journal of Nutrition. 2013;**52**(1):85-95

[46] Rajasekaran D, Manoharan S, Silvan S, Vasudevan K, Baskaran N, Palanimuthu D. Proapoptotic, anti-cell proliferative, anti-inflammatory and anti-angiogenic potential of carnosic acid during 7,12 dimethylbenz[a]anthracene-induced hamster buccal pouch carcinogenesis. African Journal of Traditional, Complementary and Alternative Medicine. 2012;**10**(1):102-112

[47] Chakraborty S, Adhikary A, Mazumdar M, Mukherjee S, Bhattacharjee P, Guha D, Choudhuri T, Chattopadhyay S, Sa G, Sen A, Das T. Capsaicin-induced activation of p53-SMAR1 auto-regulatory loop down-regulates VEGF in non-small cell lung cancer to restrain angiogenesis. PLoS One. 2014;**9**(6):e99743

[48] Min J-K. Capsaicin inhibits in vitro and in vivo angiogenesis. Cancer Research. 2004;**64**(2):644-651

[49] Mahmoud AM, Yang W, Bosland MC. Soy isoflavones and prostate cancer: A review of molecular mechanisms. The Journal of Steroid Biochemistry and Molecular Biology. 2014;**140**:116-132

[50] Krenn L, Paper DH. Inhibition of angiogenesis and inflammation by an extract of red clover (Trifolium pratense L.). Phytomedicine. 2009;**16**(12):1083-1088

[51] Fotsis T, Pepper M, Adlercreutz H, Fleischmann G, Hase T, Montesano R, Schweigerer L. Genistein, a dietary-derived inhibitor of in vitro angiogenesis. Proceedings of the National Academy of Sciences of the United States of America. 1993;**90**(7):2690-2694

[52] Gu Y, Zhu C-F, Iwamoto H, Chen J-S. Genistein inhibits invasive potential of human hepatocellular carcinoma by altering cell cycle, apoptosis, and angiogenesis. World Journal of Gastroenterology. 2005;**11**(41):6512-6517

[53] Pratheeshkumar P, Budhraja A, Son Y-O, Wang X, Zhang Z, Ding S, Wang L, Hitron A, Lee J-C, Xu M, Chen G, Luo J, Shi X. Quercetin inhibits angiogenesis mediated human prostate tumor growth by targeting VEGFR-2 regulated AKT/mTOR/P70S6K signaling pathways. PLoS One. 2012;**7**(10): e47516. https://DOI.org/10.1371/journal.pone.0047516

[54] Kong L, Wu K, Lin H. Inhibitory effects of quercetin on angiogenesis of experimental mammary carcinoma. Chinese Journal of Clinical Oncology. 2005;**2**(3):631-636

[55] Lou C, Zhang F, Yang M, Zhao J, Zeng W, Fang X, Zhang Y, Zhang C, Liang W. Naringenin decreases invasiveness and metastasis by inhibiting TGF-β-induced epithelial to mesenchymal transition in pancreatic cancer cells. PLoS One. 2012;**7**(12):e50956

[56] Anand K, Sarkar A, Kumar A, Ambasta RK, Kumar P. Combinatorial antitumor effect of naringenin and curcumin elicit angioinhibitory activities in vivo. Nutrition and Cancer. 2012;**64**(5):714-724

[57] Fang J, Zhou Q, Liu LZ, Xia C, Hu X, Shi X, Jiang BH. Apigenin inhibits tumor angiogenesis through decreasing HIF-1α and VEGF expression. Carcinogenesis. 2007;**28**(4): 858-864

[58] Germanò MP, Certo G, D'Angelo V, Sanogo R, Malafronte N, De Tommasi N, Rapisarda A. Anti-angiogenic activity of Entada africana root. Natural Product Research. 2015;**29**(16):1551-1556

[59] Sun Z-J, Chen G, Zhang W, Hu X, Huang C-F, Wang Y-F, Jia J, Zhao Y-F. Mammalian target of rapamycin pathway promotes tumor-induced angiogenesis in adenoid cystic carcinoma: Its suppression by isoliquiritigenin through dual activation of c-Jun NH2-terminal kinase and inhibition of extracellular signal-regulated kinase. Journal of Pharmacology and Experimental Therapeutics. 2010;**334**(2):500-512

[60] Jhanji V, Liu H, Law K, Lee VY-W, Huang S-F, Pang C-P, Yam GH-F. Isoliquiritigenin from licorice root suppressed neovascularisation in experimental ocular angiogenesis models. British Journal of Ophthalmology. 2011;**95**(9):1309-1315

[61] Raina K, Agarwal C, Agarwal R. Effect of silibinin in human colorectal cancer cells: Targeting the activation of NF-κB signaling. Molecular Carcinogenesis. 2013;**52**(3):195-206

[62] Yang S-H, Lin J-K, Huang C-J, Chen W-S, Li S-Y, Chiu J-H. Silibinin inhibits angiogenesis via Flt-1, but not KDR, receptor up-regulation. Journal of Surgical Research. 2005;**128**(1):140-146

[63] Tyagi A, Singh RP, Ramasamy K, Raina K, Redente EF, Dwyer-Nield LD, Radcliffe RA, Malkinson AM, Agarwal R. Growth inhibition and regression of lung tumors by silibinin: Modulation of angiogenesis by Macrophage-Associated cytokines and nuclear

Factor- B and signal transducers and activators of transcription 3. Cancer Prevention Research. 2009;**2**(1):74-83

[64] Marimpietri D, Brignole C, Nico B, Pastorino F, Pezzolo A, Piccardi F, Cilli M, Di Paolo D, Pagnan G, Longo L, Perri P, Ribatti D, Ponzoni M. Combined therapeutic effects of vinblastine and rapamycin on human neuroblastoma growth, apoptosis, and angiogenesis. Clinical Cancer Research. 2007;**13**(13):3977-3988

[65] Park K-J, Yu MO, Park D-H, Park J-Y, Chung Y-G, Kang S-H. Role of vincristine in the inhibition of angiogenesis in glioblastoma. Neurology Research. 2016; 38(10):871-9. doi: 10.1080/01616412.2016.1211231

[66] Michaelis M, Hinsch N, Michaelis UR, Rothweiler F, Simon T, ilhelm Doerr HW, Cinatl J, Cinatl J. Chemotherapy-associated angiogenesis in neuroblastoma tumors. The American Journal of Pathology. 2012;**180**(4):1370-1377

[67] Schirner M, Hoffmann J, Menrad A, Schneider MR. Antiangiogenic chemotherapeutic agents: Characterization in comparison to their tumor growth inhibition in human renal cell carcinoma models. Clinical Cancer Research. 1998;**4**(5):1331-1336.

[68] Dehelean CA, Feflea S, Molnár J, Zupko I, Soica C. Betulin as an antitumor agent tested in vitro on A431, hela and MCF7, and as an angiogenic inhibitor in vivo in the CAM assay. Natural Product Communications. 2012;**7**(8):981-985

[69] Chintharlapalli S, Papineni S, Ramaiah SK, Safe S. Betulinic acid inhibits prostate cancer growth through inhibition of specificity protein transcription factors. Cancer Research. 2007;**67**(6):2816-2823

[70] Chen Q-J, Zhang M-Z, Wang L-X. Gensenoside Rg3 inhibits hypoxia-induced VEGF expression in human cancer cells. Cellular Physiology and Biochemistry. 2010;**26**(6):849-858

[71] Xiu Yu JL, Xu H, Hu M, Luan X, Wang K, Fu Y, Zhang D. Ginsenoside Rg3 bile Salt-Phosphatidylcholine-Based mixed micelles: Design, characterization, and evaluation. Chemical and Pharmaceutical Bulletin. 2015;**63**(5):361-368

[72] Kim J-W, Jung S-Y, Kwon Y-H, Lee J-H, Lee YM, Lee B-Y, Kwon S-M. Ginsenoside Rg3 attenuates tumor angiogenesis via inhibiting bioactivities of endothelial progenitor cells. Cancer Biology & Therapy. 2012;**13**(7):504-515

[73] Cathcart M-C, Useckaite Z, Drakeford C, Semik V, Lysaght J, Gately K, O'Byrne KJ, Pidgeon GP. Anti-cancer effects of baicalein in non-small cell lung cancer in-vitro and in-vivo. BMC Cancer. 2016;**16**(1):707

[74] Liu J-J, Huang T-S, Cheng W-F, Lu F-J. Baicalein and baicalin are potent inhibitors of angiogenesis: Inhibition of endothelial cell proliferation, migration and differentiation. International Journal of Cancer. 2003;**106**(4):559-565

[75] Zhang K, Lu J, Mori T, Smith-Powell L, Synold TW, Chen S, Wen W. Baicalin increases VEGF expression and angiogenesis by activating the ERR /PGC-1 pathway. Cardiovascular Research. 2011;**89**(2):426-435

[76] Xin W, Tian S, Song J, He G, Mu X, Qin X. Research progress on pharmacological actions and mechanism of baicalein and baicalin. Current Opinion In Complementary and Alternative Medicine. 2014;**1**(2):e00010

[77] Vanden Berghe W, Sabbe L, Kaileh M, Haegeman G, Heyninck K. Molecular insight in the multifunctional activities of Withaferin A. Biochemical Pharmacology. 2012;**84**(10):1282-1291

[78] Mathur R, Gupta SK, Singh N, Mathur S, Kochupillai V, Velpandian T. Evaluation of the effect of Withania somnifera root extracts on cell cycle and angiogenesis. Journal of Ethnopharmacology. 2006;**105**(3):336-341

[79] Fanaei H, Khayat S, Kasaeian A, Javadimehr M. Effect of curcumin on serum brain-derived neurotrophic factor levels in women with premenstrual syndrome: A randomized, double-blind, placebo-controlled trial. Neuropeptides. 2016;**56**:25-31

[80] Mall M, Kunzelmann K. Correction of the CF defect by curcumin: Hypes and disappointments. BioEssays. 2005;**27**(1):9-13

[81] Garcea G, Jones DJL, Singh R, Dennison AR, Farmer PB, Sharma RA, Steward WP, Gescher AJ, Berry DP. Detection of curcumin and its metabolites in hepatic tissue and portal blood of patients following oral administration. British Journal of Cancer. 2004;**90**(5):1011-1015

[82] Epelbaum R, Schaffer M, Vizel B, Badmaev V, Bar-Sela G. Curcumin and gemcitabine in patients with advanced pancreatic cancer. Nutrition and Cancer. 2010;**62**(8):1137-1141

[83] Bayet-Robert M, Kwiatkowski F, Leheurteur M, Gachon F, Planchat E, Abrial C, Mouret-Reynier M-A, Durando X, Barthomeuf C, Chollet P. Phase I dose escalation trial of docetaxel plus curcumin in patients with advanced and metastatic breast cancer. Cancer Biology & Therapy. 2010;**9**(1):8-14

[84] Chen L, Zhang HY. Cancer preventive mechanisms of the green tea polyphenol (-)-epigallocatechin-3-gallate. Molecules. 2007;**12**(5):946-957

[85] Davalli P, Rizzi F, Caporali A, Pellacani D, Davoli S, Bettuzzi S, Brausi M, D'Arca D. Anticancer activity of green tea polyphenols in prostate gland. Oxidative Medicine and Cellular Longevity. 2012; 2012. DOI:10.1155/2012/984219

[86] Soulieres D, Senzer NN, Vokes EE, Hidalgo M, Agarwala SS, Siu LL. Multicenter phase II study of erlotinib, an oral epidermal growth factor receptor tyrosine kinase inhibitor, in patients with recurrent or metastatic squamous cell cancer of the head and neck. Journal of Clinical Oncology. 2004;22

[87] Lee U-L, Choi S-W. The chemopreventive properties and therapeutic modulation of green tea polyphenols in oral squamous cell carcinoma. ISRN Oncology. 2011;**2011**:1-7

[88] Yang X, Thomas DP, Zhang X, Culver BW, Alexander BM, Murdoch WJ, Rao MN, Tulis DA, Ren J, Sreejayan N. Curcumin inhibits platelet-derived growth factor-stimulated vascular smooth muscle cell function and injury-induced neointima formation. Arteriosclerosis Thrombosis and Vascular Biology. 2006;**26**

[89] Shimizu M, Shirakami Y, Sakai H, Kubota M, Kochi T, Ideta T, Miyazaki T, Moriwaki H. Chemopreventive potential of green tea catechins in hepatocellular carcinoma. International Journal of Molecular Sciences. 2015;**16**(3):6124-6139

Chapter 4

Chemical, Antioxidant, and Cytotoxic Properties of Native Blue Corn Extract

Rosa Guzmán-Gerónimo, Edna Alarcón Aparicio, Oscar García Barradas, Jose Chávez-Servia and Tania Alarcón-Zavaleta

Additional information is available at the end of the chapter

http://dx.doi.org/10.5772/67574

Abstract

In recent years, natural products such as dietary phytoconstituents have been the focus of scientific studies for cancer prevention. Among these are polyphenols, which have shown anticancer properties. Pigmented cereals such as blue maize are a rich source of polyphenols such as anthocyanins. Therefore, the aim of this work is to determine the chemical composition and cytotoxic activity of blue maize extract in several cancer cell lines. The total polyphenol content, total anthocyanins, and antioxidant activity of 16 blue corn samples from the Mixteco race were analyzed. From these, the sample with the highest content of polyphenols, anthocyanins, and antioxidant activity was selected and its anthocyanin fraction was isolated using an amberlite column and analyzed by means of HPLC-ESI-MS. The total polyphenol content ranged from 142.8 to 203.2 mg GAE/100g. The total anthocyanin contents varied between 19.02 and 66.92 mg C3G/100g. The antioxidant activity ranged from 18.5 to 27.8 μmol TE/g. The anthocyanin profile showed eight different compounds, mainly acylated anthocyanins. Cytotoxicity of blue corn extract on cancer cell lines was determined at concentrations of 100 and 500 μg/mL using the SRB assay. A cytotoxic effect was mainly observed on SKLU-1 and HTC-15 cell lines.

Keywords: blue corn extract, dietary phytoconstituents, anthocyanin profile, cancer cell lines, cytotoxic activity

1. Introduction

Molecules derived from natural sources, such as plants, marine organisms, and microorganisms, have become important sources of active compounds in the development of drugs for the treatment of human chronic diseases. In recent years, natural products such as dietary phytoconstituents have been the focus of scientific studies for cancer prevention [1]. Epidemiological and preclinical research indicates that dietary compounds possess chemopreventive properties, for example, garlic consumption has been associated with a lower risk of cancer [2–4]. In addition, supplementation of dietary phytochemicals for chemoprevention is gaining increased attention due to their chemical diversity, biological activity, and good availability.

Currently, more than 1000 dietary compounds belonging to different chemical classes have shown potential chemopreventive activities [5]. Among dietary constituents, polyphenols such as anthocyanins have demonstrated to exert many biological activities including anticancer properties [6]. From the chemical standpoint, anthocyanins are phenolic substances that belong to the group of flavonoids derived from the 2-phenylbenzopyrilic cation found in nature in a glycosylated or acylated form [7]. These compounds are particularly abundant in pigmented cereals such as red, purple, and black rice, black sorghum, and red, blue, or purple maize [8–10].

Mexico is the center of origin and biodiversity of maize (*Zea mays* L.). Species have an extensive genetic diversity, with 59 different races described with different shapes and colors ranging from white to yellow, red, purple, and blue [11]. Pigmented maize genotypes are used in the production of tortillas, tamales, atoles, and other traditional Mexican foods. These maize varieties have been the focus of scientific studies because they are a rich source of polyphenols such as anthocyanins. Recent data indicate that blue maize contains monomeric anthocyanins as well as acylated anthocyanins [12, 13].

Even though blue maize is an important part of the Mexican diet, there is little scientific information regarding its anthocyanin profile and anticancer properties. Chemical composition is a factor that must be considered in the selection of blue maize genotypes due to its impact on biological activity, and thus its potential applications for the treatment of disease such as cancer. For this reason, prior to embarking on cancer phytochemical trials, it is important to carry out a preclinical research in order to evaluate the potential application of phytochemicals from blue maize. It is well known that *in vitro* studies examine preliminary efficacy of phytochemicals for cancer prevention or therapy [14].

Given the above, the aim of this work is to evaluate the total content of polyphenols, anthocyanins, and the antioxidant activity of blue corn from the Mixteco race, and to determine its anthocyanin profile and the cytotoxic activity of the anthocyanin fraction in several cancer cell lines.

2. Research methods

2.1. Plant material

Sixteen samples of blue maize from the Mixteco race (**Figure 1**) were donated by the Interdisciplinary Research Center for Integral Regional Development (CIDIIR as per the

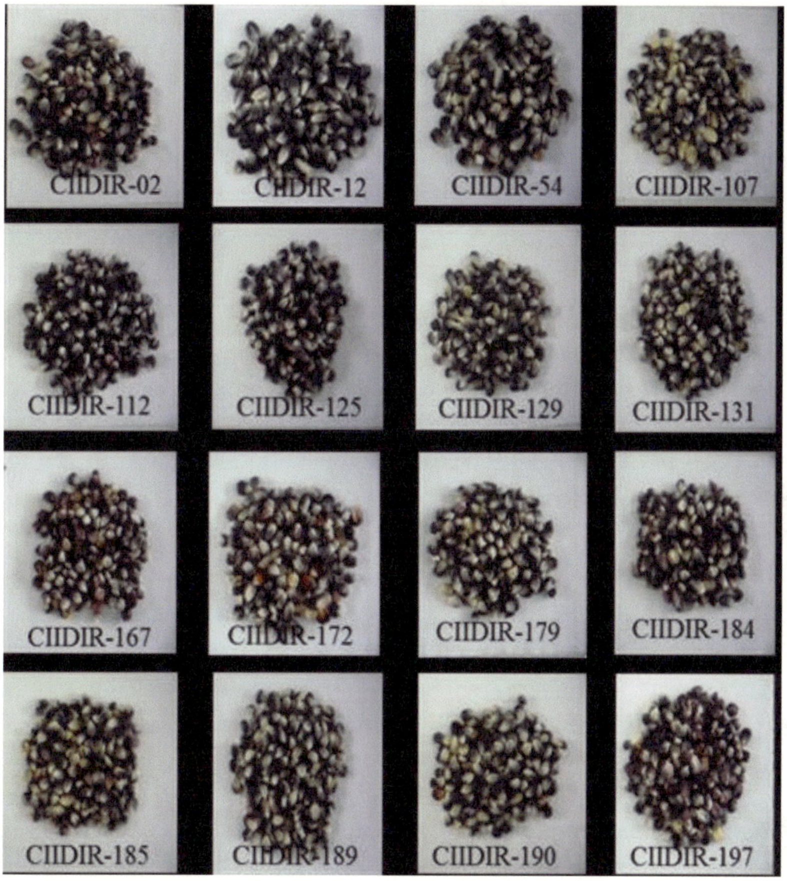

Figure 1. Grains of blue maize from Mixteco race.

Spanish acronym) of the National Polytechnic Institute, Oaxaca Unit in Mexico. Maize kernels were grounded and placed in amber bottles for analysis.

2.2. Blue corn extracts

Ground blue corn kernels (1:5 p:v) were homogenized for 20 min with ethanol acidified with citric acid 1M (85:15 v:v). This was performed using an ultrasonic homogenizer at a frequency of 20 kHz and 750 W power (Cole-Palmer Instrument Company, VCX-750, USA) with a tip diameter of 13 mm at an amplitude of 25 μm with a pulse of 5 s in the 'On' position and 5 s in the 'Off' position. The sample was placed under refrigeration for 24 h and centrifuged at 4000 rpm for 15 min at a temperature of 5°C. The process was repeated twice and the extract was concentrated using a rotary evaporator under vacuum. The conditions of extraction have been included in a patent request, MX/A/20131011202.

2.3. Total phenolic content

For analytical purposes, total polyphenols were evaluated using the colorimetric method previously described by Folin-Ciocalteu and modified by Singleton and Rossi [15]. In this study,

0.2 mL of the extract was mixed with 3.0 mL of distilled water and 0.2 mL of Folin-Ciocalteu reagent. Next, a calcium carbonate saturated solution of 0.75 mL was added. Then the mixture was incubated for 60 min at 37°C in darkness; absorbance was read at 750 nm. This measurement was compared to a standard curve prepared with a gallic acid solution (20–120 mg/L) (Sigma Chemical). The total phenolic content was expressed as milligram equivalents of gallic acid/100 g of fresh weight (mg GAE/100g).

2.4. Total monomeric anthocyanin content

Monomeric anthocyanin content was evaluated using the differential pH method [16]. Absorbance was measured in a UV-VIS spectrophotometer (Perkin Elmer, Inc., Shelton, CT, USA). For the analysis, samples were diluted in potassium chloride buffer (pH 1.0) and sodium acetate buffer (pH 4.5). The difference in absorption at 510 and 700 nm was determined in buffers at pH 1.0 and 4.5. The monomeric anthocyanin content was expressed as cyanidin 3-glucoside mg/100g.

2.5. Antioxidant activity

The antioxidant assay was performed according to the DPPH (2,2-Diphenyl-1-picrylhydrazyl) method [17]. Trolox was used to make a calibration curve (100–800 μmol). About 2.9 mL of DPPH solution was mixed with 0.1 mL of blue corn extract, and then kept in the dark for 1 h. The sample was incubated for 30 min and it absorbance was read at 517 nm. The result was expressed as μmol eq. trolox/g of sample.

2.6. Isolation and chromatographic analysis of anthocyanins

For the isolation of anthocyanins, a column was packed with amberlite XAD-7 preconditioned with 5% acetic acid [18]. Then, 1 mL of the blue corn concentrated extract was placed into the column and eluted with acidified ethanol (5% acetic acid). The eluate was then concentrated to dryness using a Buchi rotary evaporator (Heidolph Digital Laborota pump 4011) coupled to Pimo Vacum Buchi V-700. Anthocyanins were analyzed by HPLC-ESI-MS. The HPLC system was coupled to a Brüker MicrOTOF II spectrometer. The column was C-18 ZORBAX eclipse plus column with 100 mm × 2.1 mm, 3.5 μm. The isocratic elution was done with a mix of methanol:water (2:8 v:v). Mass spectra analysis was carried out in negative ion mode, scan range: 50–3000 amu, capillary voltage 3.8 kV, dry gas flow at 4.0 L/min.

2.7. Cell culture and assay for cytotoxic activity

Prostate cancer cell lines (PC-3), neoplastic myelogenous leukemic cell lines (K-562), human colon cancer cell lines (HCT-15), human breast cancer cell lines (MCF-7), and lung cancer cell lines were provided by the National Cancer Institute (NCI), USA, and the Center of HIV/AIDS Services Center in Mexico City. Cytotoxicity of blue corn extract on tumor cells was determined at different concentrations (50, 100, and 500 μg/mL), using the protein-binding dye sulforhodamine B (SRB) assay in microculture to determine cell growth [19]. Cell lines were cultured in RPMI-1640 (Sigma Chemical Co., Ltd., St. Louis, MO, USA), supplemented with 10% of fetal bovine serum purchased from Invitrogen Corporation, 2 mM L-glutamine, 100 IU/mL, penicillin G, 100 mg/mL streptomycin sulfate, and 0.25 mg/mL amphotericin B (Gibco). They were maintained at 37°C in a 5% CO_2 atmosphere and 95% humidity. For the assay, the following suspensions were prepared: 5 × 10^4 cell mL (K-562, MCF-7), 7.5 × 10^4 cell/mL (PC-3), and 10 × 10^4 cell/mL (HCT-15, SKLU-1); 100 μL of these cells in suspension were seeded in 96-well micro-titer plates and incubated in order to achieve cell attachment to the plates. After 24 h of incubation, 100 μL of each test compound and positive substances (Cisplatin) were added to each well. After 48 h of incubation, adherent cell cultures were fixed '*in situ*' by adding 50 mL of cold 50% (wt/vol) trichloroacetic acid (TCA) and incubated for 60 min. at 4°C. The supernatant was discarded and the plates were washed three times with water and then air-dried. Cultures fixed with TCA were stained for 30 min. with 100 mL of 0.4% SRB solution. Protein-bound dye was extracted with 10 μmol of unbuffered tris base and the optical densities were measured by an Ultra Microplate Reader (Elx808, BIO-TEK Instruments, Inc.) with a test wavelength of 515 nm.

3. Results and discussion

3.1. Total content of polyphenols, monomeric anthocyanins, and antioxidant activity

The first aim of this research is to evaluate the total content of polyphenols, anthocyanins, and the antioxidant activity of blue corn extracts. Ethanol acidified with citric acid was used in the preparation of the extracts, since organic acids decrease the decomposition of anthocyanins during the following concentration step [20].

The total polyphenol content was observed in the range of 143–203 mg equivalent of gallic acid/100 g sample (**Table 1**), while the concentration of monomeric anthocyanins varied from 21 to 69 mg cyanidin-3-glucoside/100 g sample. In this study, the total polyphenol and anthocyanin levels were lower than values previously reported for American and Mexican blue corn [21]. Antioxidant activity evaluated with the DPPH method showed values between 18.5 and 26.8 μmol/100 g.

Results for the total content of polyphenols, monomeric anthocyanins, and antioxidant activity were plotted in a polygons graph in order to identify the sample with the best characteristics. **Figure 2** shows that sample CIIDIR-125 had the largest content of anthocyanins and antioxidant activity; therefore, it was selected to undergo the anthocyanin profile analysis and biological tests.

3.2. Anthocyanin profile of blue corn extract

Figure 3 shows the profile of anthocyanins isolated from blue corn using amberlite XAD-resin. The MS data analysis for blue corn anthocyanins is summarized in **Table 2**. It shows ions at *m*/*z* = 287 and 271, suggesting that anthocyanins are derived mainly from cyanidin and pelargonidin. Eight anthocyanins were identified such as: cyanidin-3-(3″,6″-dimalonyl-glucoside), pelargonidin-3-glucoside dimalonate, pelargonidin-3-(sinapoyl glucoside)-5-glucoside,

Sample	Total polyphenols[1]	Monomeric anthocyanins[2]	Antioxidant activity[3]
CIIDIR-02	$154.4^{f,g,h,i}$	32.5^{de2}	18.5^{e1}
CIIDIR-12	$176.7^{c,d}$	48.5^{b}	$21.2^{d,e}$
CIIDIR-54	$158.4^{f,g}$	31.2^{e}	18.6^{e}
CIIDIR-107	$173.3^{d,e}$	53.4^{b}	$26.7^{a,b,c}$
CIIDIR-112	142.8^{j}	30.7^{e}	18.5^{e}
CIIDIR-125	203.2^{a}	66.9^{a}	$24.4^{ab,c,d}$
CIIDIR-129	$164.3^{e,f}$	$47.5^{b,c}$	$23.6^{b,c,d}$
CIIDIR-131	$173.4^{d,e}$	53.4^{b}	27.8^{a}
CIIDIR-167	$187.1^{b,c}$	32.3^{e}	$24.4^{a,b,c,d}$
CIIDIR-172	$147.4^{g,h,i}$	28.6^{ef}	$22.7^{c,d}$
CIIDIR-179	162.1^{f}	30.7^{e}	$21.5^{d,e}$
CIIDIR-184	$146.5^{i,j}$	21.4^{f}	20.6^{d},^{e}
CIIDIR-185	$192.9^{a,b}$	35.1^{de}	$26.8^{a,b}$
CIIDIR-189	$157.7^{f,g,h}$	40.3^{cd}	$22.8^{c,d}$
CIIDIR-190	$148.1^{g,h,i}$	33.1^{de}	$23.5^{b,c,d}$
CIIDIR-197	175.3^{d}	35^{de}	$26.7^{a,b,c}$

Samples with the same letters are not significant statistically ($p < 0.05$).
[1]mg GAE/100g.
[2]mg C3G/100 g.
[3]μmol TE/g.

Table 1. Content of total polyphenols, monomeric anthocyanins and antioxidant activity in blue corn samples.

pelargonidin 3-(3″,6‴-dimalonylglucoside), pelargonidin 3-(6″-malonyl glucoside)-5-(6″ acetyl glucoside), pelargonidin 3-glucoside-5-(6″-acetyl-glucoside), pelargonidin 3-(6″-malonylglucoside), and pelargonidin 3,5-diacetylglucoside. The data indicates that only acylated anthocyanins are present in blue corn from the Mixteco race. This could be due to genetic factors, farming practices, weather conditions, and soil type, which have an influence on the chemical composition of maize varieties.

3.3. Cytotoxic activity of the anthocyanin fraction from blue corn

In this study, the SRB assay was used to evaluate cytotoxic activity, and it was selected in order to avoid any interference of anthocyanins in the final reading. The effect of the blue corn extract at different concentrations on the prostate cancer cell line (PC3), neoplastic myelogenous leukemic cell line (K562), human colon cancer cell line (HCT-15), human breast cancer cell line (MCF-7), and lung cancer (SKLU-1) are shown in **Figure 4**. Generally speaking, it was observed that for blue maize extract, the percentage of growth inhibition of cancer cell lines improved with increased concentration; the analysis indicates that the blue corn extract causes growth inhibition in all cancer cell lines in a dose-dependent manner (**Figure 4**).

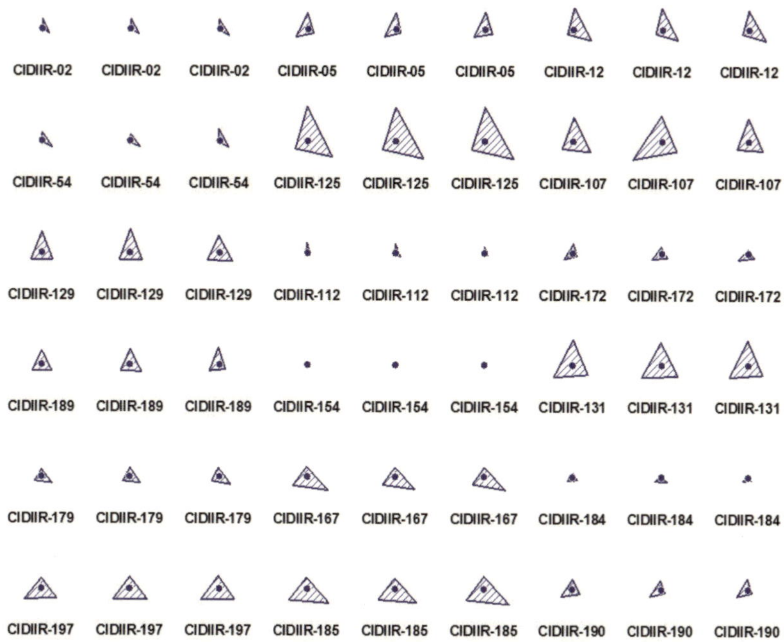

Figure 2. Polygon graph of total polyphenols, monomeric anthocyanins and antioxidant activity.

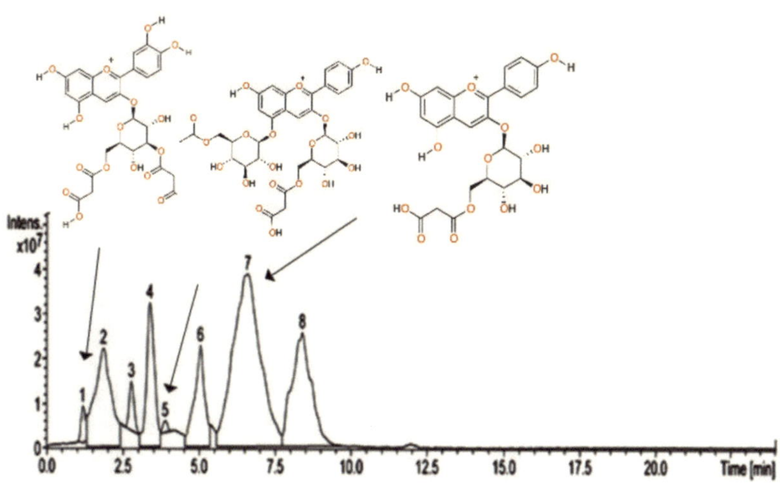

Figure 3. Anthocyanin profile of blue corn.

PC3 cells were selected due to their highly aggressive nature. Data showed 2.43% inhibition on prostate cancer cells at 500 μg/mL. Previous studies have analyzed the anticancer properties of the anthocyanin fraction from potato extracts in prostate cancer cells (PC-3) showing cytotoxicity [22]. It has been reported that the anthocyanin profile has an effect on anticancer activity. For example, pomegranate extract has an abundance of delphinidin derivatives, a compound with anticancer activity on human prostate [23]. In the present

Peak	Retention time (min)	*m/z*	Tentative identification
1	1.2	621–287	Cyanidin-3-(3″, 6″-dimalonyl-glucoside)
2	1.9	358–271	Pelargonidin-3-glucoside dimalonate
3	2.8	639–271	Pelargonidin-3-(sinapoyl glucoside)-5-glucoside
4	3.4	605–271	Pelargonidin 3-(3″,6‴-dimalonylglucoside)
5	3.9	740–519–433–271	Pelargonidin 3-(6″-malonyl glucoside)-5-(6″ acetyl glucoside)
6	5.0	654–595–434–271	Pelargonidin 3-glucoside-5-(6″-acetyl-glucoside)
7	6.6	519–271	Pelargonidin 3-(6″-malonylglucoside)
8	8.4	595–271	Pelargonidin 3,5-diacetylglucoside

Table 2. Chromatographic and mass spectral data of anthocyanins.

research, the anthocyanin profile of blue corn was composed only of cyanidin and pelargonidin derivatives; delphinidin was not detected.

In addition, the analysis indicates that the blue corn extract showed higher inhibition of cellular growth in MCF-7 cancer cells than SKLU-1 (**Figure 4**) at the same concentration

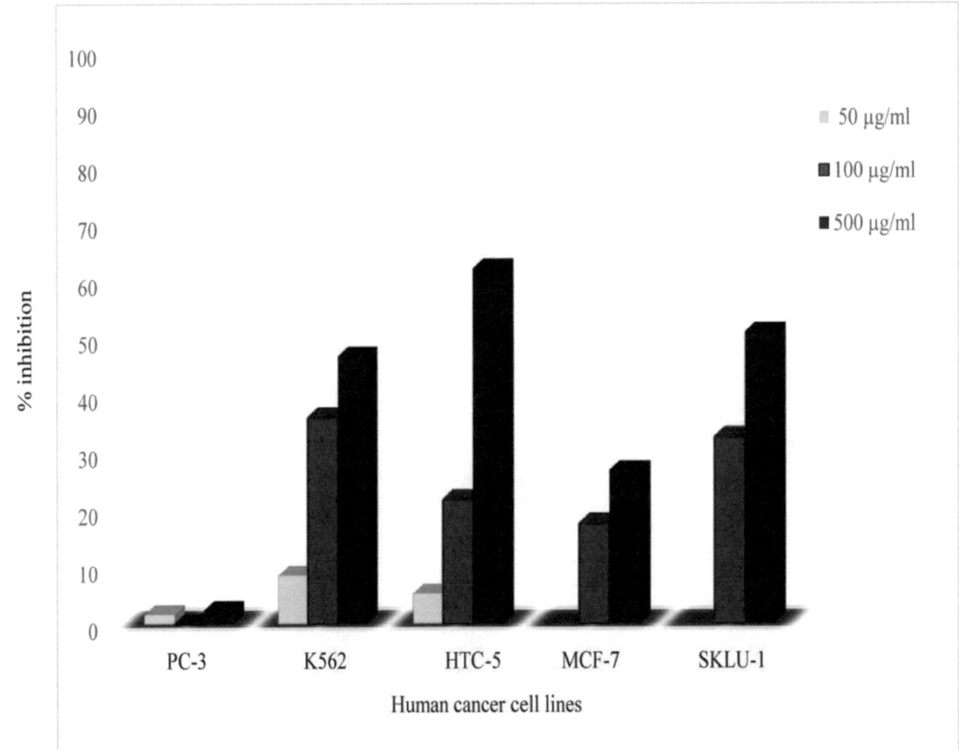

Figure 4. *In vitro* cytotoxicity of blue corn extract on several human cancer lines.

(500 μg/mL). Anthocyanin-rich extracts of cereals such as black rice and black sorghum have also showed the anticancer effects on MCF-7 cells. On the other hand, reports on the effects of anthocyanins on SKLU-1 cells are scarce; a study performed on kenaf seed extract showed cytotoxic activity toward SKLU-1 [24].

Interestingly, blue corn extract was able to inhibit 50.9% of lung cancer cells at 500 μg/mL, which suggests a potential for application in lung cancer treatment, one of the five cancer types most frequently diagnosed in male population worldwide; however, studies *in vivo* (animal experiments) and clinical trials are needed. In this regard, studies on blueberries report the presence of anthocyanins in lung tissue of mice fed with this anthocyanin-rich fruit (5% w/w) for 10 days, suggesting that fruits, vegetables, and cereals such as blue corn may be an important source of chemopreventive dietary components [25].

Likewise, blue corn extract also inhibited the growth of neoplastic myelogenous leukemic cells (K562) and colon cancer (HCT-15) cell lines on 46.7 and 62 % at 500 μg/mL, respectively. Given the above, the blue corn extract was more effective on the growth inhibitory activity on HCT-15 colon cancer cell lines as compared to other cancer cell lines. Current statistics indicate that in 2012 colorectal cancer was the third most common cancer in the world. For this reason, there is an increasing interest for chemoprevention as a cancer prevention strategy. Dietary agents such as anthocyanins have been explored for their chemopreventive effects against colon cancer [26]. *In vitro* data obtained in this research provides information for the future application of blue corn extract as a chemopreventive agent in colon cancer.

In summary, blue corn possesses antioxidant properties and its anthocyanin profile is constituted solely by acylated anthocyanins. These results are particularly important since corn is the basis of the Mexican diet; they suggest that corn anthocyanins may have anticancer activity. Further research is necessary to obtain deeper knowledge on specific molecular targets of blue corn and to ensure the safe use of these active compounds as therapeutic agents on lung and colon cancer.

Acknowledgements

The authors would like to thank the SINAREFI (BEI-MAI-10-32) from México.

Author details

Rosa Guzmán-Gerónimo[1]*, Edna Alarcón Aparicio[1], Oscar García Barradas[2], Jose Chávez-Servia[3] and Tania Alarcón-Zavaleta[1]

*Address all correspondence to: roguzman@uv.mx

1 Basic Sciences Institute, University of Veracruz, Xalapa, Veracruz, México

2 Services in Analytical Resolution, SARA, University of Veracruz, Xalapa, Veracruz, México

3 The Interdisciplinary Research Center for Integrated Regional Development, Oaxaca Unit, National Polytechnic Institute, Oaxaca, México

References

[1] Kotesha R, Takami A, Espiniza JL. Dietary phytochemicals and cancer chemoprevention: a review. Oncot. 2016;7:52517-52529. DOI: 10.18632/oncotarget.9593

[2] Mehta M, Shike M. Diet and physical activity in the prevention of colorectal cancer. J Natl Compr Canc Netw. 2014;**12**:1721-1726.

[3] Howes MJ, Simmonds MS. The role of phytochemicals as micronutrients in health and disease. Curr Opin Clin Nutr. 2014;**17**:558-566. DOI: 10.1097/MCO.0000000000000115.

[4] Li H, Li HQ, Wang Y, Xu HX, Fan WT, Wang ML, Sun PH, Xie XY. An intervention study to prevent gastric cancer by micro-selenium and large dose of allitridum. Chin Med J. 2004;**117**:1155-1160.

[5] Priyadarsini RV, Nagini S. Cancer chemoprevention by dietary phytochemicals: promises and pitfalls. Curr Pharm Biotechnol. 2012;**13**:125-136. DOI: 10.2174/138920112798868610

[6] Wang LS1, Stoner GD. Anthocyanins and their role in cancer prevention. Cancer Lett. 2008;**269**:281-290. DOI: 10.1016/j.canlet.2008.05.020

[7] Delgado-Vargas F, Jiménez AR, Paredes-López O. Natural pigments: carotenoids, anthocyanins, and betalains—characteristics, biosynthesis, processing, and stability. 1st ed. Boca Raton, Florida: CRC Press; 2003. 313 p. DOI: 10.1080/10408690091189257

[8] Goufo, Trindade H. Rice antioxidants: phenolic acids, flavonoids, anthocyanins, proanthocyanidins, tocopherols, tocotrienols, γ-oryzanol, and phytic acid. Food Sci Nutr. 2014;**2**:75-104. DOI: 10.1002/fsn3.86

[9] Awika JM1, Rooney LW.. Sorghum phytochemicals and their potential impact on human health. Phytochemistry. 2004;**65**:1199-1221. DOI: 10.1016/j.phytochem.2004.04.001

[10] Guzmán-Gerónimo RI, Alarcón-Zavaleta TM, Oliart-Ros RM, Meza-Alvarado JE, Herrera-Meza S, Chávez-Servia JL. Blue maize extract improves blood pressure, lipid profiles, and adipose tissue in high-sucrose diet-Induced metabolic syndrome in rats. J Med Food. Forthcoming. DOI: 10.1089/jmf.2016.0087

[11] Kato T, Mapes C, Mera, Serratos J, Bye R. Origin and diversification of maize: an analytical review. National Autonomous University of Mexico. 1st ed. Mexico, D.F.: CONABIO; 2009. 116 p.

[12] Salinas-Moreno Y, Pérez-Alonso JJ, Vázquez-Carrill, G, Aragón-Cuevas F. Anthocyanins and antioxidant activity in maize grains (Zea mays L.) of chalqueño, elotes cónicos and bolita races. Agroc. 2012;**46**:693-706.

[13] Salinas MY, Salas SG, Rubio HD, Ramos LN. Characterization of anthocyanin extracts from maize kernels. J Chromatogr Sci. 2005;**43**:483-487.

[14] Ross NT, Wilson CJ. In vitro clinical trials: the future of cell-based profiling. Front Pharmacol. 2014;**5**:1-6. DOI: 10.3389/fphar.2014.00121

[15] Singleton VL, Rossi, JA. Colorimetry of total phenolics with phosphomolybdic-phosphotungstic acid reagents. Am J Enol Vitic. 1965;**16**:144-150.

[16] Giusti MM, Wrolstad RE. Characterization and measurement of anthocyanins by UV-visible spectroscopy. In: Wrolstad RE, Acree, TE; An H, Decker EA, Penner MH, Reid DS, Schwartz SJ, Shoemaker CF, Sporns P. (Eds.). Current protocols in food analytical chemistry. New York, N.Y.: John Wiley and Sons, Inc.; 2001. p. F1.2.1-F1.2.9. DOI: 0.1002/0471142913

[17] Brand-Williams W, Cuvelier ME, Berset C. Use of a free radical method to evaluate antioxidant activity. LWT—Food Sci Techn. 1995;**28**:25-30. DOI: 10.1016/S0023-6438(95)80008-5

[18] Welch CR, Wu Q, Simon JE. Recent advances in anthocyanin analysis and characterization. Curr Anal Chem. 2008;**4**:75-101. DOI: 10.2174/157341108784587795

[19] Skehan P1, Storeng R, Scudiero D, Monks A, McMahon J, Vistica D, Warren JT, Bokesch H, Kenney S, Boyd MR. New colorimetric cytotoxicity assay for anticancer-drug screening. J Natl Cancer Inst. 1990;**82**:1107-1112.

[20] Dao LT, Takeoka GR, Edwards RH, Berrios JDJ. Improved method for the stabilization of anthocyanidins. J Agric Food Chem. 1998;**46**:3564-3569.

[21] Del Pozo-Insfran D, Brenes CH, Serna SO, Talcott ST. Polyphenolic and antioxidant content of white and blue corn (Zea mays L.) products. Food Res Int. 2006;**39**:696-703. DOI: 10.1016/j.foodres.2006.01.014

[22] Reddivari L, Vanamala J, Chintharlapalli S, Safe SH, Miller JC. Anthocyanin fraction from potato extracts is cytotoxic to prostate cancer cells through activation of caspase-dependent and caspase-independent pathways. Carcinog. 2007;**28**:2227-2235. DOI: 10.1093/carcin/bgm117

[23] Hafeez BB, Siddiqui IA, Asim M, Malik A, Afaq F, Adhami VM, Saleem M, Din M, Muhtar H. A dietary anthocyanidin delphinidin induces apoptosis of human prostate cancer PC3 cells in vitro and in vivo: involvement of nuclear factor-kappaB signaling. Cancer Res. 2008;**68**:8564-8572. DOI: 10.1158/0008-5472.CAN-08-2232

[24] Wong YH, Tan WY, Tan CP, Long K., Nyam KL. Cytotoxic activity of kenaf (Hibiscus cannabinus L.) seed extract and oil against human cancer cell lines. Asian Pac J Trop Biomed. 2014;**4**:S510-S515. DOI: 10.12980/APJTB.4.2014C1090

[25] Aqil F, Vadhanam MV, Jeyabalan J, Cai J, Singh IP, Gupta RC.. Detection of anthocyanins/anthocyanidins in animal tissues. J Agric Food Chem. 2014;**62**:3912-3918. DOI: 10.1021/jf500467b

[26] Tramer F, Moze S, Ademosun AO, Passamonti S, Cvorovic J. Dietary anthocyanins: impact on colorectal cancer and mechanisms of action. In: Rajunor Ettarh, editor. Colorectal cancer—from prevention to patient care. 1st ed. Rijeka, Croatia: Intech; 2012. pp. 123-158. DOI: 10.5772/27678

Chapter 5

Lycopene: Multitargeted Applications in Cancer Therapy

Kazim Sahin, Shakir Ali, Nurhan Sahin,
Cemal Orhan and Omer Kucuk

Additional information is available at the end of the chapter

http://dx.doi.org/10.5772/68131

Abstract

Cancer is an uncontrolled growth and division of cells, leading to significant morbidity and mortality and economic burden to the society. Natural products as anti-cancer molecules have drawn the attention of researchers and have resulted in the development of many successful anticancer drugs, which include camptothecins, epipodophyllotoxins, vinca alkaloids, and taxanes. Another group of compounds with anti-cancer effects include botanicals (phytochemicals) found in the diet. In recent years, a tomato carotenoid lycopene (LYC) has gained attention for its potential health benefits, especially in prevention and treatment of cancer. The studies suggest that the consumption LYC in food or by itself may reduce cancer risk. However, there are insufficient clinical trial data to support the hypothesis. LYC may play a preventive role in a variety of cancers, especially in prostate cancer. It acts by multiple mechanisms including the regulation of growth factor signalling, cell cycle arrest and/or apoptosis induction, metastasis and angiogenesis, as well as by modulating the anti-inflammatory and phase II detoxification enzymes activities. The effects can be attributed to the unique chemical structure of the carotenoid which confers it a strong antioxidant property. In this chapter, we discuss the chemopreventive and anti-cancer properties of LYC, a dietary carotenoid."

Keywords: phytochemicals, lycopene, cancer, molecular, signaling pathway

1. Introduction

Natural products, which can be defined as simple or complex molecules (primary and secondary metabolites) produced naturally by any organism, constitute a diverse group of substances some of which are part of our food, and others have medicinal properties. Over the past few decades, there has been a tremendous increase in research on isolation and purification of compounds of botanical origin and establishing the efficacy of these compounds as potential therapeutic and preventive agents. The natural products have received considerable attention as potential drugs, and a large number of medicinal plants and their formulations have been investigated and found useful in cancer chemotherapy [1]. According to an estimate, more than half of potent anticancer drugs have natural product origin [2]. Some of the plant species that have been used for medicinal purpose and suggested for their beneficial effect in cancer are listed in **Table 1**.

Plant species	Preparation	Effect
Acacia nilotica	Aqueous extracts of bark, gum, flower, and leaves	Effective in chemically-induced hepatocellular carcinoma (HCC) [3] and skin papillomagenesis [4]
Aegle marmelos	Hydro-alcoholic extract of leaf	Remission in Ehlirch ascites carcinoma (EAC) [5]
Aloe vera	Extract	Skin carcinoma [6]
Alstonia scholaris	Alkaloid fraction from bark	UV-induced carcinogenesis [7], DMBA-induced skin carcinogenesis [8] and UV-induced hematological disorder [9]
Azadirchata indica	Ethyl acetate and methanolic fractions of the leaves	DMBA-induced mammary carcinogenesis [10] and prostate cancer [11]
Biophytum sensitivum	Alcoholic extract	Dalton's lymphoma ascites (DLA) and EAC [12]
Boswellia serrata	Triterpenediol preparation	Caspase-8 activation and apoptosis [13]
Butea monosperma	Flower extract	Liver cancer [14]
Cassia auriculata	leaf extract	Decrease Bcl-2/Bax ratio [15]
Cassia occidentalis	Aqueous extracts	Inhibit growth of HCT-15, SW-620, PC-3, MCF-7, SiHa and OVCAR-5 cancer cells [16]
Cassia tora	Methanolic extract	Enhance caspase-3 activity of HeLa cells [17]
Cedrus deodara	Lignan mixture	Effect on leukemia cells [18]
Cheilanthes farinose	Fern	HCC [19]
Cinnamomum cassia		Cervical cancer cells (SiHa) [20]
Garcinia indica	Methanolic extract	Colon, breast and liver cancer [21]
Inula racemosa	Ethanolic extract of roots	Colon, ovary, prostate, lung, CNS and leukemia cells [22]
Lygodium flexuosum	Extract	Induce apoptosis in hepatoma cells [23]
Ocimum viride	Essential oils	Colorectal adenocarcinoma [24]
Oryza sativa	Methanolic extracts	C6 glioma cells [25]
Phyllanthus niruri	Hydro-alcoholic extract	Skin carcinoma [26]
Piper longum	Methanolic extract	Colon cancer [27]

Plant species	Preparation	Effect
Polyalthia longifolia	Ethanolic stem, bark and leave extracts	EAC and DLA [28]
Rhodiola imbricate	Aqueous extract	Increase ROS and arrest cell cycle progression at G2/M phase in K562 cells [29]
Semecarpus anacardium	Nut milk extract	Effect on leukemic cells from the bone marrow [30], induce apoptosis in breast cancer cells through mitochondria mediated apoptosis [31]
Sesbania grandiflora	Sesbania fraction 2, extracted from the flower	Down-regulate NF-kB, Bcl-2, p-Akt, cyclooxygenase-2, inhibits proliferation and induced apoptosis in DLA and SW-480 cells [32]
Terminalia arjuna	Ethanolic extract	Liver cancer [33]
Tinospora cordifolia	Extract	Antitumor and chemopreventive [34]
Trachyspermum ammi	Seed extract	Skin and forestomach tumor multiplicity [35]
Withania somnifera	Hydro-alcoholic extract	Colon cancer model [36], cell cycle disruption and antiangiogenic, property [37]
Zingiber officinale	Extract	Suppressed cell proliferation [38]

Table 1. List of some medicinal plants suggested for beneficial effects in cancer.

2. Natural compounds as lead molecules for cancer therapy and their mechanisms of action

Natural substances such as paclitaxel [39], alkaloids and other substances [1] have demonstrated encouraging antitumor activity in human cancer cells in vivo and in vitro. These molecules act by a variety of mechanisms. For example, paclitaxel, a complex diterpene having a taxane ring with a four-membered oxetane ring and an ester side chain at position C-13, enhances the polymerization of tubulin to stable microtubules and also interacts directly with the microtubules [39]. Other mechanisms of action of antitumor agents include the inhibition of S phase-specific topoisomerase-I (camptothecin) and S and G2 phase-specific topoisomerase-II (etoposide), blockade of G2/M and M/G1 check points (paclitaxel), and prevention of microtubule depolymerization (vinblastine). A new class, commonly known as the vascular disrupting agents (VDA) (e.g., combretastatin A4 phosphate), targets tumor blood vessels. Combretastatin A4 phosphate is a VAD isolated from Combretum caffrum and has been reported to be antimitotic and antiangiogenic, along with the microtubule-depolymerizing property [40]. Substances like berberine, a protoberberine alkaloid found in the roots, rhizomes, stems and bark of berberis, goldenseal (*Hydrastis canadensis*) and *Coptis chinensis*, have also been reported to inhibit different types of cancer [41–49]. They act by inhibiting angiogenesis and by other mechanisms in different cancer models. Mahanine, a purified lead molecule derived from the leaves of Murraya koenigii, which showed antiproliferative activity in leukemic cells, primary cells of leukemic and myeloid patients and inhibited K562 xenograft growth, activates reactive oxygen species (ROS)-mediated mitochondrial apoptotic pathway, death receptor-mediated signaling differentially in MOLT-3 and K562 cells. Piper betle, reported to decrease the mitochondrial membrane potential and induce apoptosis in primary leukemia cells from CML patients in vitro and K562 xenografts in vivo, can also augment the early ROS production [50]. Withaferin A, which induces apoptosis in HL-60 cells through multiple pathways, also enhances early ROS accumulation leading to loss of mitochondrial membrane potential and cytochrome c release, Bax translocation, caspase activation, and PARP cleavage [51]. It enhanced caspase-8 activity, caspase 3-mediated nuclear cleavage of p65/Rel, which was inhibited by N-acetylcysteine, an antioxidant, suggesting the role of early ROS production in withaferin A-mediated apoptotic signaling. The anticancer molecules, such as betulinic acid, a pentacyclic triterpene, have also been reported to directly activate mitochondria-mediated intrinsic pathway and exhibit antitumor activity [50, 52]. Resveratrol, a phytoalexin found in various food products, induces human promyelocytic leukemia cell differentiation, inhibits cyclooxygenase and hydroperoxidase functions and the development of pre-neoplastic lesions in carcinogen-treated mouse mammary glands as well as tumorigenesis in a mouse skin cancer model [53]. Various other substances isolated from plant material and found to be effective in cancer include: 2-deacetoxytaxinine (from the bark of Himalayan yew, *Taxus wallichiana*) [54], curcumin (from *Curcuma longa*) [55], quercetin 3-O-rutinoside (from the fruits of *Barringtonia racemosa*) [56], 13-epi-sclareol (from the roots of *Coleus forskohlii*) [57], corchorusin-D (from *Corchorus acutangulus*) [58], tetranortriterpenoid methyl angolensate (from the root callus extract *Soymida febrifuga*) [59], oleanonic acid (from *Lantana camara*) [60], longitriol and longimide (from the leaves of *Polyalthia longifolia*) [61], 1-hydroxytectoquinone (from *Rubia cordifolia*) [62], 3-(8′(Z),11′(Z)-pentadecadienyl catechol (from *Semecarpus anacardium* nut) [63], β-sitosterol (from *Asclepias curassavica*) [64], sulfonoquinovosyl diacylglyceride (isolated from leaves of *Azadirachta indica*) and nimbolide (from the leaves and flowers of *A. indica*) [65], diallyl disulfide (from *Allium sativum*) [66], arjunic acid (from *Terminalia arjuna*) [67], L-asparaginase, withaferin A, and ashwagandhanolide from (from *Withania somnifera*) [68–70]. Organosulfur from *Allium sativum* (diallyl disulfide and S-allylcysteine) also exhibits good antiproliferative activity [71]. S-allylcysteine is reported to inhibit N-methyl-N′-nitro-N-nitrosoguanidine-induced gastric cancer in rats when administered with tomato carotenoid LYC in a combinatorial approach [72]. A glycoprotein isolated from the bulbs of *Urginea indica* has also been reported to show antitumor activity against an ascites tumor and mouse mammary carcinoma. It inhibited NF-kB, VEGF-induced DNA fragmentation and caspase-3 activation [73].

3. Lycopene

Diets high in fruits and vegetables may reduce the risk of cancers [74–78]. Tomato and tomato-based products have been found to be effective in the stomach, lung and pleural, colorectal, oral/laryngeal/pharyngeal, esophageal, pancreatic, prostate, bladder, breast, cervical and ovarian cancers [79]. Lycopene (LYC) (C40H56; Molar mass, 536.873 g/mol) is a bright red-colored carotenoid pigment found in red fruits and vegetables particularly

http://dx.doi.org/10.5772/68131

tomato, carrot, watermelon, guava, etc., (but not in all red fruits, like strawberries, or cherries) and also in some vegetables that are not red, such as parsley and asparagus. The beneficial effects of tomato on health have been attributed to the presence of LYC. LYC is a highly unsaturated, straight-chain hydrocarbon containing 11 conjugated and two non-conjugated double bonds (**Figure 1**).

It is a non-provitamin A carotenoid. The biological significance of carotenoids has been well established and documented. The β-carotene, for example, is converted into retinal, retinoic acid, and apocarotenoids, which plays a very important role in human/animal

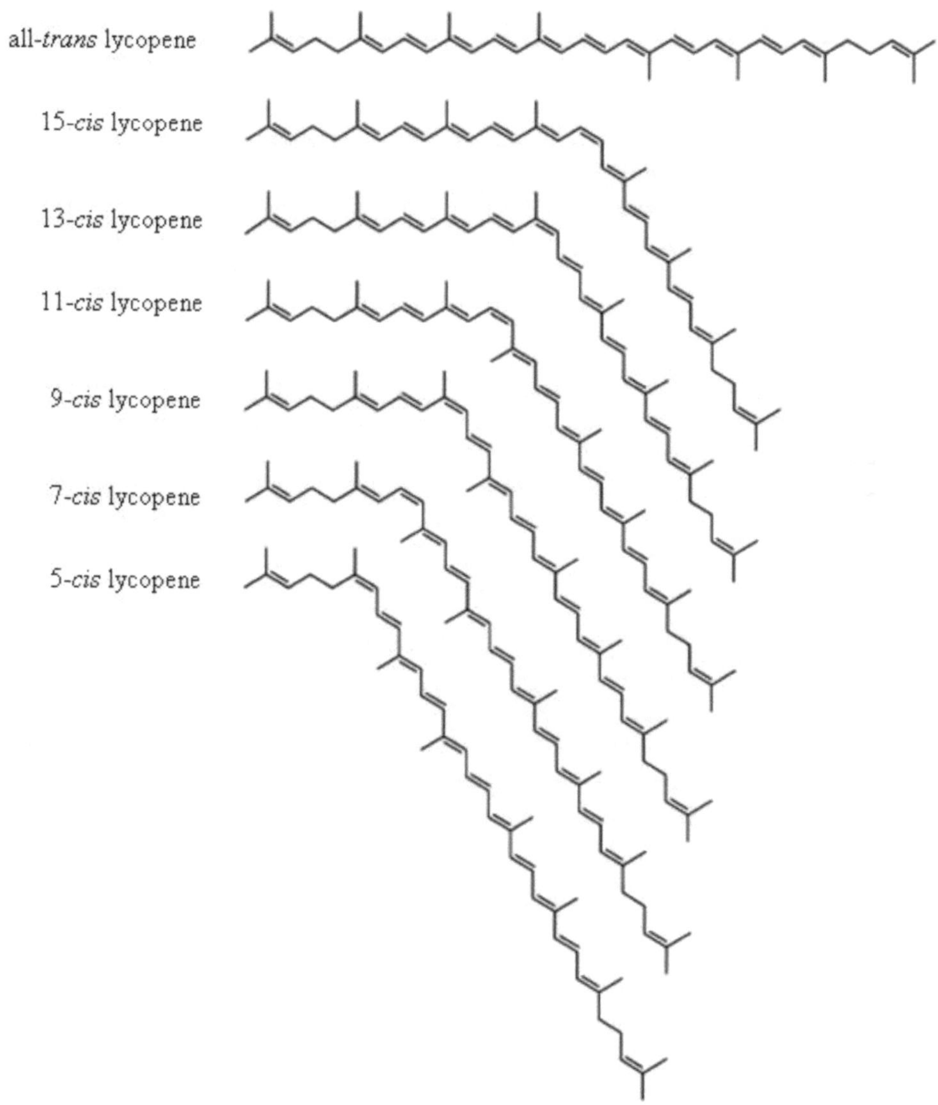

Figure 1. Chemical structures of lycopene isomers.

physiology [80]. LYC is non-provitamin A carotenoid which is not converted to vitamin A. It is a major component found in the serum and other tissues and has been inversely related to cancer and cardiovascular diseases [81]. The molecule acts as an antioxidant and has been reported to have beneficial effects, which can be attributed to its unique chemical structure [82]. LYC can modulate the intercellular gap junction communication, hormonal and immune system, and metabolic pathways.

LYC exists predominantly in trans-configuration, the most thermodynamically stable form, and as a polyene, it undergoes cis-trans isomerization induced by light, thermal energy or chemical reactions. In human plasma, LYC is an isomeric mixture containing 50% of total LYC as cis isomers. All-trans, 5-cis, 9-cis, 13-cis, and 15-cis are most commonly identified isomeric forms of LYC. LYC is poorly absorbed when ingested in its natural trans-form found in tomatoes. Heat processing of tomatoes and tomato products increases the bioavailability of LYC by inducing isomerization of LYC to the cis form [83]. LYC, which when oxidized with potassium permanganate and by atmospheric oxygen catalyzed by a metalloporphyrin, is converted into apo-lycopenals and apo-lycopenones [84]. In addition, a number of other apo-lycopenals have been suggested in fruits, vegetables, and human plasma [85–87].

4. Lycopene: its role and mechanisms of action in cancer

Carotenoid-rich foods have been associated with reduced risk of cancer, such as the prostate and other cancers by various mechanisms [81, 88–95]. The enhanced cytotoxic and apoptosis inducing the activity of LYC has been recorded in different cancer cell lines [96]. The influence of LYC and its oxidation products on the levels of intracellular ROS in three different cell lines has been studied, and in all the cases, the oxidation products increased the ROS levels than the LYC- and control-treated cells. In MCF-7 cells, ROS in control- and LYC-treated groups was lower by 16.3 and 15.5% than in oxidation product treated cells [96].

A number of mechanisms of action have been proposed to explain the anticarcinogenic action of LYC. These include: (i) the inhibition of cancer cell proliferation and induction of differentiation (of cancer cells) by modulating the expression of cell cycle regulatory proteins, (ii) modulation of the IGF-1/IGFBP-3 system, (iii) inhibition of oxidative DNA damage, (iv) modulation of redox signaling, (v) upregulation of gap-junctional gene connexin 43 (Cx43) and increased gap junctional intercellular communication, (vi) inhibition of 5-lipoxygenase, (vii) modulation of carcinogenic metabolizing enzymes, (viii) modulation of immune function, (ix) modulation of IL-6 and androgen, (x) inhibition of IL-6 and androgen, (xi) inhibition of 5-lipoxygenase, (xii) modulation of carcinogen metabolizing enzymes and (xiii) modulation of immune function [97], (xiv) reduction of oxidative stress by modulating ROS-producing enzymes (CYP-P450 enzymes, NADPH oxidase, iNOS, COX-2 and 5-LOX), (xv) inducing antioxidant/detoxifying phase II enzymes (also chemical interaction with radioactive materials), NQO1 and GST [98], (xvi) regulation of nuclear factor E2-related factor 2-antioxidant response element (Nrf2-ARE) system [99], and (xvii) inactivation of growth factor (PDGF, VEGF and IGF)-induced PI3K/AKT/PKB and Ras/RAF/MAPK signaling pathways [100] (**Figure 2**)

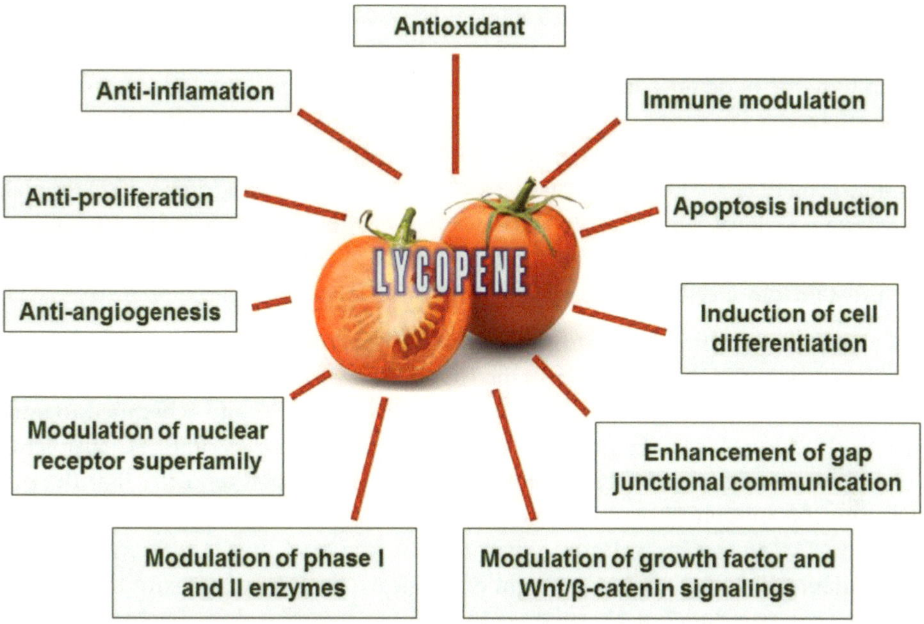

Figure 2. Mechanisms of cancer chemoprevention by lycopene.

4.1. Prostate cancer

The beneficial effects of LYC in prostate cancer (PC) have been extensively reported. A significant inverse correlation between PC and plasma LYC concentration [odds ratio (OR) = 0.17, P-trend = 0.005] has been found between the highest and lowest quintiles of intake [101]. In several experimental studies, LYC has been suggested to suppress PC in vitro and in vivo [102, 103]. It was found to down-regulate the expression of protein kinase B (AKT2) and up-regulate miR-let-7f-1 expression in PC3 cells. Reintroduction of miR-let-7f-1 into PC3 cells was able to inhibit cell proliferation and induce apoptosis. Further research has shown that up-regulation of miR-let-7f-1-targeted AKT2 and AKT2 in PC3 cells can alleviate the effects induced by miR-let-7f-1 [104]. In a recent study published by Tan et al. [105], mice fed semi-purified diets containing 10% tomato powder or 0.25% LYC beadlets up to 18 weeks had higher serum concentrations of total, 5-cis, other cis and all-trans as compared with control in β-carotene 9′,10′-oxygenase (BCO2) +/+ mice. The incidence of PC was lower in animals fed with tomato and LYC when compared with control group. The ability of LYC and tomato to inhibit prostate carcinogenesis was significantly attenuated by loss of BCO2 (P-interaction = 0.0004 and 0.0383, respectively), although the BCO2 genotype did not significantly alter the PC outcome in mice fed with the control AIN-93G diet alone. In another study, the treatment with LYC or metabolite with apo-10-lycopenal increased the BCO2 expression and decreased cell proliferation in androgen-sensitive cell lines, but did not alter BCO2 expression or cell growth in LYC androgen-resistant cells. In particular, restoration of BCO2 expression in PC cells prevented cell proliferation and colony formation independent of LYC exposure [106]. Yang et al. [107] reported that a low or high dose of LYC (4 and 16 mg/kg) and a single β-carotene (16 mg/kg) twice weekly for 7 weeks strongly inhibited the tumor growth, as evidenced by the decrease in tumor volume and tumor weight in thimeric nude mice implanted subcutaneously with human androgen-independent prostate carcinoma PC-3 cells. At high dose level, LYC and β-carotene significantly reduced the expression of PCNA (proliferating cellular nuclear antigen) in tumor tissues and increased insulin-like growth factor-binding protein-3 levels in the plasma. In addition, LYC supplementation at high dose level significantly reduced vascular endothelial growth factor (VEGF) in the plasma. Tang et al. [94] also showed that supplemental LYC inhibited the growth of DU145, a human prostate tumor cell line, transplanted into BALB/c nude mice.

Several studies supporting the relationship between consumption of tomato products and a reduced incidence of PC have come from the Health Professionals Follow-Up Study. In a randomized two-arm clinical trial, patients who have diagnosed PC and scheduled to undergo radical prostatectomy were randomly assigned to either 30 mg of oral LYC supplementation or no intervention for 3 weeks prior to surgery. The study reported that the plasma prostate-specific antigen (PSA) level decreased by 18% in the intervention group, while it increased by 14% in the control group over the study period. In the intwervention group, 11 of 15 patients (73%) had no involvement of surgical margins and/or extraprostatic tissues with cancer, compared to 2 of 11 patients (18%) in the control group. Twelve of 15 patients (80%) in the LYC group had tumors that measured 4 cc or less, compared to 5 of 11 (45%) in the control group [108]. In the same study, Kucuk et al. noted that the expression of Cx43 in the malignant part of the prostate glands was higher in LYC group than the control group. Prostatic tissue LYC levels were 47% higher in the intervention group compared to control group [108]. Phase II randomized clinical trial of 15 mg of LYC supplementation twice a day for 3 days before radical prostatectomy showed a decrease in plasma IGF-I levels, but no significant change in Bax and Bcl-2 [109]. Recently, Paur et al. [110] showed that post hoc, exploratory analyses within intermediate risk patients based on tumor classification and grade and Gleason post-surgery revealed that median PSA decreased in the tomato group as compared to controls (−2.9 and +6.5%). Separate post hoc analyses showed that the median PSA values reduced by 1% in patients with the highest increase in plasma LYC, selenium and C20:5 n-3 fatty acid, compared with the 8.5% increase in patients with the lowest increase in LYC, selenium, and C20:5 n-3 fatty acid. In addition, PSA decreased in patients with the highest increase in LYC (p = 0.009). In addition, it was showed that neither pre-diagnosis nor post-diagnosis dietary LYC intake was associated with PC-specific mortality (PCSM) (fourth and first quartile HR = 1.00, 95% GA 0.78–1.28, HR = 1.22, 95% GA 0.91–1.64, respectively). Also, neither pre-diagnosis nor post-diagnosis consumption of tomato products was associated with PCSM. Among subjects with high-risk cancers (T3-T4 or Gleason score 8–10 or nodal involvement) consistently reporting LYC intake ≥median on both postdiagnosis surveys was associated with lower PCSM (HR = 0.41, 95% GA 0.17–0.99, based on ten PCSM cases consistently ≥median intake compared to consistently reporting intake <median [111].

4.2. Breast cancer

In vitro and in vivo studies suggest that intake of LYC-containing foods may reduce breast cancer risk. Assar et al. [112] have recently reported that LYC inhibits prostate as well as breast cancer cell growth at physiologically relevant concentrations ≥1.25 μM. Similar concentrations also caused a 30–40% reduction in IκB phosphorylation (which regulates the activity of NF-κB [113] as determined by Western blot analysis. However, immunofluorescence staining of LYC-treated cells showed a significant suppression of NF-κB p65 subunit nuclear translocation (≥25%) caused by TNF. In another in vitro study reported by Gloria et al. [114], a significant decrease in the number of viable breast cancer cells treated with LYC and beta-carotene carotenoids were observed. Carotenoids promoted cell cycle arrest and then decreased cell viability in the majority of cell lines after 96 h from the controls. In addition, when cells were treated with carotenoids, an increase in apoptosis was observed in cell lines. Cui et al. [115] reported that LYC intake was inversely associated with estrogen and progesterone receptor positive breast cancer risk in postmenopausal women (n = 84,805), averaging 7.6 years (RR = 0.85 for high quartile of intake as compared with the lowest quartile of intake, P-trend = 0.064). In an animal study, the incidence of breast cancer was found to be inhibited by LYC (70%), genistein (60%) and their combination (40%). Tumor weight was reduced by 48, 61 and 67% with LYC, genistein and LYC + genistein, respectively, and the mean tumor volume decreased by 18, 35, and 65%, respectively. Administration of the combination of LYC and genistein suppressed breast cancer development and was associated with a decrease in malondialdehyde (MDA), 8-isoprostane and 8-OHDG levels, and increase in serum LYC and genistein. Animals treated with DMBA developed breast cancer associated with increased expression of Bcl-2 in breast tissues and decreased expression of Bax, caspase-3, and caspase-9. The combination of genistein and LYC was more effective than either agent alone to inhibit DMBA-induced breast tumors and to modulate the expression of apoptosis-associated proteins [116]. Recently, in a randomized, placebo-controlled, double-blind, cross-over study, Voskuil et al. [117] found that tomato extract supplementation (30 mg/day LYC) for 2 months reduced free insulin-like growth factor-I (IGF-I) in premenopausal women with a high risk of breast cancer (n = 36) I) by 7.0%. Al-Malki et al. [118] demonstrated that combined treatment of LYC and tocopherol (LYC-Toco) caused a reduction in MDA and nitric oxide (NO) in serum and breast tissues in LYC-Toco group than the LYC alone group. Superoxide dismutase, catalase, and glutathione peroxidase activities were significantly higher when compared to rats treated with LYC alone. Serum alanine transaminase, aspartate aminotransferase, total bilirubin and malondialdehyde, which increased in the group of rats treated with diethylnitrosamine (DEN), and hepatic antioxidant enzymes (catalase, superoxide dismutase, and glutathione peroxidase) and glutathione, which decreased in the cancerous group, improved in LYC-treated animals [119]. LYC also caused a reversal and reduced NF-κB and cyclooxygenase-2, consequently increasing Nrf2/HO-1 expression and inhibition of inflammatory cascade, thereby activating the antioxidant signaling. LYC also reduced increases in phosphorylated mammalian targets for phosphorylated rapamycin (p-mTOR), phosphorylated p70 ribosomal protein S6 kinase 1, phosphorylated 4E-binding protein 1, and protein kinase B.

4.3. Gastric and colorectal cancer

Studies have also reported a positive correlation between LYC or tomato product consumption and gastric and colorectal cancers [120, 121]. Although there has been a series of epidemiological studies investigating the relationship between LYC or LYC-rich food and serum/plasma LYC concentration and colorectal cancer risk, the results of these studies have not been consistent [79, 122]. Teodoro et al. [123] have demonstrated a significant reduction in the number of viable cells in human colon adenocarcinoma cells (HT-29), human colon carcinoma cells (T-84), and breast cancer cell line (MCF-7) after 48 h of treatment with LYC. LYC stimulated cell cycle arrest followed by reduced cell viability in the majority of cell lines after 96 h as compared to controls. In addition, when cells were treated with LYC, an increase in apoptosis was observed in four cell lines (T-84, HT-29, MCF-7, and DU145). LYC has also been reported to inhibit cell proliferation in human colon cancer HT-29 cells with IC50 value of 10 μM. LYC treatment also suppressed Akt activation and non-phosphorylated β-catenin protein levels in human colon cancer cells. In addition, LYC significantly increased the nuclear cyclin-dependent kinase inhibitor p27(kip) abundance and inhibited the phosphorylation of retinoblastoma tumor suppressor protein in human colon cancer cells [124]. In another study, it was shown that inhibition of cell growth by tomato digestate was dose dependent and resulted from cell cycle arrest at G0/G1 and G2/M phase and progression by apoptosis induction. Down-regulation of Cyclin D1, Bcl-2, and Bcl-x1 expression has also been observed [125]. In a study conducted by our research group [126], we showed that 5% of the tomato powder added to the diet reduced the aberrant crypt foci (ACF) ratio and also reduced adenocarcinoma development and azoxymethane (AOM)-induced colorectal cancer formation in rats. In addition, the addition of tomato powder indicated that it exhibits chemopreventive activity by regulating Nrf2/HO-1 signaling pathway in colorectal tissue while inhibiting cyclooxygenase-2 (COX-2) expression and inducing apoptosis via the NF-κB pathway. Dias et al. [127] reported that treatment with LYC, synbiotics or a combination thereof significantly increased apoptosis, decreased PCNA and p53 labeling indices, and classical ACF and mucin-negative ACF development. In addition, a lower genotoxicity of fecal water was also detected in groups treated with the chemopreventive agents. The additive/synergistic effect of combined treatment with LYC/synbiotics was observed only for the fecal water genotoxicity and mucin-negative ACF parameters. In a study in a mouse xenograft model, Tang et al. [128] reported that LYC suppressed the nuclear expression of PCNA and β-catenin proteins in tumor tissues. LYC consumption may also increase the nuclear levels of the E-cadherin adherent molecule and the cell cycle inhibitor p21 (CIP1/WAF1) protein. The inhibitory effects of LYC were associated with the suppression of COX-2, PGE (2) and phosphorylated ERK1/2 proteins. In addition, the inhibitory effects of LYC were inversely correlated with plasma levels of matrix metalloproteinase 9 (MMP-9) in tumor-bearing mice.

In a randomized, placebo-controlled, double-blind crossover study, the tomato-based LYC supplementation (Lyc-o-Mato®, 30 mg/day LYC) for 8 weeks has been reported to increase serum insulin-like growth factor binding protein-1 (IGFBP-1) concentration in men and women with high risk for colorectal cancer [129]. The group also reported that the serum IGFPB-2 concentration in men and women increased by 8.2 and 7.8%, respectively. In a double-blind, randomized, placebo-controlled trial, Walfisch et al. [130], a reduction of 25% in plasma IGF-I concentration was reported in 30 patients waiting for colectomy surgery, supplemented with Lyc-o-Mato®. In the same study, a 24% reduction in IGF-I/IGFBP-3 ratio was also observed. In another study, 20 healthy individuals participated in a double-blind crossover dietary intervention and consumed a tomato juice drink (250 ml Lyc-o-Mato® beverage, 5.7 mg LYC, 3.7 mg phytoene, 2.7 mg phytoplankton, 1.8 mg α-tocopherol) and a 26-day wash between each placebo drink [131] for 26 days each. The blood plasma levels of IGF-I were found to be inversely correlated with the consumption of LYC. In yet another study, 20 healthy subjects participated in a double-blind crossover dietary intervention and consumed a tomato juice beverage (250 ml of Lyc-o-Mato® drink) and a 26-day wash between each placebo drink, the plasma IGF-I levels were inversely correlated with the intake of LYC [131].

LYC has also been reported to inhibit *Helicobacter pylori*-induced increases in ROS, 8-OH-dG, and apoptosis by increasing Bax and decreasing Bcl-2 expression as well as PARP-1 cleavage, changes in cell cycle distribution, double-stranded DNA breaks, activation of ataxia-telangiectasia-mutated (ATM) and ATM and Rad3-related (ATR)-mediated DNA damage response in gastric epithelial AGS cells [132]. The administration of LYC (50, 100 and 150 mg/kg body weight) in gastric carcinoma-induced rats up-regulated the redox status and immune activities and was useful in reducing the gastric cancer risk [133].

4.4. Liver cancer

The frequent consumption of tomatoes and tomato-based products has been suggested to lower the risk of other cancers, such as the liver, renal and ovarian cancers. LYC can block the growth on human Hep3B hepatoma cells in a dose-dependent manner and at the same time has been shown to inhibit metastasis in SK-Hep 1 human hepatoma cell line [134, 135]. In a study conducted by our research group, we reported a decrease in serum alanine transaminase, aspartate aminotransferase, total bilirubin and malondialdehyde by LYC in the diethylnitrosamine (DEN)-treated animals. LYC increased the hepatic antioxidant enzymes (catalase, superoxide dismutase, and glutathione peroxidase) and glutathione and reduced the NF-κB/cyclooxygenase-2. The Nrf2/HO-1 expression increased, and the inflammatory cascade inhibited by LYC, suggesting an activation of the antioxidant signaling by LYC. In this study, LYC reduced the increases in phosphorylated mammalian targets of phosphorylated rapamycin (p-mTOR), phosphorylated p70 ribosomal protein S6 kinase 1, phosphorylated 4E binding protein 1, and protein kinase B [119]. In another study on DEN-induced hepatocarcinogenesis in rats, LYC was reported to be effective against preneoplastic foci in the liver by decreasing the size of the liver; whereas LYC administration in another animal study did not reduce the risk of spontaneous liver cancer [136, 137]. The LYC-added tomato paste has been reported to be protective against oxidative stress induced by N-nitrosodiethylamine (NDEA) in rats. It decreases the microsomal lipid peroxidation in the liver and significantly reduced plasma protein carbonyl levels [138]. LYC supplementation also prevents liver-specific carcinogenic DEN-induced of hepatic preneoplastic foci and macroscopic nodules in rat hepatic glutathione S-transferase placental-form positive foci in rats that developed spontaneous liver tumors and ameliorated DEN-initiated, HFD (high-fat diet)-promoted precancerous lesions [139, 140]. It was effective in decreasing NASH-promoted, DEN-initiated hepatocarcinogenesis in rats [136]. Apo-10′-lycopenoic acid, a LYC metabolite produced by β-carotene-9′,10′-oxygenase (BCO2) inhibited hepatic inflammation and liver inflammation induced by carcinogen-initiated high-fat diets [98, 141] showed that LYC supplementation (100 mg/kg diet) for 24 weeks decreased hepatic proinflammatory signal (phosphorylation of NK-κB p65 and STAT3, IL6 protein) and inflammatory foci in wild-type mice. In contrast, the protective effects of LYC in BCO2-KO were related to reduce hepatic endoplasmic reticulum stress-mediated unfolded protein response, the ER(UPR), through decreasing ER(UPR)-mediated protein kinase RNA-activated like kinase-eukaryotic initiation factor 2α activation, and inositol-requiring 1α-X-box-binding protein 1 signaling. LYC treatment in BCO2-KO mice inhibited carcinogenic signals, including Met mRNA, β-catenin protein and mTOR complex 1 activation associated with increased liver microRNA (miR)-199a/b and miR214 levels [141]. The connection between LYC and aflatoxin B1 (AFB1) initiated HCC has also been examined [142], and in recent studies [143], the hepatocarcinogenesis pathway has been linked to the activation of the oxidative stress-inflammatory pathway in rat liver.

4.5. Renal cancer

Previous research has shown that micronutrients consumed through diet or dietary supplementation, including vitamin E and carotenoids, can inhibit oxidative DNA damage, mutagenesis and tumor growth [144, 145]. However, many studies have shown that there is no significant association between RCC and antioxidant micronutrient intake [146], while others suggest supportive evidence that some micronutrients may have a protective effect [147]. Increased uptake of LYC in postmenopausal women in the Women's Health Initiative (WHI) was inversely associated with RCC risk ($p = 0.015$); compared with the lowest quartile of LYC intake, the highest quartile of intake was associated with a 39% lower risk for RCC (hazard ratio, 0.61, 95% confidence interval, 0.39–0.97) when compared with the lowest quartile of LYC intake [145]. It was also reported that no other micronutrient was significantly associated with RCC risk [145]. Another case-control study reported that the intake of vegetables was associated with a reduction in the risk of RCC (OR 0.5; 95% CI 0.3, 0.7; P trend = 0.002) [148]). In the same study, it was reported that both β-cryptoxanthin and LYC were associated with reduced risks, but when both were included in a mutually adjusted backward stepwise regression model, only β-cryptoxanthin remained significant (OR 0.5; 95% CI 0.3, 0.8). When other micronutrients and fiber types were investigated together, only vegetable fiber and β-cryptoxanthin showed significant trends. They also reported that these findings are stronger for people over 65 years of age. Additionally, among nonsmokers, low intake of cruciferous vegetables and fruit fiber was also associated with increased risk of RCC (P interaction = 0.03); similar reverse relationships were found for β-cryptoxanthin, LYC and vitamin C [148]. LYC has also been found to decrease the tumor presence and the average number of renal carcinomas in a small animal model (rat) for studying renal cell carcinoma (RCC) [149]. In the LYC group, the tumor counts decreased and as the LYC supplement increased from 0 to 200, the numbers tended to decrease linearly. Control rats fed only on a basal diet had a greater length of tumors (23.98 mm) than those fed to LYC supplementation groups (12.90 and 2.90 mm) (11.07 mm). In addition, when LYC increased from 0 to 200 mg/kg, tumor length decreased. It tended to decrease linearly. All tumors showed strong staining with antibodies to mTOR, phospho-S6, and EGFR.

4.6. Bladder cancer

LYC supplementation has been reported to exhibit a non-significant trend after administration of N-butyl-N-(4-hydroxybutyl) nitrosamine to reduce the number of bladder transitional cell carcinomas in rats [150]. In a case-control study involving 569 bladder cancer cases and 3123 controls, the relative risk for bladder cancer was 1.08, which compared the highest and lowest rates of LYC uptake [151]. However, in a cohort study, serum LYC levels in bladder cancer cases were found to be lower than those of compatible controls [152]. In another case-control study with 84 cases and 173 controls, OR for bladder cancer was 0.94 (95% CI 0.89–0.99) in the highest quartile of plasma LYC intake when compared to lowest after controlling for age, sex, education, and pack-years of smoking [153].

4.7. Lung cancer

Many studies have shown that smokers and lung cancer patients tend to be lower plasma concentrations of b-carotene, retinol, LYC, b-cryptoxanthin and a-tocopherol [154]. Graham et al. [155] have treated LYC solutions with human plasma and isolated LDL with cigarette smoke and observed the depletion of all(E)-chylopen, 5 (Z)-chylonopen and beta-carotene. Depletion of all-(E)-lycopenin (15.0 ± 11.0%, n = 10) was greater than 5 (Z)-lycopenin (10.4 ± 9.6%) or beta-carotene (12.4 ± 10.5%) in plasma. LDL was found to be more sensitive to both all(E)- and 5 (Z)-clycopenia than beta-carotene (20.8 ± 11.8, 15.4 ± 11.5 and 11.5 ± 12.5%, n = 3). It was also reported that smoke exposure reduced the concentrations of LYC in plasma and lung tissue of LYC supplemented ferrets, which was consistent with the National Health and Nutrition Examination survey III finding that smokers had lower serum levels of LYC compared to nonsmokers [156]. In one study, the concentration of LYC in lungs was 1.2 μmol/kg lung tissue in ferrets fortified with LYC at a dose of 60 mg/day, and this did not cause a harmful effect, instead it prevented the induction of lung squamous metaplasia and cell proliferation induced by smoke exposure [157]. On the other hand, intake of tomato or tomato products including LYC has been associated with a lower risk of lung cancer [158]. In cell culture, LYC has been shown to inhibit the nitration of proteins and DNA strand breakage caused by peroxynitrite treatment of hamster lung fibroblasts [159]. Apo-100-lycopenoic acid has been reported to inhibit the growth of the normal human bronchial epithelial cells, BEAS-2B immortalized normal bronchial epithelial cells, and A549 non-small cell lung cancer cells [158]. LYC dissolved in drinking water at a dose of 50 ppm significantly reduced diethylnitrosamine (DEH), methylnitrosourea (MNU), and dimethylhydrazine (DMD)-induced lung adenomas along with carcinomas in male mice [160]. The inhibitory effect of apo-100-lycopenoic acid was associated with decreased cyclin E, inhibition of cell cycle progression and an increase in cell cycle regulator p21 and p27 protein levels. In addition, apo-100-lycopenoic acid trans-activated the retinoic acid receptor β (RARβ) promoter and initiated the expression of RARβ. In another animal study, the incidence of lung adenomas and carcinomas in male mice receiving 50 ppm LYC in addition to diethylnitrosamine (DEN), N-methyl-N-(MNU) and 1,2-dimethylhydrazine (DMH) was lower than the incidence seen in non-LYC recipients (18.8 versus 75.0%) [161].

5. Concluding remarks

Some plant and plant-based products and their active ingredients exhibit significant antitumor properties. They may act by blocking the cell cycle checkpoints (paclitaxel) and specific enzymes, such as the S-phase specific topoisomerase-I (camptothecins) and S and G2 phase-specific topoisomerase-II (etoposide), and by preventing the microtubule polymerization (vinblastine), as well as by various other mechanisms. Diallyl disulfide, limonoids, azadirachtin, pentacyclic triterpenediol, theaflavins, curcumin, lupeol, and AECHL-1 [162–169], for example, modulate the p53-regulated pathways. Bromelain, theaflavin, thearubigin, curcumin, E-piplartine (trans-piplartine), 3β-hydroxylup-20(29)-ene-27,28-dioic acid, withanolide D, withaferin A [70, 170–176] affect MAPK-regulated pathways. The other pathways include death receptors (example, theaflavins [177] and ROS-mediated pathways (isointermedeol, mahanine, chlorogenic acid, withaferin A [50, 51, 178]. The β-sitosterol, which has a significant anticancer activity against colon cancer, acts by scavenging ROS and suppressing the expression of PCNA [62]. Sesquiterpene isointermedeol (ISO), which is a major constituent of *Cymbopogon flexuosus* (lemon grass) and inhibitor of proliferation of human leukaemia HL-60 cells, also induces ROS production with the concomitant loss of mitochondrial membrane potential, DNA laddering, and apoptotic body formation.

LYC, which is a highly unsaturated, straight-chain hydrocarbon, is reported to be beneficial in cancers, especially the prostate cancer. It can reduce oxidative stress by modulating ROS-producing enzymes (CYP-P450 enzymes, NADPH oxidase, iNOS, COX-2, and 5-LOX) and inducing antioxidant/detoxifying phase II enzymes [98]. These phase II enzymes are regulated by the nuclear factor E2-related factor 2-antioxidant response element (Nrf2-ARE) system. The Nrf2/HO-1 signaling is suggested to be an important primary target for chemoprevention (cisplatin-induced nephrotoxicity) by LYC. LYC can also decrease inflammation by inhibiting NF-κB [99]. It can inhibit the proliferation and induction of differentiation of cancer cells by modulating the expression of cell cycle regulatory proteins, modulating the IGF-1/IGFBP-3 system and other mechanisms including the prevention of oxidative DNA damage and modulation of the immune function, as well as the inactivation of growth factor (PDGF, VEGF, and IGF) induced PI3K/AKT/PKB and Ras/RAF/MAPK signaling pathways [100].

6. Future perspective

Overall, the research articles reviewed in this chapter provide convincing evidence suggesting a role for LYC in cancer, particularly in prostate cancer. LYC may act by a variety of mechanisms, some of which could be linked to the antioxidant activity of this non-pro-vitamin-A carotenoid. Lycopene supplementation could be a potential candidate for future clinical trials in prostate cancer and other cancers both as a preventive and therapeutic agent and in combination with other therapies. This phytochemical offers great promise in integrative oncology and warrants further clinical evaluation with careful attention to individualized dose escalation until an effective and safe dose is found.

Acknowledgements

This work was supported by the Turkish Academy of Sciences (KS).

Author details

Kazim Sahin[1*], Shakir Ali[2], Nurhan Sahin[1], Cemal Orhan[1] and Omer Kucuk[3]

*Address all correspondence to: nsahinkm@yahoo.com

1 Veterinary Faculty, Firat University, Elazig, Turkey

2 Department of Biochemistry, School of Chemical and Life Sciences, Jamia Hamdard, New Delhi, India

3 Winship Cancer Institute, Emory University, Atlanta, Georgia, USA

References

[1] Newman DJ. Natural products as leads to potential drugs: an old process or the new hope for drug discovery?. Journal of Medicinal Chemistry. 2008;**51**:2589-2599. DOI: 10.1021/jm0704090

[2] Mondal S, Bandyopadhyay S, Ghosh MK, Mukhopadhyay S, Roy S, Mandal C. Natural products: promising resources for cancer drug discovery. Anti-Cancer Agents in Medicinal Chemistry. 2012;**12**:49-75. DOI: 10.2174/187152012798764697

[3] Singh BN, Singh BR, Sarma BK, Singh HB. Potential chemoprevention of N-nitrosodiethylamine-induced hepatocarcinogenesis by polyphenolics from *Acacia nilotica* bark. Chemico-Biological Interactions. 2009;**181**:20-28. DOI: 10.1016/j.cbi.2009.05.007

[4] Meena PD, Kaushik P, Shukla S, Soni AK, Kumar M, Kumar A. Anticancer and antimutagenic properties of *Acacia nilotica* (Linn.) on 7,12-dimethylbenz(a)anthracene-induced skin papillomagenesis in Swiss albino mice. Asian Pacific Journal of Cancer Prevention. 2006;**7**:627-632

[5] Jagetia GC, Venkatesh P, Baliga MS. *Aegle marmelos* (L.) Correa inhibits the proliferation of transplanted Ehrlich ascites carcinoma in mice. Biological and Pharmaceutical Bulletin. 2005;**28**:58-64

[6] Saini M, Goyal PK, Chaudhary G. Anti-tumor activity of *Aloe vera* against DMBA/croton oil-induced skin papillomagenesis in Swiss albino mice. Journal of Environmental Pathology, Toxicology and Oncology. 2010;**29**:127-135

[7] Jahan S, Goyal PK. Protective effect of *Alstonia scholaris* against radiation-induced clastogenic and biochemical alterations in mice. Journal of Environmental Pathology, Toxicology and Oncology. 2010;**29**:101-111

[8] Jahan S, Chaudhary R, Goyal PK. Anticancer activity of an Indian medicinal plant, *Alstonia scholaris*, on skin carcinogenesis in mice. Integrative Cancer Therapies. 2009;**8**:273-279. DOI: 10.1177/1534735409343590

[9] Gupta U, Jahan S, Chaudhary R, Goyal PK. Amelioration of radiation-induced hematological and biochemical alterations by *Alstonia scholaris* (a medicinal plant) extract. Integrative Cancer Therapies. 2008;**7**:155-161. DOI: 10.1177/1534735408322850

[10] Vinothini G, Manikandan P, Anandan R, Nagini S. Chemoprevention of rat mammary carcinogenesis by *Azadirachta indica* leaf fractions: modulation of hormone status, xenobiotic-metabolizing enzymes, oxidative stress, cell proliferation and apoptosis. Food and Chemical Toxicology. 2009;**47**:1852-1863. DOI: 10.1016/j.fct.2009.04.045

[11] Kumar S, Suresh PK, Vijayababu MR, Arunkumar A, Arunakaran J. Anticancer effects of ethanolic neem leaf extract on prostate cancer cell line (PC-3). Journal of Ethnopharmacology. 2006;**105**:246-250. DOI: 10.1016/j.jep.2005.11.006

[12] Guruvayoorappan C, Kuttan G. Immunomodulatory and antitumor activity of *Biophytum sensitivum* extract. Asian Pacific Journal of Cancer Prevention. 2007;**8**(1):27-32

[13] Bhushan S, Kumar A, Malik F, Andotra SS, Sethi VK, Kaur IP, Taneja SC, Qazi GN, Singh J. A triterpenediol from *Boswellia serrata* induces apoptosis through both the intrinsic and extrinsic apoptotic pathways in human leukemia HL-60 cells. Apoptosis. 2007;**12**(10):1911-1926. DOI: 10.1007/s10495-007-0105-5

[14] Choedon T, Shukla SK, Kumar V. Chemopreventive and anticancer properties of the aqueous extract of flowers of *Butea monosperma*. Journal of Ethnopharmacology. 2010;**129**(2):208-213. DOI: 10.1016/j.jep.2010.03.011

[15] Prasanna R, Harish CC, Pichai R, Sakthisekaran D, Gunasekaran P. Anti-cancer effect of *Cassia auriculata* leaf extract in vitro through cell cycle arrest and induction of apoptosis in human breast and larynx cancer cell lines. Cell Biology International. 2009;**33**(2):127-134. DOI: 10.1016/j.cellbi.2008.10.006

[16] Bhagat M, Saxena AK. Evaluation of *Cassia occidentalis* for in vitro cytotoxicity against human cancer cell lines and antibacterial activity. Indian Journal of Pharmacology. 2010;**42**(4):234-237. DOI: 10.4103/0253-7613.68428

[17] Rejiya CS, Cibin TR, Abraham A. Leaves of *Cassia tora* as a novel cancer therapeutic—an in vitro study. Toxicology in Vitro. 2009;**23**(6):1034-1038. DOI: 10.1016/j.tiv.2009.06.010

[18] Saxena A, Saxena AK, Singh J, Bhushan S. Natural antioxidants synergistically enhance the anticancer potential of AP9-cd, a novel lignan composition from *Cedrus deodara* in human leukemia HL-60 cells. Chemico-Biological Interactions. 2010;**188**(3):580-590. DOI: 10.1016/j.cbi.2010.09.029

[19] Radhika NK, Sreejith PS, Asha VV. Cytotoxic and apoptotic activity of *Cheilanthes farinosa* (Forsk.) Kaulf. against human hepatoma, Hep3B cells. Journal of Ethnopharmacology. 2010;**128**(1):166-171. DOI: 10.1016/j.jep.2010.01.002

[20] Koppikar SJ, Choudhari AS, Suryavanshi SA, Kumari S, Chattopadhyay S, Kaul GR. Aqueous cinnamon extract (ACE-c) from the bark of *Cinnamomum cassia* causes apoptosis in human cervical cancer cell line (SiHa) through loss of mitochondrial membrane potential. BMC Cancer. 2010;**10**:210. DOI: 10.1186/1471-2407-10-210

[21] Kumar S, Chattopadhyay SK, Darokar MP, Garg A, Khanuja SP. Cytotoxic activities of xanthochymol and isoxanthochymol substantiated by LC-MS/MS. Planta Medica. 2007;**73**(14):1452-1456. DOI: 10.1055/s-2007-990255

[22] Pal HC, Sehar I, Bhushan S, Gupta BD, Saxena AK. Activation of caspases and poly (ADP-ribose) polymerase cleavage to induce apoptosis in leukemia HL-60 cells by *Inula racemosa*. Toxicology in Vitro. 2010;**24**(6):1599-1609. DOI: 10.1016/j.tiv.2010.06.007

[23] Wills PJ, Asha VV. Chemopreventive action of *Lygodium flexuosum* extract in human hepatoma PLC/PRF/5 and Hep 3B cells. Journal of Ethnopharmacology. 2009;**122**(2):294-303. DOI: 10.1016/j.jep.2009.01.006

[24] Sharma M, Agrawal SK, Sharma PR, Chadha BS, Khosla MK, Saxena AK. Cytotoxic and apoptotic activity of essential oil from Ocimumviride towards COLO 205 cells. Food and Chemical Toxicology. 2010;**48**(1):336-344. DOI: 10.1016/j.fct.2009.10.021

[25] Rao AS, Reddy SG, Babu PP, Reddy AR. The antioxidant and antiproliferative activities of methanolic extracts from Njavara rice bran. BMC Complementary and Alternative Medicine. 2010;**10**:4. DOI: 10.1186/1472-6882-10-4

[26] Sharma P, Parmar J, Verma P, Sharma P, Goyal PK. Antitumor activity of *Phyllanthus niruri* (a medicinal plant) on chemicalinduced skin carcinogenesis in mice. Asian Pacific Journal of Cancer Prevention. 2009;**10**(6):1089-1094

[27] Nalini N, Manju V, Menon VP. Effect of spices on lipid metabolism in 1,2-dimethylhydrazine-induced rat colon carcinogenesis. Journal of Medicinal Food. 2006;**9**(2):237-245. DOI: 10.1089/jmf.2006.9.237

[28] Manjula SN, Kenganora M, Parihar VK, Kumar S, Nayak PG, Kumar N. Ranganath Pai KS, Rao CM. Antitumor and antioxidant activity of *Polyalthia longifolia* stem bark ethanol extract. Pharmaceutical Biology. 2010;**48**(6):690-696. DOI: 10.3109/13880200903257974

[29] Mishra KP, Padwad YS, Dutta A, Ganju L, Sairam M, Banerjee PK, Sawhney RC. Aqueous extract of Rhodiola imbricata rhizome inhibits proliferation of an erythroleukemic cell line K-562 by inducing apoptosis and cell cycle arrest at G2/M phase. Immunobiology. 2008;**213**(2):125-131. DOI: 10.1016/j.imbio.2007.07.003

[30] Sugapriya D, Shanthi P, Sachdanandam P. Restoration of energy metabolism in leukemic mice treated by a siddha drug *Semecarpus anacardium* Linn. nut milk extract. Chemico-Biological Interactions. 2008;**173**(1):43-58. DOI: 10.1016/j.cbi.2008.01.013

[31] Mathivadhani P, Shanthi P, Sachdanandam P. Apoptotic effect of *Semecarpus anacardium* nut extract on T47D breast cancer cell line. Cell Biology InternationalCell Biology International. 2007;**31**(10):1198-1206

[32] Laladhas KP, Cheriyan VT, Puliappadamba VT, Bava SV, Unnithan RG, Vijayammal PL, Anto RJ. A novel protein fraction from *Sesbania grandiflora* shows potential anticancer and chemopreventive efficacy, in vitro and in vivo. Journal of Cellular and Molecular Medicine. 2010;**14**(3):636-646 . DOI: 10.1111/j.1582-4934.2008.00648.x

[33] Sivalokanathan S, Ilayaraja M, Balasubramanian MP. Antioxidant activity of *Terminalia arjuna* bark extract on Nnitrosodiethylamine induced hepatocellular carcinoma in rats. Molecular and Cellular Biochemistry. 2006;**281**(1-2):87-93

[34] Chaudhary R, Jahan S, Goyal PK. Chemopreventive potential of an Indian medicinal plant (*Tinospora cordifolia*) on skin carcinogenesis in mice. Journal of Environmental Pathology, Toxicology and Oncology. 2008;**27**(3):233-243

[35] Singh B, Kale RK. Chemomodulatory effect of *Trachyspermum ammi* on murine skin and forestomach papillomagenesis. Nutrition and Cancer. 2010;**62**(1):74-84 . DOI: 10.1080/01635580903191478

[36] Muralikrishnan G, Amanullah S, Basha MI, Dinda AK, Shakeel F. Modulating effect of *Withania somnifera* on TCA cycle enzymes and electron transport chain in azoxymethane-induced colon cancer in mice. Immunopharmacology and Immunotoxicology. 2010;**32**(3):523-527. DOI: 10.3109/08923970903581540

[37] Mathur R, Gupta SK, Singh N, Mathur S, Kochupillai V, Velpandian T. Evaluation of the effect of *Withania somnifera* root extracts on cell cycle and angiogenesis. Journal of Ethnopharmacology. 2006;**105**(3):336-341

[38] Vijaya PV, Arul DCS, Ramkuma KM. Induction of apoptosis by ginger in HEp-2 cell line is mediated by reactive oxygen species. Basic & Clinical Pharmacology & Toxicology. 2007;**100**(5):302-307

[39] Horwitz SB. Taxol (paclitaxel): mechanisms of action. Annals of Oncology. 1994;**5**(Suppl 6):S3-6

[40] Chin YW, Balunas MJ, Chai HB, Kinghorn AD. Drug discovery from natural sources. The AAPS Journal. 2006;**8**(2):E239-253

[41] Serafim TL, Oliveira PJ, Sardao VA, Perkins E, Parke D, Holy J. Different concentrations of berberine result in distinct cellular localization patterns and cell cycle effects in a melanoma cell line. Cancer Chemotherapy and Pharmacology. 2008;**61**(6):1007-1018

[42] Pinto-Garcia L, Efferth T, Torres A, Hoheisel JD, Youns M. Berberine inhibits cell growth and mediates caspase-independent cell death in human pancreatic cancer cells. Planta Medica. 2010;**76**(11):1155-1161. DOI: 10.1055/s-0030-1249931

[43] Auyeung KK, Ko JK. *Coptis chinensis* inhibits hepatocellular carcinoma cell growth through nonsteroidal anti-inflammatory drug-activated gene activation. International Journal of Molecular Medicine. 2009;**24**(4):571-577

[44] Sun Y, Xun K, Wang Y, Chen X. A systematic review of the anticancer properties of berberine, a natural product from Chinese herbs. Anticancer Drugs. 2009;**20**(9):757-769. DOI: 10.1097/CAD.0b013e328330d95b

[45] Sindhu G, Manoharan S. Anti-clastogenic effect of berberine against DMBA-induced clastogenesis. Basic & Clinical Pharmacology & Toxicology. 2010;**107**(4):818-824. DOI: 10.1111/j.1742-7843.2010.00579.x.

[46] Kim S, Choi JH, Kim JB, Nam SJ, Yang JH, Kim JH, Lee JE. Berberine suppresses TNF-alpha-induced MMP-9 and cell invasion through inhibition of AP-1 activity in MDA-MB-231 human breast cancer cells. Molecules. 2008;**13**(12):2975-2985. DOI: 10.3390/molecules13122975

[47] Choi MS, Oh JH, Kim SM, Jung HY, Yoo HS, Lee YM, Moon DC, Han SB, Hong JT. Berberine inhibits p53-dependent cell growth through induction of apoptosis of prostate cancer cells. International Journal of Oncology. 2009;**34**(5):1221-1230

[48] Lin CC, Lin SY, Chung JG, Lin JP, Chen GW, Kao ST. Down-regulation of cyclin B1 and up-regulation of Wee1 by berberine promotes entry of leukemia cells into the G2/M-phase of the cell cycle. Anticancer Research. 2006;**26**(2A):1097-1104

[49] Tang J, Feng Y, Tsao S, Wang N, Curtain R, Wang Y. Berberine and *Coptidis rhizoma* as novel antineoplastic agents: a review of traditional use and biomedical investigations. Journal of Ethnopharmacology. 2009;**126**(1):5-17. DOI: 10.1016/j.jep.2009.08.009

[50] Rakshit S, Mandal L, Pal BC, Bagchi J, Biswas N, Chaudhuri J, Chowdhury AA, Manna A, Chaudhuri U, Konar A, Mukherjee T, Jaisankar P, Bandyopadhyay S. Involvement of ROS in chlorogenic acid-induced apoptosis of Bcr-Abl+ CML cells. Biochemical Pharmacology. 2010;**80**(11):1662-1675. DOI: 10.1016/j.bcp.2010.08.013

[51] Malik F, Kumar A, Bhushan S, Khan S, Bhatia A, Suri KA, Qazi GN, Singh J. Reactive oxygen species generation and mitochondrial dysfunction in the apoptotic cell death of human myeloid leukemia HL-60 cells by a dietary compound withaferin A with concomitant protection by N-acetyl cysteine. Apoptosis. 2007;**12**(11):2115-2133

[52] Fulda S. and Kroemer G. Targeting mitochondrial apoptosis by betulinic acid in human cancers. Drug Discovery Today. 2009;**14**(17-18):885-890. DOI: 10.1016/j.drudis.2009.05.015

[53] Athar M, Back JH, Tang X, Kim KH, Kopelovich L, Bickers DR and Kim AL. Resveratrol: a review of preclinical studies for human cancer prevention. Toxicology and Applied Pharmacology. 2007;**224**(3):274-283.

[54] Reddy KP, Bid HK, Nayak VL, Chaudhary P, Chaturvedi JP, Arya KR, Konwar R, Narender T. In vitro and in vivo anticancer activity of 2-deacetoxytaxinine J and synthesis of novel taxoids and their in vitro anticancer activity. European Journal of Medicinal Chemistry. 2009;**44**(10):3947-3953. DOI: 10.1016/j.ejmech.2009.04.022

[55] Singh M, Pandey A, Karikari CA, Singh G, Rakheja D. Cell cycle inhibition and apoptosis induced by curcumin in Ewing sarcoma cell line SK-NEP-1. Medical Oncology. 2009;**27**(4):1096-1101. DOI: 10.1007/s12032-009-9341-6

[56] Samanta SK, Bhattacharya K, Mandal C, Pal BC. Identification and quantification of the active component quercetin 3-Orutinoside from Barringtonia racemosa, targets mitochondrial apoptotic pathway in acute lymphoblastic leukemia. Journal of Asian Natural Products Research. 2010;**12**(8):639-648. DOI: 10.1080/10286020.2010.489040

[57] Sashidhara KV, Rosaiah JN, Kumar A, Bid HK, Konwar R, Chattopadhyay N. Cell growth inhibitory action of an unusual labdane diterpene, 13-epi-sclareol in breast and uterine cancers in vitro. Phytotherapy Research. 2007;**21**(11):1105-1108

[58] Mallick S, Ghosh P, Samanta SK, Kinra S, Pal BC, Gomes A, Vedasiromoni JR. Corchorusin-D, a saikosaponin-like compound isolated from *Corchorus acutanglus* Lam., targets mitochondrial apoptotic pathways in leukemic cell lines (HL-60 and U937). Cancer Chemotherapy and Pharmacology. 2010;**66**(4):709-719. DOI: 10.1007/s00280-009-1214-3

[59] Chiruvella KK, Kari V, Choudhary B, Nambiar M, Ghanta RG, Raghavan SC. Methyl angolensate, a natural tetranortriterpenoid induces intrinsic apoptotic pathway in leukemic cells. FEBS Letters. 2008;**582**(29):4066-4076. DOI: 10.1016/j.febslet.2008.11.001

[60] Ghosh S, Das Sarma M, Patra A, Hazra B. Anti-inflammatory and anticancer compounds isolated from Ventilago madraspatana Gaertn., *Rubia cordifolia* Linn. and *Lantana camara* Linn. Journal of Pharmacy and Pharmacology. 2010;**62**(9):1158-1166. DOI: 10.1111/j.2042-7158.2010.01151.x

[61] Sashidhara KV, Singh SP, Kant R, Maulik PR, Sarkar J, Kanojiya S, Ravi KK. Cytotoxic cycloartane triterpene and rare isomeric bisclerodane diterpenes from the leaves of *Polyalthia longifolia* var. pendula. Bioorganic & Medicinal Chemistry Letters. 2010;**20**(19):5767-5771. DOI: 10.1016/j.bmcl.2010.07.141

[62] Lajkó E, Bányai P, Zámbó Z, Kursinszki L, Szőke É, Kőhidai L. Targeted tumor therapy by *Rubia tinctorum* L.: analytical characterization of hydroxyanthraquinones and investigation of their selective cytotoxic, adhesion and migration modulator effects on melanoma cell lines (A2058 and HT168-M1). Cancer Cell International. 2015;**18**(15):119. DOI: 10.1186/s12935-015-0271-4

[63] Nair PK, Melnick SJ, Wnuk SF, Rapp M, Escalon E, Ramachandran C. Isolation and characterization of an anticancer catechol compound from *Semecarpus anacardium*. Journal of Ethnopharmacology. 2009;**122**(3):450-456. DOI: 10.1016/j.jep.2009.02.001

[64] Baskar AA, Ignacimuthu S, Paulraj GM, Al Numair KS. Chemopreventive potential of beta-Sitosterol in experimental colon cancer model—an in vitro and in vivo study. BMC Complementary and Alternative Medicine. 2010;**10**:24. DOI: 10.1186/1472-6882-10-24

[65] Chatterjee R, Singh O, Pachuau L, Malik SP, Paul M, Bhadra K, Paul S, Kumar GS, Mondal NB, Banerjee S. Identification of a sulfonoquinovosyldiacylglyceride from *Azadirachta indica* and studies on its cytotoxic activity and DNA binding properties. Bioorganic & Medicinal Chemistry Letters. 2010;**20**(22):6699-6702. DOI: 10.1016/j.bmcl.2010.09.007

[66] Arunkumar A, Vijayababu MR, Kanagaraj P, Balasubramanian K, Aruldhas MM, Arunakaran J. Growth suppressing effect of garlic compound diallyl disulfide on prostate cancer cell line (PC-3) in vitro. Biological and Pharmaceutical Bulletin. 2005;**28**(4):740-743

[67] Joo H, Lee HJ, Shin EA, Kim H, Seo KH, Baek NI, Kim B, Kim SH. c-Jun N-terminal kinase-dependent endoplasmic reticulum stress pathway is critically involved in arjunic acid induced apoptosis in non-small cell lung cancer cells. Phytotherapy Research. 2016;**30**(4):596-603. DOI: 10.1002/ptr.5563

[68] Puliyappadamba VT, Cheriyan VT, Thulasidasan AK, Bava SV, Vinod BS, Prabhu PR, Varghese R, Bevin A, Venugopal S, Anto RJ. Nicotine-induced survival signaling in lung

cancer cells is dependent on their p53 status while its downregulation by curcumin is independent. Molecular Cancer. 2010;**9**:220. DOI: 10.1186/1476-4598-9-220

[69] Ravindran J, Prasad S, Aggarwal BB. Curcumin and cancer cells, how many ways can curry kill tumor cells selectively?. The AAPS Journal. 2009;**11**(3):495-510. DOI: 10.1208/s12248-009-9128-x

[70] Bhui K, Tyagi S, Prakash B, Shukla Y. Pineapple bromelain induces autophagy, facilitating apoptotic response in mammary carcinoma cells. Biofactors. 2010;**36**(6):474-482. DOI: 10.1002/biof.121

[71] Babica P, Čtveráčková L, Lenčešová Z, Trosko JE, Upham BL. Chemopreventive agents attenuate rapid inhibition of gap junctional intercellular communication induced by environmental toxicants. Nutrition and Cancer. 2016;**68**(5):827-837. DOI: 10.1080/01635581.2016.1180409

[72] Velmurugan B, Mani A, Nagini S. Combination of Sallylcysteine and lycopene induces apoptosis by modulating Bcl-2, Bax, Bim and caspases during experimental gastric carcinogenesis. European Journal of Cancer Prevention. 2005;**14**(4):387-393.

[73] Deepak AV, Salimath BP. Antiangiogenic and proapoptotic activity of a novel glycoprotein from *U. indica* is mediated by NFkappaB and Caspase activated DNase in ascites tumor model. Biochimie. 2006;**88**(3-4):297-307

[74] U.S. National Research Council, Committee on Diet and Health. Diet and health: implications for reducing chronic disease risk. Washington (DC): National Academy Press. 1989

[75] American Cancer Society. Nutrition and cancer: causation and prevention. An American Cancer Society special report. CA: A Cancer Journal for Clinicians. 1984;**34**:5-10

[76] Steinmetz KA, Potter JD. Vegetables, fruit, and cancer. I. Epidemiology. Cancer Causes Control. 1991;**2**(5):325-357

[77] Block G, Patterson B, Subar A. Fruit, vegetables, and cancer prevention: a review of the epidemiological evidence. Nutrition and Cancer. 1992;**18**(1):1-29

[78] Glade MJ. Food, nutrition, and the prevention of cancer: a global perspective. American Institute for Cancer Research/World Cancer Research Fund, American Institute for Cancer Research, 1997. Nutrition. 1999;**15**(6):523-526

[79] Giovannucci E. Tomatoes, tomato-based products, lycopene, and cancer: review of the epidemiologic literature. Journal of the National Cancer Institute. 1999;**91**(4):317-331

[80] Eroglu A, Harrison EH. Carotenoid metabolism in mammals, including man: formation, occurrence, and function of apocarotenoids. The Journal of Lipid Research. 2013;**54**(7):1719-1730. DOI: 10.1194/jlr.R039537

[81] Rao AV, Agarwal S. Role of antioxidant lycopene in cancer and heart disease. The Journal of the American College of Nutrition. 2000;**19**(5):563-569

[82] Nguyen ML, Schwartz SJ. Lycopene: chemical and biological properties. Food Technology. 1999;**53**:38-45

[83] Stahl W, Sies H. Uptake of lycopene and its geometrical isomers is greater from heat-processed than from unprocessed tomato juice in humans. Journal of Nutrition. 1992;**122**:2161-2166

[84] Caris-Veyrat C, Schmid A, Carail M, Böhm V. Cleavage products of lycopene produced by in vitro oxidations: characterization and mechanisms of formation. Journal of Agricultural and Food Chemistry. 2003;**51**(25):7318-7325

[85] Ferreira AL, Yeumb KJ, Russell RM, Krinsky NI, Tang G. Enzymatic and oxidative metabolites of lycopene. The Journal of Nutritional Biochemistry. 2004;**14**(9):531-540

[86] Gajic M, Zaripheh S, Sun F, Erdman JW Jr. Apo-80-lycopenal and apo-120-lycopenal are metabolic products of lycopene in rat liver. Journal of Nutrition. 2006;**136**(6):1552-1557

[87] Kopec RE, Riedl KM, Harrison EH, Curley Jr, RW, Hruszkewycz DP, Clinton SK, Schwartz SJ. Identification and quantification of apolycopenals in fruits, vegetables, and human plasma. Journal of Agricultural and Food Chemistry. 2010;**58**(6):3290-3296. DOI: 10.1021/jf100415

[88] Giovannucci E, Rimm EB, Liu Y, Stampfer MJ, Willett WC. A rospective study of tomato products, lycopene, and prostate cancer risk. Journal of the National Cancer Institute. 2002;**94**(5):391-398

[89] Etminan M, Takkouche B, Caamaño-Isorna F. The role of tomato products and lycopene in the prevention of prostate cancer: a meta-analysis of observational studies. Cancer Epidemiology, Biomarkers & Prevention. 2004;**13**(3):340-345

[90] Talvas J, Caris-Veyrat C, Guy L, Rambeau M, Lyan B, Minet-Quinard R, Lobaccaro JM, Vasson MP, Georgé S, Mazur A, Rock E. Differential effects of lycopene consumed in tomato paste and lycopene in the form of a purified extract on target genes of cancer prostatic cells. The American Journal of Clinical Nutrition. 2010;**91**(6):1716-1724. DOI: 10.3945/ajcn.2009.28666

[91] Nahum A, Hirsch K, Danilenko M, Watts CK, Prall OW, Levy Y, Sharoni Y. Lycopene inhibition of cell cycle progression in breast and endometrial cancer cells is associated with reduction in cyclin D levels and retention of p27Kip1 in the cyclin E-cdk2 complexes. Oncogene. 2001;**20**(26):3428-3436

[92] Livny O, Kaplan I, Reifen R, Polak-Charcon S, Madar Z, Schwartz B. Lycopene inhibits proliferation and enhances gap-junction communication of KB-1 human oral tumor cells. Journal of Nutrition. 2002;**132**(12):3754-3759.

[93] Liu C, Lian F, Smith DE, Russell RM, Wang XD. Lycopene supplementation inhibits lung squamous metaplasia and induces apoptosis via upregulating insulin-like growth factor-binding protein 3 in cigarette smoke exposed ferrets. Cancer Research. 2003;**63**(12):3138-3144

[94] Tang L, Jin T, Zeng X, Wang JS. Lycopene inhibits the growth of human androgen-independent prostate cancer cells in vitro and in BALB/c nude mice. Journal of Nutrition. 2005;**135**(2):287-290

[95] Herzog A, Siler U, Spitzer V, Seifert N, Denelavas A, Hunziker PB, Hunziker W, Goralczyk R, Wertz K. Lycopene reduced gene expression of steroid targets and inflammatory markers in normal rat prostate. The FASEB Journal. 2005;**19**(2):272-274

[96] Arathi BA, Sowmya PR, Kuriakose GC, Vijay K, Baskaran V, Jayabaskaran C, Lakshminarayana R. Enhanced cytotoxic and apoptosis inducing activity of lycopene oxidation products in different cancer cell lines. Food and Chemical Toxicology. 2016;**97**:265-276. DOI: 10.1016/j.fct.2016.09.016

[97] Seren S, Lieberman R, Bayraktar UD, Heath E, Sahin K, Andic F, Kucuk O. Lycopene in cancer prevention and treatment. American Journal of Therapeutics. 2008;**15**(1):66-81. DOI: 10.1097/MJT.0b013e31804c7120

[98] Ip BC, Wang XD. Non-alcoholic steatohepatitis and hepatocellular carcinoma: implications for lycopene intervention. Nutrients. 2013;**6**(1):124-162. DOI: 10.3390/nu6010124

[99] Sahin K, Tuzcu M, Sahin N, Ali S, Kucuk O. Nrf2/HO-1 signaling pathway may be the prime target for chemoprevention of cisplatin-induced nephrotoxicity by lycopene. Food and Chemical Toxicology . 2010;**48**(10):2670-2674. DOI: 10.1016/j.fct.2010.06.038

[100] Trejo-Solís C, Pedraza-Chaverrí J, Torres-Ramos M, Jiménez-Farfán D, Cruz Salgado A, Serrano-García N, Osorio-Rico L, Sotelo J. Multiple molecular and cellular mechanisms of action of lycopene in cancer inhibition. Evidence-Based Complementary and Alternative Medicine. 2013;**2013**:705121. DOI: 10.1155/2013/705121

[101] Lu QY, Hung JC, Heber D, Go VL, Reuter VE, Cordon-Cardo C, Scher HI, Marshall JR, Zhang ZF. Inverse associations between plasma lycopene and other carotenoids and prostate cancer. Cancer Epidemiology, Biomarkers & Prevention. 2001;**10**(7):749-756

[102] Hwang ES, Bowen PE. Cell cycle arrest and induction of apoptosis by lycopene in LNCaP human prostate cancer cells. Journal of Medicinal Food. 2004;**7**:284-289

[103] Ford NA, Elsen AC, Zuniga K, Lindshield BL, Erdman JW Jr. Lycopene and apo-12′-lycopenal reduce cell proliferation and alter cell cycle progression in human prostate cancer cells. Nutrition and Cancer. 2011;**63**:256-263. DOI: 10.1080/01635581.2011.523494

[104] Li D, Chen L, Zhao W, Hao J, An R. MicroRNA-let-7f-1 is induced by lycopene and inhibits cell proliferation and triggers apoptosis in prostate cancer. Molecular Medicine Reports. 2016;**13**(3):2708-2714. DOI: 10.3892/mmr.2016.4841

[105] Tan HL, Thomas-Ahner JM, Moran NE, Cooperstone JL, Erdman JW Jr, Young GS, Clinton SK. β-Carotene 9′,10′ oxygenase modulates the anticancer activity of dietary tomato or lycopene on prostate carcinogenesis in the TRAMP model. Cancer Prevention Research (Phila). 2016;**2**. DOI: 10.1158/1940-6207.CAPR-15-0402

[106] Gong X, Marisiddaiah R, Zaripheh S, Wiener D, Rubin LP. Mitochondrial β-carotene 9′,10′ oxygenase modulates prostate cancer growth via NF-κB inhibition: a lycopene-independent function. Molecular Cancer Research. 2016;**14**(10):966-975

[107] Yang CM, Yen YT, Huang CS, Hu ML. Growth inhibitory efficacy of lycopene and β-carotene against androgen-independent prostate tumor cells xenografted in nude mice. Molecular Nutrition & Food Research. 2011;**55**(4):606-612. DOI: 10.1002/mnfr.201000308

[108] Kucuk O, Sarkar F, Sakr W, Djuric Z, Khachik F, Pollak M, Bertram J, Grignon D, Banerjee M, Crissman J, Pontes E, Wood DP Jr. Phase II randomized clinical trial of lycopene supplementation before radical prostatectomy. Cancer Epidemiology, Biomarkers & Prevention. 2001;**10**(8):861-868

[109] Gupta S. Review prostate cancer chemoprevention current status and future prospect. Toxicology and Applied Pharmacology. 2007;**224**(3):369-376. DOI: 10.1016/j.taap.2006.11.008

[110] Paur I, Lilleby W, Bøhn SK, Hulander E, Klein W, Vlatkovic L, Axcrona K, Bolstad N, Bjøro T, Laake P, Taskén KA, Svindland A, Eri LM, Brennhovd B, Carlsen MH, Fosså SD, Smeland SS, Karlsen AS, Blomhoff R. Tomato-based randomized controlled trial in prostate cancer patients: effect on PSA. Clinical Nutrition. 2016;**pii: S0261-5614**(16):30147-30149. DOI: 10.1016/j.clnu.2016.06.01

[111] Wang Y, Jacobs EJ, Newton CC, McCullough ML. Lycopene, tomato products and prostate cancer-specific mortality among men diagnosed with nonmetastatic prostate cancer in the Cancer Prevention Study II Nutrition Cohort. International Journal of Cancer. 2016;**138**(12):2846-2855. DOI: 10.1002/ijc.30027

[112] Assar EA, Vidalle MC, Chopra M, Hafizi S. Lycopene acts through inhibition of IκB kinase to suppress NF-κB signaling in human prostate and breast cancer cells. Tumour Biology. 2016;**37**(7):9375-9385. DOI: 10.1007/s13277-016-4798-3

[113] Ali S, Mann DA. Signal transduction via the NF-κB pathway: a targeted treatment modality for infection, inflammation and repair (Review). Cell Biochemistry and Function. 2004;**22**(2):67-79. DOI: 10.1002/cbf.1082

[114] Gloria NF, Soares N, Brand C, Oliveira FL, Borojevic R, Teodoro AJ. Lycopene and beta-carotene induce cell-cycle arrest and apoptosis in human breast cancer cell lines. Anticancer Research. 2014;**34**(3):1377-1386

[115] Cui Y, Shikany JM, Liu S, Shagufta Y, Rohan TE. Selected antioxidants and risk of hormone receptor-defined invasive breast cancers among postmenopausal women in the Women's Health Initiative Observational Study. The American Journal of Clinical Nutrition. 2008;**87**(4):1009-1018

[116] Sahin K, Tuzcu M, Sahin N, Akdemir F, Ozercan I, Bayraktar S, Kucuk O. Inhibitory effects of combination of lycopene and genistein on 7,12-dimethyl benz(a)anthracene-induced breast cancer in rats. Nutrition and Cancer. 2011;**63**(8):1279-1286. DOI: 10.1080/01635581.2011.606955

[117] Voskuil DW, Vrieling A, Korse CM, Beijnen JH, Bonfrer JM, van Doorn J, Kaas R, Oldenburg HS, Russell NS, Rutgers EJ, Verhoef S, van Leeuwen FE, van't Veer LJ, Rookus MA. Effects of lycopene on the insulin-like growth factor (IGF) system in premenopausal breast cancer survivors and women at high familial breast cancer risk. Nutrition and Cancer. 2008;**60**(3):342-353. DOI: 10.1080/01635580701861777

[118] Al-Malki AL, Moselhy SS, Refai MY. Synergistic effect of lycopene and tocopherol against oxidative stress and mammary tumorigenesis induced by 7,12-dimethyl[a] benzanthracene in female rats. Toxicology and Industrial Health. 2012;**542**(6):542-548. DOI: 10.1177/0748233711416948

[119] Sahin K, Orhan C, Tuzcu M, Sahin N, Ali S, Bahcecioglu IH, Guler O, Ozercan I, Ilhan N, Kucuk O. Orally administered lycopene attenuates diethylnitrosamine-induced hepatocarcinogenesis in rats by modulating Nrf-2/HO-1 and Akt/mTOR pathways. Nutrition and Cancer. 2014;**66**(4):590-598. DOI: 10.1080/01635581.2014.894092

[120] Kim MJ, Kim H. anticancer effect of lycopene in gastric carcinogenesis. Journal of Cancer Prevention. 2015;**20**(2):92-96. DOI: 10.15430/JCP.2015.20.2.92

[121] Wang X, Yang HH, Liu Y, Zhou Q, Chen ZH. Lycopene consumption and risk of colorectal cancer: a meta-analysis of observational studies. Nutrition and Cancer. 2016;**68**(7):1083-1096. DOI: 10.1080/01635581.2016.1206579

[122] Liu C, Russell RM. Nutrition and gastric cancer risk: an update. Nutrition Reviews. 2008;**66**(5):237-249. DOI: 10.1111/j.1753-4887.2008.00029.x

[123] Teodoro AJ, Oliveira FL, Martins NB, Maia Gde A, Martucci RB, Borojevic R. Effect of lycopene on cell viability and cell cycle progression in human cancer cell lines. Cancer Cell International. 2012;**12**(1):36. DOI: 10.1186/1475-2867-12-36

[124] Tang FY, Shih CJ, Cheng LH, Ho HJ, Chen H. Lycopene inhibits growth of human colon cancer cells via suppression of the Akt signaling pathway. Molecular Nutrition & Food Research. 2008;**52**(6):646-654. DOI: 10.1002/mnfr.200700272

[125] Palozza P, Bellovino D, Simone R, Boninsegna A, Cellini F, Monastra G, Gaetani S. Effect of beta-carotene-rich tomato lycopene beta-cyclase (tlcy-b) on cell growth inhibition in HT-29 colon adenocarcinoma cells. British Journal of Nutrition. 2009;**102**(2):207-214. DOI: 10.1017/S0007114508169902

[126] Tuzcu M, Aslan A, Tuzcu Z, Yabas M, Bahcecioglu IH, Ozercan IH, Kucuk O, Sahin K. Tomato powder impedes the development of azoxymethane-induced colorectal cancer in rats through suppression of COX-2 expression via NF-κB and regulating Nrf2/HO-1 pathway. Molecular Nutrition & Food Research. 2012;**56**(9):1477-1481. DOI: 10.1002/mnfr.20120013

[127] Dias MC, Vieiralves NF, Gomes MI, Salvadori DM, Rodrigues MA, Barbisan LF. Effects of lycopene, synbiotic and their association on early biomarkers of rat colon carcinogenesis. Food and Chemical Toxicology . 2010;**48**(3):772-780. DOI: 10.1016/j.fct.2009.12.003

[128] Tang FY, Pai MH, Wang XD. Consumption of lycopene inhibits the growth and progression of colon cancer in a mouse xenograft model. Journal of Agricultural and Food Chemistry. 2011;**59**(16):9011-9021. DOI: 10.1021/jf2017644

[129] Vrieling A, Voskuil DW, Bonfrer JM, Korse CM, van Doorn J, Cats A, Depla AC, Timmer R, Witteman BJ, van Leeuwen FE, Van't Veer LJ, Rookus MA, Kampman E. Lycopene supplementation elevates circulating insulin-like growth factor binding protein-1 and -2 concentrations in persons at greater risk of colorectal cancer. American Journal of Clinical Nutrition. 2007;**86**(5):1456-1462

[130] Walfisch S, Walfisch Y, Kirilov E, Linde N, Mnitentag H, Agbaria R, Sharoni Y, Levy J. Tomato lycopene extract supplementation decreases insulin-like growth factor-I levels in colon cancer patients. European Journal of Cancer Prevention. 2007;**16**(4):298-303

[131] Riso P, Brusamolino A, Martinetti A, Porrini M. Effect of a tomato drink intervention on insulin-like growth factor (IGF)-1 serum levels in healthy subjects. Nutrition and Cancer. 2006;**55**(2):157-162

[132] Jang SH, Lim JW, Morio T, Kim H. Lycopene inhibits Helicobacter pylori-induced ATM/ATR-dependent DNA damage response in gastric epithelial AGS cells. Free Radical Biology & Medicine. 2012;**52**(3):607-615. DOI: 10.1016/j.freeradbiomed.2011.11.010

[133] Liu C, Russell RM, Wang XD. Lycopene supplementation prevents smoke-induced changes in p53, p53 phosphorylation, cell proliferation, and apoptosis in the gastric mucosa of ferrets. Journal of Nutrition. 2006;**136**(1):106-111

[134] Park YO, Hwang ES, Moon TW. The effect of lycopene on cell growth and oxidative DNA damage of Hep3B human hepatoma cells. Biofactors. 2005;**23**(3):129-139

[135] Hwang ES, Lee HJ. Inhibitory effects of lycopene on the adhesion, invasion, and migration of SK-Hep1 human hepatoma cells. Experimental Biology and Medicine (Maywood). 2006;**231**(3):322-327

[136] Astorg P, Gradelet S, Berges R, Suschetet M. Dietary lycopene decreases the initiation of liver preneoplastic foci by diethylnitrosamine in the rat. Nutrition and Cancer. 1997;**29**(1):60-68

[137] Watanabe S, Kitade Y, Masaki T, Nishioka M, Satoh K, Nishino H. Effects of lycopene and Sho-saiko-to on hepatocarcinogenesis in a rat model of spontaneous liver cancer. Nutrition and Cancer. 2001;**39**(1):96-101

[138] Kujawska M, Ewertowska M, Adamska T, Sadowski C, Ignatowicz E, Jodynis-Liebert J. Antioxidant effect of lycopene-enriched tomato paste on N-nitrosodiethylamine-induced oxidative stress in rats. Journal of Physiology and Biochemistry. 2014;**70**(4):981-990. DOI: 10.1007/s13105-014-0367-7

[139] Wang Y, Ausman LM, Greenberg AS, Russell RM, Wang XD. Dietary lycopene and tomato extract supplementations inhibit nonalcoholic steatohepatitis-promoted hepatocarcinogenesis in rats. International Journal of Cancer. 2010;**126**(8):1788-1796. DOI: 10.1002/ijc.24689

[140] Toledo LP, Ong TP, Pinho AL, Jordão A Jr, Vanucchi H, Moreno FS. Inhibitory effects of lutein and lycopene on placental glutathione S-transferase-positive preneoplastic lesions and DNA strand breakage induced in Wistar rats by the resistant hepatocyte model of hepatocarcinogenesis. Nutrition and Cancer. 2003;**47**(1):62-69

[141] Ip BC, Liu C, Ausman LM, von Lintig J, Wang XD. Lycopene attenuated hepatic tumorigenesis via differential mechanisms depending on carotenoid cleavage enzyme in mice. Cancer Prevention Research (Phila). 2014;**7**(12):1219-1227. DOI: 10.1158/1940-6207.CAPR-14-0154

[142] Nishino H. Cancer prevention by natural carotenoids. Journal of Cellular Biochemistry. 1997;**67**(27):86-91. DOI: 10.1002/(SICI)1097-4644(1997)27+<86::AID-JCB14>3.0.CO;2-J

[143] Maurya BK, Trigun SK. Fisetin modulates antioxidant enzymes and inflammatory factors to inhibit aflatoxin-B1 induced hepatocellular carcinoma in rats. Oxidative Medicine and Cellular Longevity. 2016;**2016**:1972793. DOI: .org/10.1155/2016/1972793

[144] Sharoni Y, Linnewiel-Hermoni K, Khanin M, Salman H, Veprik A, Danilenko M, Levy J. Carotenoids and apocarotenoids in cellular signaling related to cancer: a review. Molecular Nutrition & Food Research. 2012;**56**(2):259-269. DOI: 10.1002/mnfr.201100311

[145] Ho WJ, Simon MS, Yildiz VO, Shikany JM, Kato I, Beebe-Dimmer JL, Cetnar JP, Bock CH. Antioxidant micronutrients and the risk of renal cell carcinoma in the Women's Health Initiative cohort. Cancer. 2015;**121**(4):580-588. DOI: 10.1002/cncr.29091

[146] Bertoia M, Albanes D, Mayne ST, Männistö S, Virtamo J, Wright ME. No association between fruit, vegetables, antioxidant nutrients and risk of renal cell carcinoma. International Journal of Cancer. 2010;**126**(6):1504-1512. DOI: 10.1002/ijc.24829

[147] Bosetti C, Scotti L, Maso LD, Talamini R, Montella M, Negri E, Ramazzotti V, Franceschi S, La Vecchia C. Micronutrients and the risk of renal cell cancer: a case-control study from Italy. International Journal of Cancer. 2007;**120**(4):892-896

[148] Brock KE, Ke L, Gridley G, Chiu BC, Ershow AG, Lynch CF, Graubard BI, Cantor KP. Fruit, vegetables, fibre and micronutrients and risk of US renal cell carcinoma. British Journal of Nutrition. 2012;**108**(6):1077-1085. DOI: 10.1017/S0007114511006489

[149] Sahin K, Cross B, Sahin N, Ciccone K, Suleiman S, Osunkoya AO, Master V, Harris W, Carthon B, Mohammad R, Bilir B, Wertz K, Moreno CS, Walker CL, Kucuk O. Lycopene in the prevention of renal cell cancer in the TSC2 mutant Eker rat model. Archives of Biochemistry and Biophysics. 2015;**572**:36-39. DOI: 10.1016/j.abb.2015.01.006

[150] Okajima E, Ozono S, Endo T, Majima T, Tsutsumi M, Fukuda T, Akai H, Denda A, Hirao Y, Okajima E, Nishino H, Nir Z, Konishi Y. Chemopreventive efficacy of piroxicam administered alone or in combination with lycopene and ß-carotene on the development of rat urinary bladder carcinoma after N-butyl-N-(4-hydroxybutyl) nitrosamine treatment. Japanese Journal of Cancer Research. 1997;**88**(6):543-552

[151] Zeegers MP, Goldbohm RA, van den Brandt PA. Are retinol, vitamin C, folate and carotenoids intake associated with bladder cancer risk? Results from the Netherlands Cohort Study. British Journal of Cancer. 2001;**28**(7):977-983.

[152] Helzlsouer KJ, Comstock GW, Morris JS. Selenium, lycopene, alpha-tocopherol, beta-carotene, retinol, and subsequent bladder cancer. Cancer Research. 1989;**49**(21):6144-6148

[153] Hung RJ, Zhang ZF, Rao JY, Pantuck A, Reuter VE, Heber D, Lu QY. Protectivev effects of plasma carotenoids on the risk of bladder cancer. Journal of Urology. 2006; **176**(3):1192-1197

[154] Klarod K, Hongsprabhas P, Khampitak T, Wirasorn K, Kiertiburanakul S, Tangrassameeprasert R, Daduang J, Yongvanit P, Boonsiri P. Serum antioxidant levels and nutritional status in early and advanced stage lung cancer patients. Nutrition. 2011;**27**(11-12):1156-1160. DOI: 10.1016/j.nut.2010.12.019

[155] Graham DL, Carail M, Caris-Veyrat C, Lowe GM. Cigarette smoke and human plasma lycopene depletion. Food and Chemical Toxicology. 2010;**48**(8-9):2413-2420. DOI: 10.1016/j.fct.2010.06.001

[156] Liu C, Russell RM, Seitz HK, Wang XD. Ethanol enhances retinoic acid metabolism into polar metabolites in rat liver via induction of cytochrome P4502E1. Gastroenterology. 2001;**120**(1):179-189

[157] Liu C, Russell RM, Wang XD. Exposing ferrets to cigarette smoke and a pharmacological dose of beta-carotene supplementation enhance in vitro retinoic acid catabolism in lungs via induction of cytochrome P450 enzymes. Journal of Nutrition. 2003;**133**(1):173-179

[158] Lian F, Smith DE, Ernst H, Russell RM, Wang XD. Apo–100–lycopenoic acid inhibits lung cancer cell growth in vitro, and suppresses lung tumorigenesis in the A/J mouse model in vivo. Carcinogenesis. 2007;**28**(7):1567-1574

[159] Muzandu K, Ishizuka M, Sakamoto KQ, Shaban Z, El Bohi K, Kazusaka A, Fujita S. Effect of lycopene and beta-carotene on peroxynitrite-mediated cellular modifications. Toxicology and Applied Pharmacology. 2006;**215**(3):330-340

[160] Kim DJ, Takasuka N, Kim JM, Sekine K, Ota T, Asamoto M, Murakoshi M, Nishino H, Nir Z, Tsuda H. Chemoprevention by lycopene of mouse lung neoplasia after combined initiation treatment with DEN, MNU and DMH. Cancer Letters. 1997;**120**(1):15-22

[161] Kim DJ, Takasuka N, Nishino H, Tsuda H. Chemopreventiopn of lung cancer by 1319 lycopene. Biofactors. 2000;**13**:95-102

[162] Pratheeshkumar P, Thejass P, Kutan G. Diallyl disulfide induces caspase-dependent apoptosis via mitochondria-mediated intrinsic pathway in B16F-10 melanoma cells by up-regulating p53, caspase-3 and down-regulating pro-inflammatory cytokines and nuclear factor-κβ-mediated Bcl-2 activation. Journal of Environmental Pathology, Toxicology and Oncology. 2010;**29**(2):113-125.

[163] Priyadarsini RV, Murugan RS, Sripriya P, Karunagaran D, Nagini S. The neem limonoids azadirachtin and nimbolide induce cell cycle arrest and mitochondria-mediated apoptosis in human cervical cancer (HeLa) cells. Free Radical Research. 2010;**44**(6):624-634. DOI: 10.3109/10715761003692503

[164] Kumar HG, Priyadarsini VR, Vinothini G, Letchoumy VP, Nagini S. The neem limonoids azadirachtin and nimbolide inhibit cell proliferation and induce apoptosis in an animal model of oral oncogenesis. Investigational New Drugs. 2010;**28**(4):392-401. DOI: 10.1007/s10637-009-9263-3

[165] Bhushan S, Malik F, Kumar A, Isher HK, Kaur IP, Taneja SC, Singh J. Activation of p53/p21/PUMA alliance and disruption of PI-3/Akt in multimodal targeting of apoptotic signaling cascades in cervical cancer cells by a pentacyclic triterpenediol from *Boswellia serrata*. Molecular Carcinogenesis. 2009;**48**(12):1093-1108. DOI: 10.1002/mc.20559

[166] Adhikary A, Mohanty S, Lahiry L, Hossain DM, Chakraborty S, Das T. Theaflavins retard human breast cancer cell migration by inhibiting NF-kappaB via p53-ROS cross-talk. FEBS Letters. 2010;**584**(1):7-14. DOI: 10.1016/j.febslet.2009.10.081

[167] Singh M, Singh N. Curcumin counteracts the proliferative effect of estradiol and induces apoptosis in cervical cancer cells. Molecular and Cellular Biochemistry. 2010;**347**(1-2):1-11. DOI: 10.1007/s11010-010-0606-3

[168] Banerjee M, Singh P, Panda D. Curcumin suppresses the dynamic instability of microtubules, activates the mitotic checkpoint and induces apoptosis in MCF-7 cells. The FEBS Journal. 2010;**277**(16):3437-3448. DOI: 10.1111/j.1742-4658.2010.07750.x

[169] Lavhale MS, Kumar S, Mishra SH, Sitasawad SL. A novel triterpenoid isolated from the root bark of Ailanthus excelsa Roxb (Tree of Heaven), AECHL-1 as a potential anti-cancer agent. PLoS One. 2009;**4**(4):e5365. DOI: 10.1371/journal.pone.0005365

[170] Bhattacharya U, Halder B, Mukhopadhyay S, Giri AK. Role of oxidation-triggered activation of JNK and p38 MAPK in black tea polyphenols induced apoptotic death of A375 cells. Cancer Science. 2009;**100**(10):1971-1978. DOI: 10.1111/j.1349-7006.2009.01251.x

[171] Patel R, Krishnan R, Ramchandani A, Maru G. Polymeric black tea polyphenols inhibit mouse skin chemical carcinogenesis by decreasing cell proliferation. Cell Proliferation. 2008;**41**(3):532-553. DOI: 10.1111/j.1365-2184.2008.00528.x

[172] Prasad CP, Rath G, Mathur S, Bhatnagar D, Ralhan R. Potent growth suppressive activity of curcumin in human breast cancer cells: modulation of Wnt/beta-catenin signaling. Chemico-Biological Interactions. 2009;**181**(2):263-271. DOI: 10.1016/j.cbi.2009.06.012

[173] Jyothi D, Vanathi P, Mangala Gowri P, Rama Subba Rao V, Madhusudana Rao J, Sreedhar AS. Diferuloylmethane augments the cytotoxic effects of piplartine isolated from *Piper chaba*. Toxicology in Vitro. 2009;**23**(6):1085-1091. DOI: 10.1016/j.tiv.2009.05.023

[174] Sathya S, Sudhagar S, Vidhya Priya M, Bharathi Raja R, Muthusamy VS, Niranjali Devaraj S, Lakshmi BS. 3β-Hydroxylup-20(29)-ene-27,28-dioic acid dimethyl ester, a novel natural product from Plumbago zeylanica inhibits the proliferation and migration of MDA-MB-231 cells. Chemico-Biological Interactions. 2010;**188**(3):412-420. DOI: 10.1016/j.cbi.2010.07.019

[175] Mondal S, Mandal C, Sangwan R, Chandra S, Mandal C. Withanolide D induces apoptosis in leukemia by targeting the activation of neutral sphingomyelinase-ceramide

cascade mediated by synergistic activation of c-Jun N-terminal kinase and p38 mitogenactivated protein kinase. Molecular Cancer. 2010;**9**:239. DOI: 10.1186/1476-4598-9-239

[176] Mandal C, Dutta A, Mallick A, Chandra S, Misra L, Sangwan RS, Mandal C. Withaferin A induces apoptosis by activating p38 mitogen-activated protein kinase signaling cascade in leukemic cells of lymphoid and myeloid origin through mitochondrial death cascade. Apoptosis. 2008;**13**(12):1450-1464. DOI: 10.1007/s10495-008-0271-0

[177] Lahiry L, Saha B, Chakraborty J, Adhikary A, Mohanty S, Hossain DM, Banerjee S, Das K, Sa G, Das T. Theaflavins target Fas/caspase-8 and Akt/pBad pathways to induce apoptosis in p53-mutated human breast cancer cells. Carcinogenesis. 2010;**31**(2):259-268. DOI: 10.1093/carcin/bgp240

[178] Kumar A, Malik F, Bhushan S, Sethi VK, Shahi AK, Kaur J, Taneja SC, Qazi GN, Singh J. An essential oil and its major constituent isointermedeol induce apoptosis by increased expression of mitochondrial cytochrome c and apical death receptors in human leukaemia HL-60 cells. Chemico-Biological Interactions. 2008;**171**(3):332-347

Section 3

Anticancer Compounds from Cannabinoids and Endophytic Fungi

Chapter 6

Phytochemical Aspects and Therapeutic Perspective of Cannabinoids in Cancer Treatment

Sanda Vladimir-Knežević, Biljana Blažeković, Maja Bival Štefan and Marija Kindl

Additional information is available at the end of the chapter

http://dx.doi.org/10.5772/67746

Abstract

Cannabinoids comprise the plant-derived compounds and their synthetic derivatives as well as endogenously produced lipophilic mediators. Phytocannabinoids are terpenophenolic secondary metabolites predominantly produced in *Cannabis sativa* L. The principal active constituent is delta-9-tetrahydrocannabinol (THC), which binds to endocannabinoid receptors to exert its pharmacological activity, including psychoactive effect. The other important molecule of current interest is non-psychotropic cannabidiol (CBD). Since 1970s, phytocannabinoids have been known for their palliative effects on some cancer-associated symptoms such as nausea and vomiting reduction, appetite stimulation and pain relief. More recently, these molecules have gained special attention for their role in cancer cell proliferation and death. A large body of evidence suggests that cannabinoids affect multiple signalling pathways involved in the development of cancer, displaying an anti-proliferative, proapoptotic, anti-angiogenic and anti-metastatic activity on a wide range of cell lines and animal models of cancer. These findings have led to the development of clinical studies to investigate potential anti-cancer activity in humans, but reliable clinical evidence for this therapeutic option is still missing.

Keywords: cannabinoids, phytochemistry, THC, CBD, cancer

1. Introduction

Cannabis sativa L. (Cannabaceae) is one of the first plants cultivated by man and one of the oldest plant sources of fibre, food and remedies. It has a long history of medical use in the Middle East and Asia, dating back to the sixth century BC. During a period of colonial expansion in the early nineteenth century, cannabis found a way to Western Europe as a medicine to alleviate a variety of conditions, such as pain, spasms, dysentery, depression, sleep disturbance and loss of appetite. In the beginning of the twentieth century, due to the availability of substitute drugs, absence of quality control and the risk of abuse and intoxication, cannabis medication fell into disuse. Moreover, following the UN Single Convention on Narcotic Drugs in 1961, cannabis and its products were classified as narcotics. Phytochemical analysis of cannabis in the 1940s and 1960s led to the discovery of a unique group of terpenophenolic secondary metabolites, known as cannabinoids, of which *trans*-(−)-delta-9-tetrahydrocannabinol (THC) was shown to be the primary active constituent which is responsible for the plant's psychoactive effect [1–3]. Many natural products besides cannabinoids have been isolated from cannabis, including terpenes, flavonoids, steroids and nitrogenous compounds. Up to date, 750 constituents have been identified from cannabis, out of which over 100 are classified as cannabinoids [4, 5]. Research of the cannabis medical properties has gained worldwide interest after the discovery of two types of cannabinoid receptors, which are G-protein coupled receptors specifically responding to endocannabinoids and phytocannabinoids, and related synthetic cannabimimetic compounds. Therefore, the term cannabinoids now includes not only the plant-derived compounds (phytocannabinoids), but also in laboratory synthesised derivatives (synthetic cannabinoids) and a family of endogenously produced compounds (endocannabinoids) [6]. The therapeutic properties of cannabis have been much debated from scientific and regulatory points of view over the years. The medical use of cannabis is still controversial and strongly limited by unavoidable psychotropic effects. However, solid scientific data indicated the potential of therapeutic value of cannabis in controlling some forms of pain, relieving chemotherapy-induced nausea and vomiting, treating cachexia and anorexia in AIDS patients and combating muscle spasms in multiple sclerosis with no evidence that giving cannabis to the patients would increase illicit drug use in the general population [7]. Nowadays, many countries legalised cannabis for medical purposes. To avoid abuse, numerous centres for cannabis therapy are founded worldwide and usually organised as clinics where cannabis can be prescribed in various forms, including dried plant material and cannabis extract. So far, only three cannabis-based medicines have been registered for certain indications. In the context of cancer, dronabinol (synthetically generated THC) and nabilone (a synthetic THC analogue) can be prescribed to prevent chemotherapy-induced nausea and vomiting. Nabiximols, plant extract enriched in THC and cannabidiol (CBD) at an approximate 1:1 ratio, are approved for the treatment of cancer-associated pain [8]. Apart from these palliative effects, recent preclinical studies suggest that various cannabinoids exert antitumour effects in different experimental cancer models [1]. In this chapter, we will focus on phytochemistry and pharmacology of cannabinoids as well as their current and potential roles in symptom management and cancer therapy.

2. The cannabis plant

The concept of *Cannabis* as a monotypic genus containing just a single highly polymorphic species is widely accepted, although there has been a long-standing debate among taxonomists regarding classification of the existing varieties. Other previously described species, including *C. indica* Lam. and *C. ruderalis* Janisch., are now recognised as varieties of *C. sativa* L. based on morphological, anatomical, phytochemical and genetic studies [9, 10]. *C. sativa* L. is an annual, herbaceous, taprooted and predominantly dioecious plant. Its height (0.2–6 m) and degree of branching depend on both genetic and environmental factors. Staminate (male) plants are usually taller but less robust than pistillate (female) plants. The leaves are petiolate, palmately compound, with an odd number (3–13) of coarsely serrate, lanceolate leaflets. The male inflorescence is a lax panicle or compound cyme composed of many individual, yellowish green, pedicellate flowers containing five pendulous anthers. The pistillate flowers are green, sometimes purple to red, sessile, grouped in apical leaf axils or terminals of branches. They form short, congested pseudo-spikes among leaf-like bracts and bracteoles. Each flower has a small green bract enclosing the ovary with two long, slender pistils projecting well above the bract. The male plants commence flowering slightly before the females. When mature, the sepals on the male flowers are open to enable passing air currents to transfer the released pollens to the pistillate flowers. Soon after pollination, the male plants wither and die in order to secure more space, nutrients and water to the females so that they could produce a healthy crop of viable seeds. Following fertilisation, the ovary develops into an achene, a fruit containing a single seed with a hard shell [11–13]. The surface of aerial plant parts is covered in trichomes. These are either covering (non-glandular) trichomes or glandular trichomes containing a resin (**Figure 1**). Non-glandular trichomes are numerous, unicellular, rigid and curved hairs, with a slender pointed apex. Cystolithic trichomes found on the upper surface of the cannabis leaves are swollen at the base and have calcium carbonate crystals (cystoliths), while slender non-cystolithic trichomes occur mainly on the lower side of the leaves, bracts and bracteoles. Three morphologically distinct types of glandular trichomes have been identified: (1) a long multi-cellular stalk and a multi-cellular head with approximately eight radiating club-shaped cells (capitate-stalked); (2) sessile with a multi-cellular head (capitate-sessile); (3) a short unicellular stalk and a bi-cellular, rarely four-cell, head (bulbous). These are mainly associated with the female inflorescences, but they can also be found on the underside of the leaves and occasionally on the stems of young plants. Bulbous and capitate-sessile trichomes occur on all parts of vegetative and flowering shoots. In contrast, capitate-stalked trichomes are restricted to flowering regions. The glandular trichomes are secretory structures, where the cannabinoid-laden resin is produced and stored. Besides cannabinoids, these trichomes produce terpenes, which are responsible for the typical plant aroma. The extreme variations in cannabinoid contents of the different tissues are due to markedly different distributions of glandular trichomes on the surface of the plant [14, 15]. The unfertilised flower heads and flower bracts of the female plant are the primary source of cannabinoids (**Figure 1**).

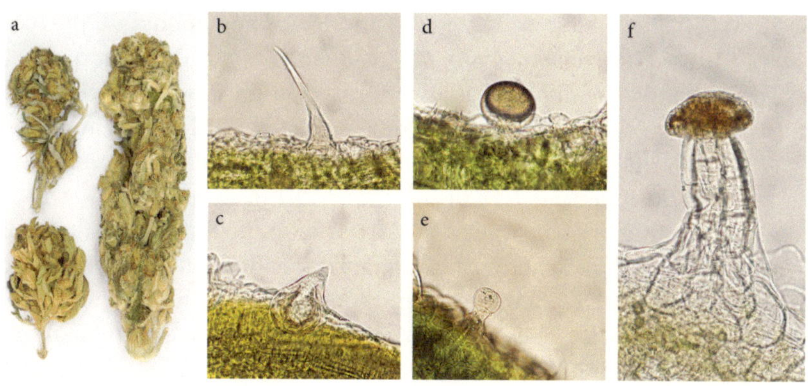

Figure 1. *Cannabis sativa* L. – dried pistillate inflorescences and trichomes on their surface. (a) dried pistillate inflorescences (50% of the size); (b) non-cystolithic trichome; (c) cystolithic trichome; (d) capitate-sessile trichome; (e) simple bulbous trichome; (f) capitate-stalked trichome (400×).

3. Biosynthesis and structure of phytocannabinoids

Phytocannabinoids represent a group of terpenophenolic compounds predominantly produced in the cannabis plant. These secondary metabolites are biosynthesised as prenylated aromatic carboxylic acids, and while almost no neutral forms can be found in fresh plants. However, cannabinoid acids may convert to their neutral homologues by spontaneous decarboxylation under the influence of light, heat or prolonged storage. The precursors of phytocannabinoids originate from two distinct biosynthetic pathways: the polyketide pathway, giving rise to olivetolic acid (OA) or divarinic acid (DA), and methylerythritol phosphate pathway, leading to the synthesis of geranyl pyrophosphate (GPP). The biogenesis of phytocannabinoids containing n-pentyl side chain starts with the condensation of OA and GPP into cannabigerolic acid (CBGA), catalysed by geranyl pyrophosphate—olivetolate geranyl transferase (GOT). The isoprenylation step is next followed by activity of three corresponding oxidative cyclases that generate tetrahydrocannabinolic acid (THCA), cannabidiolic acid (CBDA) and cannabichromenic acid (CBCA) from CBGA as the key intermediate. The phytocannabinoid acids are non-enzymatically decarboxylated into cannabigerol (CBG), delta-9-tetrahydrocannabinol (delta-9-THC), cannabidiol (CBD) and cannabichromene (CBC) [16, 17]. **Figure 2** shows the cannabinoid biosynthetic pathway and the structures of the major constituents. The biosynthesis of phytocannabinoids with C3 side-chain (propyl cannabinoids) from DA probably follows a similar pathway yielding cannabigerovarinic acid [18].

Over 100 various phytocannabinoids have been found so far, but many of them are produced in trace quantities or represent auto-oxidation artefacts [16, 19]. The structural diversity of naturally occurring cannabinoids is the result of differences in the nature of their isoprenyl residue, resorcinyl core and side chain. Based on the structural variation, Hanuš and coworkers [4] have classified phytocannabinoids as follows: cannabigerol, cannabichromene, cannabidiol, tetrahydrocannabinol, cannabinol, thymyl, cannabielsoin, cannabicyclol and 8,9-secomenthyl types. The *Cannabigerol type* compounds are one of the most structurally diversified classes of phytocannabinoids. A linear isoprenyl residue is their main feature, as exemplified by CBG, which was the first structurally elucidated and also the first natural cannabinoid to be synthesised. The isoprenyl residue of CBG is non-oxygenated, indicating its early biogenetic stage within phytocannabinoids. Other components of this type are propyl side-chain analogues (cannabigerovarin) and monomethyl ether derivative. The isoprenyl residue is oxidatively fused to the resorcinyl ring in the *cannabichromene type*. Cannabichromene (CBC) is the simplest natural cannabinoid to obtain by synthesis and the only major phytocannabinoid that shows a bluish fluorescence under UV light. CBD, as the main representative of the *cannabidiol type* compounds, was isolated in 1940, but the correct structure elucidation was reported more than two decades later. CBD and its corresponding acid are the most abundant cannabinoids in the fibre-type of cannabis (non-psychotropic). Ten CBD type phytocannabinoids with C1–C5 side-chains have been described. The *tetrahydrocannabinol type* compounds contain several bis-reduced forms of cannabinol (CBN), differing in location of the remaining double bond, the configuration of the chiral centres, or both isomeric options. The most prominent constituent of this subclass is delta-9-THC, the main psychoactive ingredient of cannabis plant, isolated in 1942, but structurally elucidated only in 1964. Other representative of this type is delta-8-THC,

http://dx.doi.org/10.5772/67746

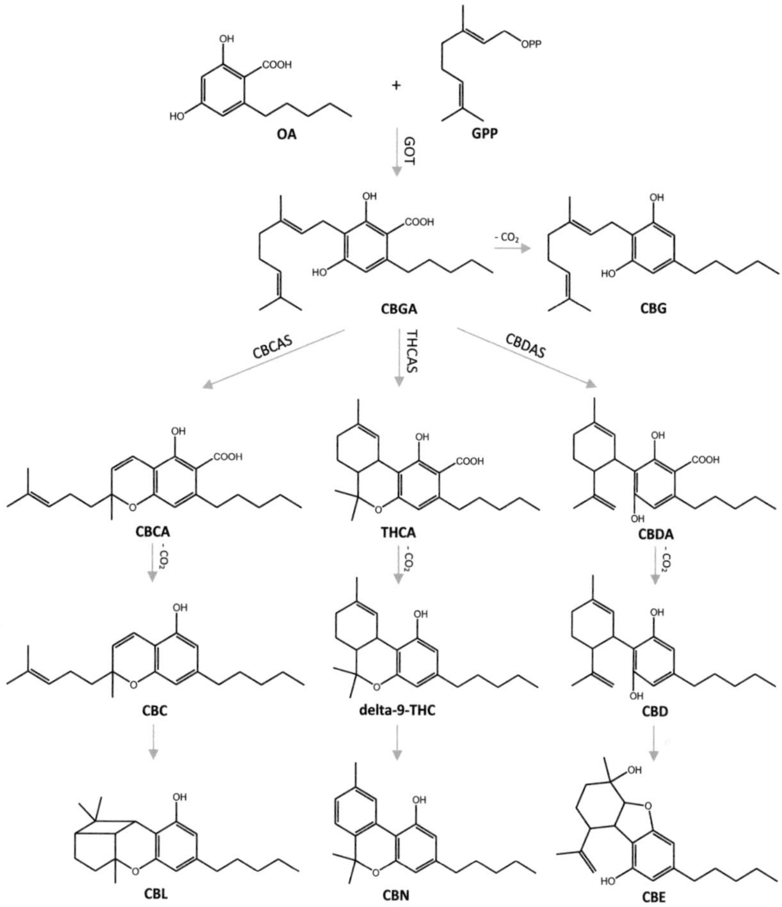

Figure 2. Biosynthesis and degradation of the major phytocannabinoids. OA—olivetolic acid; GPP—geranyl pyrophosphate; GOT—geranyl pyrophosphate—olivetolate geranyl transferase; CBGA—cannabigerolic acid; CBG—cannabigerol; CBCAS—cannabichromenic acid synthase; THCAS—tetrahydrocannabinolic acid synthase; CBDAS—cannabidiolic acid synthase; CBCA—cannabichromenic acid; THCA—tetrahydrocannabinolic acid; CBDA—cannabidiolic acid; CBC—cannabicromene; delta-9-THC—delta-9-tetrahydrocannabinol; CBD—cannabidiol; CBL—cannabicyclol; CBN—cannabinol; CBE—cannabielsoin.

most likely to be generated from delta-9-THC or CBD. It is easier to synthesise and more thermodynamically stable than delta-9-THC. CBN and its derivatives and analogues (*cannabinol type*) are considered artefacts derived from oxidative aromatisation of the corresponding THC type compounds. Their concentration in cannabis products depends on age and storage condition. CBN is highly stable towards oxidative degradation and so has been used as a marker for the identification of narcotic cannabis in archaeological findings. The structural hallmark of *thymyl type* represented by cannabinodiol and cannabifuran is the presence of thymyl group obtained by aromatisation of the menthyl moiety of CBD. The *Cannabielsoin type* compounds are the result of the intra-molecular opening of cannabidiol-type epoxides and could be isolated artefacts. Cannabielsoin (CBE) is the major pyrolytic product of CBD and therefore expected to be present in cannabis smoke. Other artefacts formed during storage of the plant material in the presence of light are *cannabicyclol* (CBL) and its derivatives, characterised by a five-atom ring and C1 bridge instead of a typical six-membered ring in the cannabinoid structure. *8,9-Secomenthyl cannabidiols* are formed by splitting of the endocyclic double bonds of delta-9-THC (cannabicoumaronone) and CBD (cannabimovone) [4, 19, 20].

4. Phytochemical characterisation of cannabinoids

Various scientific attempts have been made to classify *Cannabis* taxa based on their cannabinoid composition, which is under strong environmental influences and also depends on plant sex and maturity. The most important classification of cannabis types in forensics and legislation is that into drug type (marijuana) and fibre type (hemp). A high amount of psychoactive THC characterises the drug type, while particularly low content defines the fibre type [21, 22]. Nowadays, cannabis is divided mainly into three chemotypes (i.e. chemical phenotypes) on the basis of the content ratio of the two major cannabinoids, THC and CBD, in dried inflorescence: (1) THC > 0.3% and CBD < 0.5% (THC predominant); (2) THC ≥ 0.3% and CBD > 0.5% (intermediate); (3) THC < 0.3% and CBD > 0.5% (CBD predominant). Two rare chemotypes with prevalence of CBG and cannabinoid-free, respectively, have also been found [23, 24]. Apart from these chemotypes, de Meijer [25] has additionally described CBC, delta-9-tetrahydrocannabivarin (THCV) and other propyl cannabinoid-rich chemotypes. A large variation of cannabis strains have been developed during a long period of breeding and selection. Over 700 different cultivars of cannabis have been catalogued and many more varieties are thought to exist [26]. With the increasing use of cannabis for medical purposes, the need for a clear chemotaxonomic distinction between varieties has become even more important. Phytocannabinoids were chosen as chemotype markers as they are considered to be the main pharmacologically active constituents in cannabis [27].

Because of the complex chemistry of cannabis, advanced separation techniques, such as gas chromatography (GC) or high performance liquid chromatography (HPLC), often coupled with mass spectrometry detection (MS), are necessary for the determination of the typical phytochemical profiles of cannabis constituents [28, 29]. Thin layer chromatography (TLC) is suitable only for identification of cannabis plant material, detection of its principal cannabinoids and distinguishing between main chemotypes. The separation of phytocannabinoids is mainly achieved by using silica gel as stationary phase, reversed phase for the non-polar system and normal phase for the polar system. Two different reagents for the visualisation of cannabinoids, fast blue and vanillin-sulphuric acid, can be used [11, 30, 31]. **Figure 3** shows high performance thin layer chromatography (HPTLC) chromatogram of cannabis ethanolic extracts, representing THC and CBD predominant types, respectively.

Gas chromatography, commonly coupled to flame ionisation detection (FID) or MS, provides data only on neutral cannabinoids. Due to the high temperature of the injection port, the rapid decarboxylation of the acidic cannabinoids to the neutral forms occurs, thus the real cannabinoid profile of the plant material does not correspond to the results obtained. Derivatisation of phytocannabinoid acids to their trimethylsilyl esters before injection is one approach that can allow the separation and detection of the acidic and neutral forms. Identification of the phytocannabinoids is most readily performed by GC-MS, method of choice for creating cannabis

http://dx.doi.org/10.5772/67746

profiles and metabolic fingerprints [12, 28, 32]. GC-FID is suitable for routine identification and quantification of the major phytocannabinoids as illustrated in **Figure 4**, representing THC and CBD predominant types, respectively.

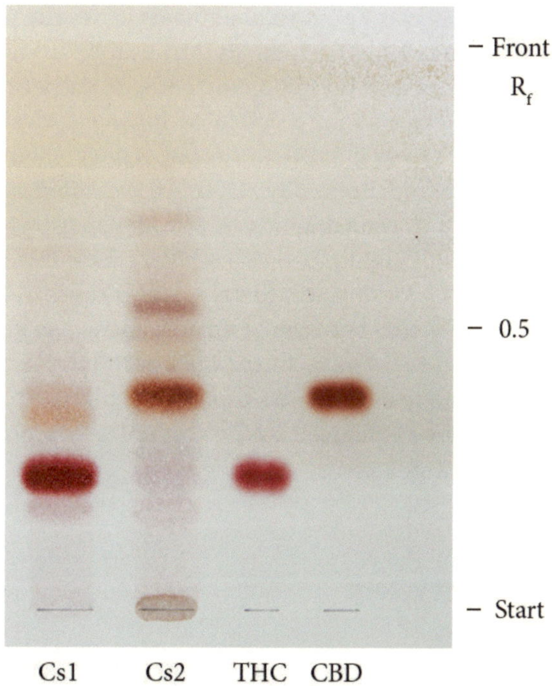

Figure 3. HPTLC chromatogram of phytocannabinoids in the concentrated ethanolic extracts of cannabis inflorescence. Cs1—THC predominant type of *Cannabis sativa* extract; Cs2—CBD predominant type of *Cannabis sativa* extract; stationary phase: HPTLC silica gel C_{18} F_{254}; mobile phase: methanol-water with 0.1% glacial acetic acid 75:25 (V/V); detection: Fast blue reagent; R_f (THC) = 0.25; R_f (CBD) = 0.38.

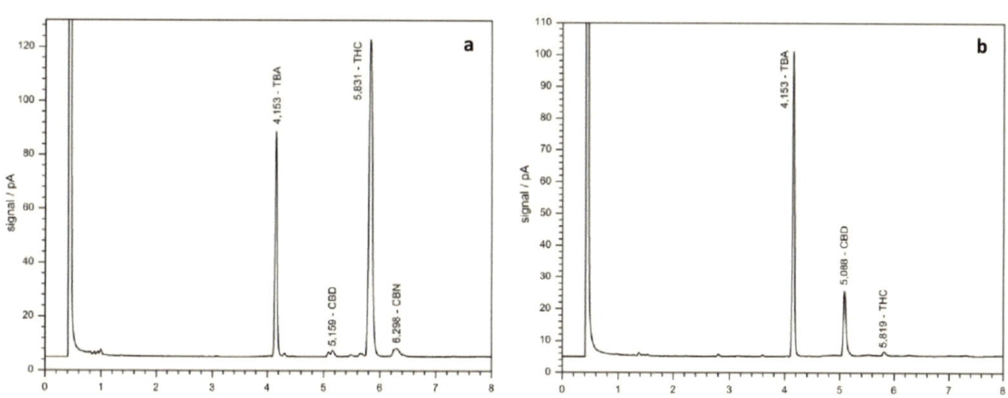

Figure 4. GC-FID chromatograms of two concentrated ethanolic extracts of cannabis inflorescence. (a) THC predominant type of cannabis extract (THC/CBD = 87;2). (b) CBD predominant type of cannabis extract (THC/CBD = 0.08). Agilent 7890A gas chromatograph equipped with FID; HP-5MS column (15 m x 0.25 mm i.d., 0.25 μm film thickness); carrier gas: helium at a constant flow rate of 2.0 mL/minute; temperature program: initial temperature 200°C for 2 minutes, increased by 10°C/minute to final temperature 240°C and held for further 2 minutes; detector temperature 300°C; injector temperature 280°C with split ratio of 20:1; injection volume 1.5 μL; i.s. – tribenzylamine (TBA).

Both acidic and neutral forms of phytocannabinoids can be directly analysed by means of HPLC without any derivatisation step. In contrast to GC, no decomposition occurs during HPLC analysis, which is the main advantage for obtaining the complete cannabinoid profiles. Analytical methods based on reversed-phase chromatography with gradient elution are commonly used. Detection of phytocannabinoids is usually performed by UV and diode array detectors (DAD), but high sensitivity can best be achieved through the use of thermospray MS. Apart from several HPLC methods, ultra performance liquid chromatography (UPLC) method has also been validated for the analysis of a wide range of phytocannabinoids in plant material [13, 29]. Moreover, a novel method of ultra-high performance supercritical fluid chromatography (UHPSFC) coupled with DAD/MS for the separation and discrimination of cannabinoids in complex matrices has been developed and validated [33]. Giese et al. [5] highlighted that typical concentration ranges for the cannabinoids vary from 0.1 to 40% of inflorescence dry weight. These data show how extreme the variations of phytocannabinoids between plant specimens can get, indicating that the cannabis for medical use should always be thoroughly profiled. Therefore, the previously mentioned analyses are of interest given the probability that both the therapeutic and adverse effects of cannabis may be dictated by the concentrations and interactions of certain phytocannabinoids.

5. The endocannabinoid system

The endocannabinoid system (ECS) consists of endogenous cannabinoids, their receptors and the enzymes responsible for their biosynthesis, transport and degradation. The endocannabinoids are lipophilic mediators, which include amides, esters and ethers of long-chain polyunsaturated fatty acids, mostly arachidonic acid. The first two identified and most studied endocannabinoids are N-arachidonylethanolamide called anandamide (AEA) and 2-arachidonoylglycerol (2-AG) (**Figure 5**). AEA and 2-AG are not pre-synthesised and stored in vesicles like classical neurotransmitters, but rather released from the cells immediately after biosynthesis. They are synthesised via enzymatic pathways from phospholipid precursors in the plasma membrane of post-synaptic cells on demand upon relevant physiological or pathological stimuli. After release, acting as retrograde messengers, AEA and 2-AG travel backwards to stimulate receptors on the pre-synaptic membrane. The main intermediate in the synthesis of AEA is *N*-acyl-phosphatidylethanolamine (NArPE), transformed into anandamide by several possible pathways among which the most investigated is the direct conversion catalysed by an enzyme of phospholipase D family. 2-AG is produced primarily by the hydrolysis of diacylglycerols (DAGs) via DAG lipases α and β. The endocannabinoids act on their receptors only locally, possibly because of their high lipophilicity, and are immediately inactivated under physiological conditions. The suggested mechanisms of endocannabinoid transport across the plasma membrane (facilitated transport, passive diffusion and/or endocytosis) are still not fully elucidated. After their cellular re-uptake, AEA is rapidly degraded by the enzyme fatty acid amide hydrolase (FAAH) while 2-AG is hydrolysed by monoacylglycerol lipase (MAGL) forming arachidonate and ethanolamine or glycerol, respectively [34, 35].

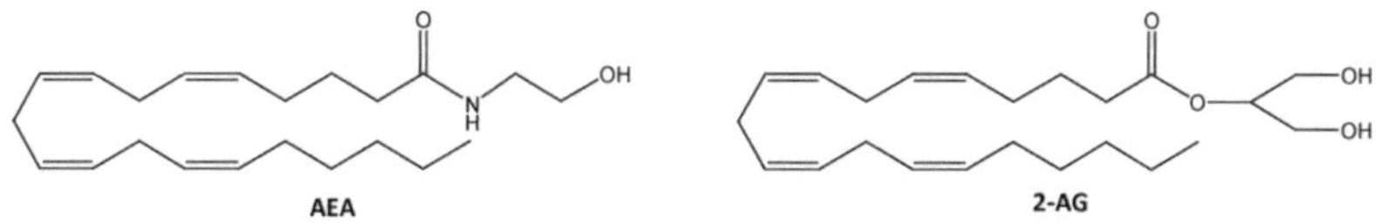

Figure 5. The structures of main endocannabinoids anandamide (AEA) and 2-arachidonoylglycerol (2-AG).

Apart from hydrolytic degradation, endocannabinoids may also be oxidised by cyclooxygenase-2, lipoxygenases and cytochrome P450 [36].

The cannabinoids exert their effects by binding to specific receptors, among which the most important are cannabinoid receptors CB1 and CB2 encoded by different genes and exhibiting 44% homology in their primary structure. They belong to the large rhodopsin family of G-protein-coupled receptors (GPCRs) with seven transmembrane domains connected by three extracellular and three intra-cellular loops, an extracellular N-terminal tail and an intra-cellular C-terminal tail. There is increasing evidence supporting the existence of additional targets for cannabinoids like transient receptor potential (TRP) ligand-gated cation channels (vanilloid type 1, TRPV1, melastatin type 8, TRPM8 and ankyrin type 1, TRPA1), certain orphan GPCRs (GPR55, GPR119 and GPR18), 5-hydroxytryptamine receptor subtype 1A (5-HT_{1A}) and peroxisome proliferator-activated receptors (PPARs). The functions of cannabinoid receptors can be modulated by endo-, phyto- or synthetic-cannabinoids which target the orthosteric or allosteric binding sites on the receptors. The cannabinoid receptors modulate adenylyl cyclase (AC) activity depending on its isoform expressed in the cells and, consequently, alter the cellular production of second messenger cyclic adenosine monophosphate (cAMP). The activation of CB1 and CB2 receptors mainly causes inhibition of AC and the subsequent reduction of intra-cellular cAMP levels leads to the inactivation of the protein kinase A (PKA) phosphorylation pathway. Studies have shown that cannabinoid receptors can also be coupled to other types of intra-cellular signals, such as the protein kinase B, phosphoinositide 3-kinase and phospholipase C pathway. Also, activation of CB1 and CB2 receptors leads to the downstream activation of mitogen-activated protein kinase (MAPK), p44/42, p38 and c-JUN amino terminal kinase as signalling pathways to regulate nuclear transcription factors. Unlike the activation of CB2 receptor, which generally has no effect on ion channels, CB1 receptors inhibit calcium channels and activate potassium channels. The cannabinoid receptors are widely distributed in the human body. CB1 receptors are localised predominantly in the CNS and mainly expressed in areas that are involved in the control of motor coordination and movement, memory, learning, emotions, sensory perception and autonomic and endocrine functions. In addition, CB1 receptors are present to a lesser extent in some organs and peripheral tissues, including endocrine glands, leukocytes, adipocytes, spleen, liver, heart and part of the reproductive, urinary and gastrointestinal systems. By contrast, the CB2 receptor was initially described as present in the immune system, but more recently it has also been shown to be expressed in additional cell types [37–40]. Since elevated expression of CB1 and CB2 receptors and higher levels of endocannabinoids have been found in many types of cancer, compared to normal tissues, the ECS has been recognised as attractive potential target for cancer therapy. The growing evidence over the past decade suggests that cannabinoids affect multiple signalling pathways involved in the development of cancer, displaying an anti-proliferative, proapoptotic, anti-angiogenic and anti-metastatic activity on a wide range of cell lines and animal models of cancer [41].

6. Preclinical evidence on cannabinoids as anti-cancer agents

Despite remarkable advances in understanding and treating cancer, finding new, more effective pharmacotherapeutics still remains a key challenge for scientists worldwide. The first study suggesting that plant-derived cannabinoids might be potential anti-cancer agents, demonstrating their ability to inhibit tumour growth *in vitro* and *in vivo* and to increase the survival of lung cancer-bearing animals, was published more than 40 years ago [42]. Later discoveries of the ECS in the human body, combined with the development of numerous preclinical testing models, have paved the way for a renaissance in the study of anti-cancer properties of cannabinoids in the last two decades. A large body of *in vitro* data has been accumulated demonstrating that cannabinoids affect a wide spectrum of tumour cells, including gliomas, neuroblastomas, lymphomas, hepatocarcinoma as well as thyroid, skin, prostate, pancreatic, breast, cervical, colon, gastric, lung and some other cancers [6, 41, 43]. Several plant-derived (THC and CBD), synthetic (e.g. JWH-133, WIN-55,212-2 and KM-233) and endogenous cannabinoids (AEA and 2-AG) were found to be potent inhibitors of both cancer growth and spreading due to their ability of modulating various cell-signalling pathways [6, 37, 43, 44]. Their anti-neoplastic action mainly relies on the activation of cannabinoid CB1 and/or CB2 receptors, although some other non-CB1/CB2 receptors, like TRPV1 and PPARs, as well as mechanisms unrelated to receptor stimulation may also be involved [43, 45, 46]. Cannabinoids might stop the uncontrolled growth of cancer cells by several different mechanisms, including inhibition of cell-cycle progression, inhibition of cell proliferation as well as induction of autophagy and apoptosis [41, 43, 44]. Due to their modulatory actions on various cell cycle regulatory molecules, like cyclin A and cyclin dependent kinase (CDK) 2, cannabinoids have been shown to cause arrest of cell cycle progression in different phases (e.g. G0/G1, G2/M), leading to growth inhibition and/or apoptotic death of cancer cells [43]. The anti-proliferative activity is based on their ability to inhibit proliferative and oncogenic pathways in cancer cells, such as adenylyl cyclase and cyclic adenosine monophosphate/protein kinase A (cAMP/PKA) pathway leading to the activation of mitogen-activated protein kinase (MAPK) pathway as well as cell cycle blockade with induction of the CDK inhibitor (CDKI) p27Kip1 and p21waf, decrease in epidermal growth factor (EGF) receptor (EGFR) expression and/or attenuation of EGFR tyrosine kinase activity, decrease in the activity and/or expression of nerve growth factor (NGF), prolactin, or vascular endothelial growth factor (VEGF) tyrosine kinase receptors. The MAPK signalling cascades, consisting of the extracellular signal-regulated kinase (ERK1/2), c-Jun N-terminal kinase (JNK) and p38 MAPK, as well as phosphatidylinositol 3 kinase (PI3K)-Akt pathways seems to have a prominent role in the control of tumour cell fate by cannabinoids [43, 45]. Cancer cell death-inducing activity of cannabinoids relies greatly on the apoptosis and, among several molecular mechanisms, the stimulation of endoplasmic reticulum (ER) stress and subsequent autophagy has been recently suggested as the most common one. Cannabinoids can induce accumulation of *de novo*–synthesised ceramide and thereby activate an ER stress-related response through up-regulation of the

http://dx.doi.org/10.5772/67746

stress-regulated protein p8 and several of its downstream targets, like activating transcription factor 4 (ATF4), C/EBP homologous protein (CHOP) and pseudokinase tribbles-homologue 3 (TRIB3), leading to the inhibition of the AKT–mammalian target of rapamycin complex 1 (mTORC1) signalling, and autophagy-mediated apoptosis. Cannabinoid-evoked and ER stress-dependent activation of calcium/calmodulin-dependent protein kinase β (CaCMKKβ) and AMP-activated protein kinase (AMPK) lead, together with the p8/TRIB3 pathway, to autophagy and apoptosis [1, 46]. Tumour angiogenesis represents additional important target for cancer therapy affected by cannabinoids. They can directly inhibit vascular endothelial cell migration and survival or act indirectly by modulating the expression of pro-angiogenic factors, like VEGF, matrix metalloproteinase-2 (MMP-2) or anti-angiogenic factors like tissue inhibitor of matrix metalloproteinase 1 (TIMP-1) as well as their receptors in tumours [41, 44]. Besides influencing the growth of different cancer cells, cannabinoids may exert their anti-cancer effects by inhibiting all the steps of tumour progression. The inhibitory effect on migration, adhesion and invasion through CB receptors is related to the blocking of key pathways such as EGF-EGFR, RhoA-RhoA kinase (ROCK), focal adhesion kinase (FAK)-Src and of MMPs and TIMP-1, which are fundamental for the invasiveness and spread of tumours [41, 43, 44]. Non-CB receptors mediated anti-metastasic effects may rely on the down-regulation of the helix-loop-helix (bHLH) transcription factor inhibitor of DNA binding 1 (ID1) [46]. **Tables 1** and **2** summarise preclinical evidence collected during the last decade about the role of two most-investigated phytocannabinoids, THC and CBD, in different type of cancers and their associated cell signalling pathways.

Recent *in vivo* studies demonstrated that cannabinoids of plant, synthetic and endogenous origin are able to decrease tumour growth and metastasis of different experimental cancers [47]. Preclinical assessments have mainly been conducted using human tumour engraft models, where human cancer cells were subcutaneously injected (ectopic model) or transplanted into the same origin site of the tumour (orthotropic model) in immunodeficient mice. The syngeneic (allograft) models, established by transplantation of mice cancer cells in immunocompetence animals, as well as carcinogen-induced spontaneous tumour models and genetically engineered mouse models (GEMM) have also been used, but rarely [47, 48]. An overview of last decades' discoveries revealed the effectiveness of THC against experimental glioma, liver, pancreatic, breast and lung cancers (**Table 1**) while CBD was found to be effective against glioma and neuroblastoma, melanoma, colon, breast, prostate and lung cancers (**Table 2**). Among other phytocannabinoids, CBG could be considered as a candidate for colon cancer prevention and treatment [49]. Beside these findings, the potential clinical interest of cannabinoids is additionally strongly suggested by their selectivity for tumour cells (and even ability to protect the non-transformed cells) as well as by their good tolerance in animal studies and the absence of normal tissue toxicities that are still the major limitations of most conventional chemotherapeutics [45]. However, several studies reported that THC and some other cannabinoids can inhibit apoptosis in the transformed-cell lines, exhibit proangiogenic effect and stimulate cancer cell proliferation or show a biphasic effect in cancer cells by increasing their proliferation at lower concentrations and decreasing at higher concentrations [37, 41]. The ability to promote the tumours growth was found in two experimental animal model cancers and attributed to their suppression of anti-tumour immune response [37]. Despite the few mentioned conflicting data, the majority of recent preclinical studies provide the supporting evidence on cannabinoids as promising anti-cancer agents, thus encouraging further clinical investigations.

Considering the possibilities for therapeutic use of cannabinoids in cancer, their combination with traditional chemotherapy or radiotherapy seems to be an interesting option. The possible advantages of combination therapy may be a synergistic effect evident as improved efficiency, lowered doses and consequently attenuated toxic side effect or reduced drug resistance. Accordingly, γ-irradiation was found to enhance CBD-induced apoptotic death in cultured leukaemia cells [50]. Synergism of plant-derived cannabinoids and radiation was confirmed *in vivo*, where the simultaneous treatment with THC and CBD enhanced the cancer-killing effects of the radiation in murine glioma model [51]. Preclinical evidence also supports the combination of phytocannabinoids and chemotherapy drug temozolomide (TMZ), commonly used in patients with glioblastoma. Torres et al. [52] proved that co-administration of TMZ with THC reduces the growth of glioma xenograft to a much higher extent than the treatment with the individual agents, observing effect in the TMZ-resistant tumours also. Interestingly, combined treatment with TMZ and submaximal doses of THC and CBD (approximate 1:1 ratio) produced similar anti-tumoural effect in both TMZ-sensitive and TMZ-resistant tumours. Usage of main cannabis constituents together may be therapeutically very attractive, since CBD has the ability to potentiate anti-cancer properties of THC and, as a non-psychotropic cannabinoid, can mitigate adverse psychoactive effects of THC that limit its clinical use [46, 52]. Recent data also revealed that CBD-enriched cannabis extract can significantly enhance the efficacy of bicalutamide or docetaxel, two standard drugs used in the treatment of prostate cancer, and taken together even prolong the survival of treated animals [53]. Overall, recent findings provide promising evidence on the benefits of cannabinoid-based combinational therapy in cancer, and suggest novel therapeutic opportunities that need to be clinically proven in future.

Cancer type	Experimental model	Findings [reference]
Brain (Glioma)	*in vitro*	
	U251MG, U87MG	Inhibited cell cycle progression (G0/1 arrest) by down-regulation of E2F transcription factor 1 and cyclin A [54]
	C6.9, U87MG	Inhibition of migration by inhibition of TIMP-1 expression via ceramide and stress protein p8 [55]
	C6.9, U87MG	Inhibition of invasion by down-regulating MMP-2 via ceramide and p8 [56]
	U87MG	Induced autophagy-mediated cell death through ER stress–evoked stimulation of ceramide synthesis *de novo*, eIF2α phosphorylation and up-regulation of p8/TRIB3 pathway leading to inhibition of Akt/mTORC1 pathway; autophagy leads to apoptosis [57]
	in vivo	
	C6.9 xenograft	Decreased tumour growth and tumoural TIMP-1 expression [55]
	U87MG xenograft	Decreased tumour grow and tumoural MMP-2 expression [56]
		Decreased tumour growth and activated autophagic mediated cell death pathway (↑TRIB3, ↑LC3-II, ↑caspase 3, ↓rpS6) [57]

Cancer type	Experimental model	Findings [reference]
Lung	*in vitro* A549, SW-1573	Inhibited proliferation, migration and invasion of tumour cells by inhibition of EGFR-mediated activation of MAPKs (ERK1/2, JNK1/2) [58]
	in vivo A549 xenograft	Reduced tumour growth and metastasis through inhibition of proliferation (↓Ki67), vascularisation (↓CD31) and decreased phosphorylation of FAK, ERK1/2 and Akt [58]
	LL2 allograft	No significant effect on tumour growth [59]
Liver	*in vitro* HepG2, HuH-7	Induced cancer cell death through autophagy stimulation via CB2 receptors by (i) inhibition of the Akt/mTORC1 axis via ER stress with TRIB3 up-regulation and (ii) stimulation of AMPK via CaMKKβ; autophagy leads to apoptosis [60]
	HepG2	Anti-proliferative action modulated by up-regulation of PPARγ-dependent pathways through TRIB3 [61]
	in vivo HepG2 xenograft HuH-7 xenograft	Reduced tumour growth relies on decreased mTORC1 activation, enhanced AMPK phosphorylation and increased autophagy and apoptosis [60]
	HepG2 orthotopic	Decreased hepatomegaly and ascites, ↓α-fetoprotein, in tumour ↑pAMPK, ↓pAkt, ↓pS6, ↓procaspase-3 [60]
	HepG2 xenograft	Reduced tumour growth via PPARγ activation [61]
Pancreas	*in vitro* MiaPaCa2, Panc1	Induced cancer cell death by apoptosis via activation of the p8-ATF-4-TRIB3 pathway (↑caspase-3, ↑ceramide) [62]
	in vivo MiaPaCa2 xenograft	Reduced tumour growth [62]
Breast	*in vitro* EVSA-T, HMEC	Reduced cancer cell proliferation through apoptosis and cell cycle blockade (G2-M arrest) by CDK1 down-regulation [63]
	in vivo MMTV-neu	Reduced tumour growth, tumour number and metastases by cell proliferation inhibition (↓Ki67), apoptosis (↑caspase 3), decreased angiogenesis and ↓MMP2 [64]
	N202.1 xenograft	Decreased tumour growth via Akt inhibition [64]
Skin	*in vitro* CHL-1, A375, SK-MEL-28	Induced cancer cell death by activating non-canonical autophagy-mediated apoptosis dependent on Atg7 but not Beclin-1 or Ambra1 [65]
	in vivo CHL-1 xenograft	Inhibited tumour growth via autophagy and apoptosis (↓Ki67, ↑TUNEL, ↑LC3) [65]
	HCmel12 xenograft	Reduced tumour growth in CB receptor-dependent manner and decreased inflammatory immune cell infiltrates in the tumour microenvironment [66]

Table 1. Effects of THC on different types of cancer.

Abbreviations are listed in **Table 2**.

Cancer type	Experimental model	Findings [reference]
Brain	*In vitro*	
	U87	Induced apoptosis of cancer cells through caspase activation (↑caspase-8, -9 and -3) and oxidative stress (↑ROS, ↓GSH, ↑GPx, ↑GRed) [67]
	in vivo	
	U87 xenograft	Reduced tumour growth through inhibition of 5-LOX (↓LTB4) and ECS—activation of FAAH (↓AEA) [68]
	U251 orthotopic xenograft	Reduced tumour progression and cancer cell invasion through down-regulation of Id-1 expression [69]
	3832, 387 orthotopic xenograft	Initial inhibition of tumour growth (↓Ki67, ↓pAkt, (↑caspase-3) followed by tumour resistance [70]
	SK-N-SH xenograft	Suppressed neuroblastoma tumour growth via apoptosis induction (↑caspase-3) [71]
Lung	*In vitro*	
	A549, H460	Anti-invasive and anti-metastatic action via up-regulation of ICAM-1 which leads to enhanced cancer cell adhesion to LAK cells and subsequent enhance of LAK cell-mediated cancer cell lysis [72]
	in vivo	
	A549 xenograft	Decreased tumour growth and inhibited tumour cell invasion via down-regulation of PAI-1 [73]
		Decreased tumour metastasis [74]
		Inhibited cancer cell invasion and metastasis by stimulation of TIMP-1 via up-regulation of ICAM-1 [75]
		Decreased tumour growth via apoptosis caused by up-regulation of COX-2 and PPAR-γ [76]
Colon	*In vivo*	
	Azoxymethane-induced cancer	Reduced preneoplastic lesions, number of polyps and tumours through apoptosis by inhibition of the PI3K-Akt pathway (↓pAkt, ↑caspase 3) [77]
Prostate	*In vitro*	
	LNCaP, DU-145	Induced cell death through apoptotic pathways (↑caspase 3, ↑PUMA, ↑CHOP, ↑intra-cellular Ca^{2+}, down-regulation of AR, p53 activation, ↑ROS) [53]
	LNCaP	Induced phosphatase-dependent apoptosis in cancer cells via CB1/CB2 [78]
	in vivo	
	LNCaP xenograft	Decreased tumour growth [53]

Cancer type	Experimental model	Findings [reference]
Breast	*In vitro*	
	MCF-7, KiMol, C6, MDA-MB-231	Inhibited cancer cell proliferation through proapoptotic effect and by cell cycle blockade at G1/S phase, acting directly via CB2 and TRPV1 receptors and indirectly via elevation of intracellular Ca^{2+} and ROS [79]
	MDA-MB-231, 4T1	Anti-proliferative and anti-invasive effect by up-regulation of ERK and ROS pathways leading to down-regulation of Id-1 protein expression [80]
	MDA-MB-231	Induced cancer cell death by both apoptosis (↑PARP) and autophagy (↑LC3-II) through induction of ER stress and inhibition of Akt/mTOR/4EBP1 signalling independently of receptor activation; important role of ROS and Beclin-1 [81]
	SUM159, 4T1.2	Inhibited tumour cell proliferation, migration and invasion through EGF/EGFR pathway inhibiting EGF-induced activation of EGFR, ERK, Akt and NF-kB signalling and actin stress fibre formation and focal adhesion formation; Anti-metastatic effect also by decreasing secretion of MMP-2 and MMP-9 as well as chemokines CCL3, GM-CSF, MIP-2 [82]
	In vivo	
	MDA-MB xenograft	Decreased tumour growth and lung metastasis [79]
	4T1 orthotopic 4T1 allograft	Reduced tumour growth and metastasis. Anti-metastatic effect by down-regulation of tumoural Id1 expression [80, 83]
	4T1.2 orthotopic MVT-1 orthotopic	Inhibited tumour growth and lung metastasis due to anti-proliferative (↓Ki67) and angiogenic (↓CD31) effects and inhibition of EGFR, Akt and ERK activation [82]

AEA—anandamide; Akt—serine/threonine protein kinase; AMPK—adenosine monophosphate-activated protein kinase; AR—androgen receptor; ATF-4—activating transcription factor 4; Atg7—autophagy-related protein 7; CaMKKβ—calcium/calmodulin-dependent protein kinase β; CCL3—chemokine (C-C motif) ligand 3; CD31—cluster of differentiation 31, syn. platelet endothelial cell adhesion molecule (PECAM-1); CDK1—Cyclin-dependent kinase 1; CHOP—transcription factor CAAT/enhancer binding homologous protein; COX-2—cyclooxygenase-2; 4EBP1—eukaryotic translation initiation factor 4E binding protein 1; ECS—endocannabinoid system; EGF—epidermal growth factor; EGFR—epidermal growth factor receptor; eIF2α—α subunit of eukaryotic initiation factor 2; ER—endoplasmic reticulum; ERK—extracellular signal-regulated kinase; FAAH—fatty acid amide hydrolase; FAK—focal adhesion kinase; GM-CSF—granulocyte-macrophage colony-stimulating factor; GPx—glutathione peroxidase; GRed—glutathione reductase; GSH—glutathione; ICAM-1—intercellular adhesion molecule 1; Id-1—helix-loop-helix protein inhibitor of DNA binding-1; JNK1/2—c-Jun N-terminal protein kinases 1 and 2; Ki67—biomarker of cancer cells proliferation LAK cells - lymphokine-activated killer cells; LC3—microtubule-associated protein 1 light chain 3; 5-LOX—arachidonate 5-lipoxygenase; LTB4—leukotriene B4; MAPK—mitogen-activated protein kinase; MIP-2—macrophage inflammatory protein 2; MMP—matrix metalloproteinase; mTOR—mechanistic target of rapamycin; mTORC1—mammalian target of rapamycin complex 1; NF-kB—nuclear factor-kappa B; p53—tumour protein 53; p8—stress-regulated protein; PAI-1—plasminogen activator inhibitor-1; pAkt—phosphorylated Akt; pAMPK—phosphorylated adenosine monophosphate-activated protein kinase; PARP—poly (ADP-ribose) polymerase; PI3K—phosphoinositide 3-kinase; PPARγ—peroxisome proliferator-activated receptor γ; pS6—phosphorylated-ribosomal protein S6; PUMA—p53 up-regulated modulator or apoptosis; ROS—reactive oxygen species; rpS6—ribosomal protein S6; TIMP-1—tissue inhibitor of matrix metalloproteinase 1; TRIB3-—tribbles pseudokinase 3; TUNEL—terminal deoxynucleotidyl transferase dUTP nick end labelling.

Table 2. Effects of CBD on different types of cancer.

7. Clinical studies of cannabinoids in cancer care

7.1. Clinical anti-cancer studies

The promising preclinical data have encouraged the development of clinical studies aimed at investigating the potential therapeutic value of cannabinoids as anti-cancer agents. The only clinical study published up to date was a pilot phase I trial in which nine patients with recurrent glioblastoma multiforme (GBM) that have previously failed standard therapy underwent intracranial THC administration. The study showed that THC delivery was safe without evident psychoactive effects and that THC neither facilitates tumour growth nor decreases patients' survival. Additionally, THC inhibited tumour-cell proliferation and induced apoptosis in samples obtained from two patients before and after treatment. However, evaluation of patients' survival requires a larger study with a different design and preferably oral or oromucosal application [46, 84]. According to the register of clinical trials [85], there are several on-going clinical trials evaluating anti-cancer activity of cannabinoids. Two phase I/II clinical studies in recurrent GBM patients are being conducted to assess the safety and effectiveness of the administration of an oromucosal spray containing cannabis extract (2.7 mg THC and 2.5 mg CBD in 100 μL) in combination with dose-intense TMZ (NCT01812603 and NCT01812616). These studies have passed their completion date, but the status has not yet been verified. Evaluation of pure CBD as a single-agent for solid tumour (NCT02255292) started in 2014 as a phase II clinical trial and still did not reveal any results. Dexanabinol, a synthetic cannabinoid, is currently undergoing phase I trial for the treatment of advanced solid tumours (NCT01489826). This non-psychotropic cannabinoid was applied in different doses with the intention to determine the maximum safe dose, to understand interactions between the body and the drug and to measure any reduction in size of patients' tumour. Data on tumour response and the number of adverse events have not yet been reported.

7.2. Studies on chemotherapy-induced nausea and vomiting

In contrast to rare clinical anti-cancer studies, clinical trials evaluating efficacy of cannabinoids in cancer symptom management have a long history. The 1970s and 1980s mark a period of intensive clinical trials dealing with chemotherapy-induced nausea and vomiting (CINV), but the interest in these investigations is not decreasing due to the influence of CINV on patients' life quality and compliance with future treatment [86, 87]. Modern anti-emetic treatment includes corticosteroids, serotonin receptor antagonists (5-HT_3) and neurokinin (NK_1) receptor antagonists, while cannabinoids (dronabinol and nabilone) are prescribed to the patients who have failed to respond to conventional anti-emetic therapy [88, 89]. Majority of clinical studies have compared efficacy of cannabinoids to dopamine receptor antagonist and neuroleptics [87], yet some recent studies have been focusing on newer generation agents such as 5-HT_3 and NK_1 receptor antagonists. Meiri and coworkers [90] have design randomised, double-blind, placebo-controlled, parallel group, five-day study for evaluating dronabinol alone and in combination with ondansetron, a 5-HT_3 receptor antagonist. They recruited 61 patients with delayed CINV, which is defined as nausea and vomiting occurring more than 24 hours after chemotherapy and lasting up to one week. Obtained results indicated that dronabinol or ondansetron was similarly effective and well tolerated, but combination of these two drugs was not more effective than either drug alone. Duran and coworkers [91] conducted a pilot, double-blind, parallel, placebo-controlled phase II clinical trial with standardised oromucosal cannabis extract containing a mixture of THC and CBD (2.7 mg THC and 2.5 mg CBD per spray) in patients with CINV. To be recruited in the study, patients had to have moderately emetogenic cancer therapy caused CINV lasting more than 24 hours despite standard anti-emetic therapy. During five days patients were allowed to add up to eight sprays per day along with their standard therapy. Combination of cannabis extract with standard anti-emetic therapy was well tolerated and provided better protection against delayed CINV. The benefits of cannabinoids in CINV are undoubtedly confirmed in numerous clinical studies, but there is lack of studies dealing with cannabis plant [92]. First scientific article about use of smoked cannabis reported it as a rescue drug in case of vomiting episodes [93]. In 2001, Musty and Rossi [94] published the review about effects of smoked cannabis and oral THC based on previously unpublished USA clinical trials with cannabis and/or THC. The investigation included 748 patients who smoked cannabis prior to and/or after cancer chemotherapy and 345 patients who used the oral THC capsules. Patients who smoked cannabis experienced 70–100% relief from nausea and vomiting, while those on THC capsules reported 76–88% relief. Although it is clear that cannabinoids can serve as anti-emetic agents in cancer therapy, clinical studies on their effectiveness on nausea and vomiting in advanced cancer and metastasis are needed since there are case-reports in which cannabinoids showed potential therapeutic use for these indications [95].

7.3. Studies on cancer-related pain

In the last decades, available clinical data on benefits of cannabinoids in chronic pain were scarce; however, currently there are many clinical studies, which include various cannabinoid preparations and test different chronic pain conditions [96]. Animal studies in a variety of nociceptive assays have confirmed that activation of CB1 receptors by exogenously applied agonists can reduce pain sensitivity, while activation of CB2 receptors may promote analgesia without psychoactive side effects usual for CB1 agonist [97]. Patients who are suffering from chronic cancer-related pain usually are put on high doses of opiates, which alter their state of consciousness. It has been reported that cancer patients down-sized opioid dose after adding cannabis in their pain regimen and when selecting cannabis extract, THC-rich cannabis extract was the first choice, though many patients experienced pain relief after using CBD-rich type [92]. In multi-centre, double-blind, randomised, placebo-controlled, parallel-group, two-week study, THC:CBD extract and THC extract were evaluated in patients with intractable cancer-related pain. Study included 177 patients with inadequate analgesia despite opioid dosing. During first week patients self-titrated dose up to maximum of 48 actuations (each 100 μL containing 2.7 mg THC and 2.5 mg CBD or just 2.7 mg THC) per day and remained on that dose till the end of the study. The mean number of THC/CBD sprays was 9.26 and of THC 8.47 per day. Analysis of change from baseline in Numeral Rating Scale score was significantly in favour of THC/CBD extract, while THC extract showed non-significant change. There was no change in dose of opioid background medication as well [98]. A long-term, open-label, follow-up study investigated the long-term tolerability of THC/CBD and THC oromucosal spray in 43 patients with terminal cancer-related pain refractory to opioid who had participated in previously mentioned trial. Patients self-administered the medication to their optimal dose, again with limitation to a maximum of 48 sprays per day. The duration of treatment with THC/CBD spray (39 patients) was from minimum of 2 and maximum of 579 days (median 25 days) while treatment with THC spray lasted from 4 up to 657 days (median 151.5 days). THC/CBD spray was found to be well tolerated in long-term use, and patients did not ask for higher dose of spray or other pain-relieving medication. Long-term use of cannabinoids did not result with loss of relieving effect on cancer pain [99]. Another randomised, placebo-controlled, graded-dose trial evaluating THC/CBD extract was conducted among opioid-treated patients with poorly-controlled chronic pain who received placebo, low (1–4 sprays/day), medium (6–10 sprays/day) or high dose (11–16 sprays/day) of 2.8 mg THC/2.5 mg CBD extract. During period of five weeks average pain, worst pain and sleep disruption were measured among 360 patients, of which 263 completed the study. Low and medium dose group of patients showed greater analgesia than placebo group and could be assumed as effective and safe, while in high-dose group dose medication was not well-tolerated and had no analgesic effect [100]. Another type of pain that usually occurs in cancer patients is chemotherapy-induced peripheral neuropathy caused by neurotoxicity of drugs such as platinum compounds, vinca alkaloids, taxols and suramin. Although chemotherapy is limited to a short period of use and to a specific tissue, there is no adequate medications for prophylaxis of this type of neuropathy and therapy is restricted to symptomatic treatment of paraesthesia and pain. Ion channel blockers and tricyclic anti-depressants are first choice for treating neuropathy symptoms [101]. Being resistant to conventional treatments, neuropathy lowers life quality in affected patients and limits dosing and duration of chemotherapy, which is crucial for extending their life. Preclinical studies implied that cannabinoid agonists can suppress neuropathy caused by chemotherapeutics, namely vincristine, paclitaxel and cisplatin; moreover, they had better efficacy than conventional treatment. For effectiveness estimation of cannabinoid extract for treating neuropathy, a randomised, placebo-controlled, cross-over pilot study with 18 patients was conducted. Patients were experiencing neuropathic pain, which persisted for three months after chemotherapy with paclitaxel, vincristine or cisplatin, and were treated with maximum of 12 oromucosal sprays (each containing 2.7 mg THC and 2.5 mg CBD) per day. First study period lasted for four weeks with the result of five patients having a decrease of 2.6 on an 11-point numeric rating scale for pain intensity, but in whole group, there was no significant difference between treated and placebo group. Ten patients have entered the extension phase for the next six months (five have completed the study), and confirmed pain reduction by average dose of 4.5 sprays per day. Despite inconsistent results, these findings support studying cannabinoids for chemotherapy-induced neuropathic pain in larger randomised controlled trials [102].

7.4. Cannabis and cancer associated anorexia/cachexia

Many cancer patients experience cachexia, anorexia as well as progressive loss of adipose tissue and skeletal muscle mass. Poor chemotherapy response and decreased survival are often connected with cachexia, a syndrome characterised by systemic inflammation, negative protein and energy balance, and an involuntary loss of body mass [103]. Majority of clinical studies dealing with cachexia and anorexia are focused on AIDS patients and as a result dronabinol was approved for treatment of anorexia associated with weight loss in patients with AIDS. Still there are some clinical evidences that show that cannabinoids could be beneficial for patients with cancer-associated anorexia/cachexia. One of earliest trials with cancer patients, in 1976, showed that oral THC in doses up to 15 mg per day stimulated appetite and produced significant weight gain [104]. Eighteen cancer patients with anorexia and life expectancy more than 4 weeks underwent a phase II study of THC under regime 2.5 mg tree times per day, one hour after meal. Thirteen patients responded positively to the appetite stimulating effects of THC, but rather surprising was the fact that nausea was common side-effect [105]. In contrast, study conducted in 2006 did not confirm these results. Multi-centre, phase II, randomised, double blind, placebo controlled clinical trial included 164 patients with advanced incurable cancer and involuntary weight loss more than 5%. Patients were divided in placebo, cannabis extract (2.5 mg THC and 1 mg CBD in a capsule) or THC (2.5 mg in a capsule) group, and they were assigned to take capsules twice per day, one hour before meal for six weeks. There were no significant differences between groups considering appetite, quality of life, cannabinoid related toxicity, mood and nausea [106]. It is rather unusual that in this large trial there were no side effects, which suggest that administrated dose of cannabinoids is suboptimal. Moreover, in case of the use of cannabinoids for anorexia and cachexia, European Palliative Care Research Collaborative noticed that dose-regimen of THC used in clinical trials may be the reason for its lack of efficacy. They concluded that for future trials individual dose titration could be more efficient [107, 108]. These theses were confirmed in another randomised, double-blind, placebo-controlled pilot trial in which influence of THC on taste improvement, smell perception, appetite, caloric intake and quality of life was explored. Twenty-one advanced cancer patients, with poor appetite and chemosensory alterations, received THC (2.5 mg, twice per day) and had the option to increase their drug dose to a maximum of 20 mg/day. Though study population was not specifically cachexic, THC-treated patients had improvement in taste, appetite, protein consumption and sleep quality [109].

To summarise, cannabinoids show positive results in various clinical trials considering treatment of nausea, vomiting, pain and anorexia/cachexia while clinical anti-cancer studies are yet to be reported. The perspective of cannabis-based therapy also depends on a paradigm shift from illicit drug to clinically proved medicine. Due to their acceptable safety profile, with side effects that are generally tolerable and reversible [92], clinical trials testing them as single drugs or in combination therapies in various types of cancer are needed, particularly with respect to their effects on tumour growth and patient survival.

Author details

Sanda Vladimir-Knežević*, Biljana Blažeković, Maja Bival Štefan and Marija Kindl

*Address all correspondence to: svladimir@pharma.hr

Department of Pharmacognosy, Faculty of Pharmacy and Biochemistry, University of Zagreb, Zagreb, Croatia

References

[1] Velasco G, Sánchez C, Guzmán M. Cancer. In: Pertwee E, editor. Handbook of Cannabis. 1st ed. Oxford: Oxford University Press; 2014. pp. 626-649. DOI: 10.1093/acprof:oso/9780199662685.003.0035

[2] Giacoppo S, Mandolino G, Galuppo M, Bramanti P, Mazzon E. Cannabinoids: New promising agents in the treatment of neurological diseases. Molecules. 2014;**19**:18781-18816. DOI: 10.3390/molecules191118781

[3] Whiting PF, Wolff RF, Deshpande S, Di Nisio M, Duffy S, Hernandez AV, Keurentjes JC, Lang S, Misso K, Ryder S, Schmidlkofer S, Westwood M, Kleijnen J. Cannabinoids for Medical Use: A Systematic Review and Meta-analysis. The Journal of the American Medical Association. 2015;**313**: 2456-2473. DOI: 10.1001/jama.2015.6358

[4] Hanuš LO, Meyer SM, Muñoz E, Taglialatela-Scafati O, Appendino G. Phytocannabinoids: A unified critical inventory. Natural Products Reports. 2016;**33**:1357-1392. DOI: 10.1039/C6NP00074F

[5] Giese MW, Lewis MA, Giese L, Smith KM. Development and validation of a reliable and robust method for the analysis of cannabinoids and terpenes in cannabis. Journal of AOAC International. 2015;**98**:1503-1522. DOI: 10.5740/jaoacint.15-116

[6] Chakravarti B, Ravi J, Ganju RK. Cannabinoids as therapeutic agents in cancer: Current status and future implications. Oncotarget. 2004;**15**:5852-5872. DOI: 10.18632/oncotarget.2233

[7] Clark PA. The ethics of medical marijuana: government restrictions vs. medical necessity. Journal of Public Health Policy. 2000;**21**:40-60. DOI: 10.2307/3343473

[8] Cffarel MM, Andradas C, Pérez-Gómez E, Guzmán M, Sánchez C. Cannabinoids: A new hope for breast cancer therapy? Cancer Therapy Rewievs. 2012;**38**:911-918. DOI: 10.1016/j.ctrv.2012.06.005

[9] Chandra S, Lata H, Khan IA, ElSohly MA. The role of biotechnology in *Cannabis sativa* propagation for the production of phytocannabinoids. In: Chandra S, Lata H, Varma A, editors. Biotechnology for Medicinal Plant. Berlin Heidelberg: Springer-Verlag; 2013. pp. 123-148. DOI: 10.1007/978-3-642-29974-2_5

[10] Small E. Evolution and classification of *Cannabis sativa* (Marijuana, Hemp) in relation to human utilization. Botanical Review. 2015;**81**:189-294. DOI: 10.1007/s12229-015-9157-3

[11] Raman A. The Cannabis plant: Botany, cultivation and processing for use. In: Brown DT, editor. Cannabis: The Genus *Cannabis*. 1st ed. Amsterdam: Harwood Academic Publishers; 1998. pp. 29-54. ISBN: 978-90-5702-291-3

[12] American Herbal Pharmacopoeia. Cannabis Inflorescence. Boca Raton: CRC Press; 2013. pp. 1-65. ISBN: 1-929425-33-3

[13] ElSohly MA, Thomas BF. The Botany of Cannabis sativa L. In: Thomas BF, editor. The analytical chemistry of cannabis: Quality assessment, assurance, and regulation of medicinal marijuana and cannabinoid preparations. 1st ed. Amsterdam: Elsevier; 2016. pp. 1-26. DOI: 10.1016/B978-0-12-804646-3.00001-1

[14] Mahlberg PG, Kim ES. Accumulation of cannabinoids in glandular trichomes of cannabis (Cannabaceae). Journal of Industrial Hemp. 2004;**9**:15-36. DOI: 10.1300/J237v09n01_04

[15] Potter DJ. Cannabis horticulture. In: Pertwee E, editor. Handbook of Cannabis. 1st ed. Oxford: Oxford University Press; 2014. pp. 65-88. DOI: 10.1093/acprof:oso/9780199662685.003.0004

[16] Aizpurua-Olaizola O, Soydaner U, Öztürk E, Schibano D, Simsir Y, Navarro P, Etxebarria N, Usobiaga A. Evolution of the cannabinoid and terpene content during the growth of *Cannabis sativa* plants from different chemotypes. Journal of Natural Products. 2016;**79**:324-331. DOI: 10.1021/acs.jnatprod.5b00949

[17] Andre CM, Hausman JF, Guerriero G. *Cannabis sativa*: the plant of the thousand and one molecules. Frontiers in Plant Science. 2016;**7**:1-19. DOI: 10.3389/fpls.2016.00019

[18] Flores-Sanchez IJ, Verpoorte R. Secondary metabolism in cannabis. Phytochemistry Reviews. 2008;**7**:615-639. DOI: 10.1007/s11101-008-9094-4

[19] ElSohly MA, Gul W. Constituents of *Cannabis sativa*. In: Pertwee E, editor. Handbook of Cannabis. 1st ed. Oxford: Oxford University Press; 2014. pp. 3-22. DOI: 10.1093/acprof:oso/9780199662685.003.0001

[20] Brenneisen R. Chemistry and analysis of phytocannabinoids and other *Cannabis* constituents. In: ElSohly MA, editor. Marijuana and the Cannabinoids. New Jersey: Humana Press; 2007. pp. 17-49. ISBN 1-58829-456-0

[21] Hazekamp A, Fischedick JT. Cannabis – from cultivar to chemovar. Drug Testing and Analysis. 2012;**4**:660-667. DOI: 10.1002/dta.407

[22] Hillig KW, Mahlberg PG. A chemotaxonomic analysis of cannabinoid variation in *Cannabis* (Cannabaceae). American Journal of Botany. 2004;**91**:966-975. DOI: 10.3732/ajb.91.6.966

[23] Galal AM, Slade D, Gul W, El-Alfy AT, Ferreira D, ElSohly MA. Naturally occurring and related synthetic cannabinoids and their potential therapeutic applications. Recent Patents on CNS Drug Discovery. 2009;**4**:112-136. DOI: 10.2174/157488909788453031

[24] Mandolino G, Carboni A. Potential of marker-assisted selection in hemp genetic improvement. Euphytica. 2004;**140**:107-120. DOI: 10.1007/s10681-004-4759-6

[25] de Meijer E. The chemical phenotypes (chemotypes) of *Cannabis*. In: Pertwee E, editor. Handbook of Cannabis. 1st ed. Oxford: Oxford University Press; 2014. pp. 89-110. DOI: 10.1093/acprof:oso/9780199662685.003.0005

[26] Erkelens JL, Hazekamp A. That which we call Indica, by any other name would smell as sweet. Cannabinoids. 2014;**9**:9-15

[27] Elzinga S, Fischedick J, Podkolinski R, Raber JC. Cannabinoids and terpenes as chemotaxonomic markers in cannabis. Natural Products Chemistry and Research. 2015;**3**:1-9. DOI: 10.4172/2329-6836.1000181

[28] Raharjo TJ, Verpoorte R. Methods for the analysis of cannabinoids in biological materials: a review. Phytochemical Analysis. 2004;**15**:79-94. DOI: 10.1002/pca.753

[29] Hazekamp A, Fischedick JT, Llano Díez M, Lubbe A, Ruhaak RL. Chemistry of cannabis. Development & modification of bioactivity. In: Mander L, Liu HW, editors. Comprehensive Natural Products II. Amsterdam: Elsevier; 2010. pp. 1033-1084. DOI: 10.1016/B978-008045382-8.00091-5

[30] Galand N, Ernouf D, Montigny F, Dollet J, Pothier J. Separation and identification of cannabis components by different planar chromatography techniques (TLC, AMD, OPLC). Journal of Chromatographic Science. 2004;**42**:130-134 DOI: 10.1093/chromsci/42.3.130

[31] Fischedick JT, Glas R, Hazekamp A, Verpoorte R. A qualitative and quantitative HPTLC densitometry method for the analysis of cannabinoids in *Cannabis sativa* L. Phytochemical Analysis. 2009;**20**:421-426. DOI: 10.1002/pca.1143

[32] Bruci Z, Papoutsis I, Athanaselis S, Nikolaou P, Pazari E, Spiliopoulou C, Vyshka G. First systematic evaluation of the potency of *Cannabis sativa* plants grown in Albania. Forensic Science International. 2012;**222**:40-46. DOI: 10.1016/j.forsciint.2012.04.032

[33] Wang M, Wang YH, Avula B, Radwan MM, Wanas AS, Mehmedic Z, van Antwerp J, ElSohly MA, Khan IA. Quantitative determination of cannabinoids in Cannabis and cannabis products using ultra-high-performance supercritical fluid chromatography and diode array/mass spectrometric detection. Journal of Forensic Sciences. 2016;**61**:1-10. DOI: 10.1111/1556-4029.13341

[34] Fezza F, Maccarrone M. Endocannabinoid biochemistry: What do we know after 50 years? In: Di Marzo V, editor. Cannabinoids. 1st ed. Chichester: John Wiley & Sons, Ltd; 2014. pp. 53-95. DOI: 10.1002/9781118451281.ch3

[35] Di Marzo V. Targeting the endocannabinoid system: to enhance or reduce? Natural Reviews Drug Discovery. 2008;**7**:438-455. DOI: 10.1038/nrd2553

[36] Urquhart P, Nicolaou A, Woodward DF. Endocannabinoids and their oxygenation by cyclo-oxygenases, lipoxygenases and other oxygenases. Biochimica et Biophysica Acta. 2015;**1851**:366-376. DOI: 10.1016/j.bbalip.2014.12.015

[37] Velasco G, Sánchez C, Guzmán M. Towards the use of cannabinoids as antitumour agents. Nature Reviews Cancer. 2012;**12**:436-444. DOI: 10.1038/nrc3247

[38] Iannotti FA, Di Marzo V, Petrosino S. Endocannabinoids and endocannabinoid-related mediators: targets, metabolism and role in neurological disorders. Progress in Lipid Research. 2016;**62**:107-128. DOI: 10.1016/j.plipres.2016.02.002

[39] Lu D, Potter DE. Cannabinoids and the cannabinoid receptors: An overview. In: Preedy VR, editor. Handbook of Cannabis and Related Pathologies: Biology, Pharmacology, Diagnosis, and Treatment, 1st ed. Amsterdam: Academic Press; 2017. pp. 553-563. DOI: 10.1016/B978-0-12-800756-3.00068-5

[40] Hill AJ, Williams CM, Whalley BJ, Stephens GJ. Phytocannabinoids as novel therapeutic agents in CNS disorders. Pharmacology & Therapeutics. 2012;**133**:79-97. DOI: 10.1016/j.pharmthera.2011.09.002

[41] Ramer R, Hinz B. Antitumorigenic targets of cannabinoids – current status and implications. Expert Opinion on Therapeutic Targets. 2016;**20**:1219-1235. DOI: 10.1080/14728222.2016.1177512

[42] Munson AE, Harris LS, Friedman MA, Dewey WL, Carchman RA. Antineoplastic activity of cannabinoids. Journal of the National Cancer Institute. 1975;**55**:597-602. DOI: 10.1093/jnci/55.3.597

[43] Hermanson DJ, Marnett LJ. Cannabinoids, endocannabinoids, and cancer. Cancer Metastasis Reviews. 2011;**30**:599-612. DOI: 10.1007/s10555-011-9318-8

[44] Pisanti S, Picardi P, D'Alessandro A, Laezza C, Bifulco M. The endocannabinoid signaling system in cancer. Trends in Pharmacological Sciences. 2013;**34**:273-282. DOI: 10.1016/j.tips.2013.03.003

[45] De Petrocellis L, Bifulco M, Ligresti A, Marzo VD. Potential use of cannabimimetics in the treatment of cancer. In: Mechoulam R, editor. Cannabinoids as Therapeutics. Basel: Birkhäuser; 2005. pp. 165-181. DOI: 10.1007/3-7643-7358-X

[46] Velasco G, Sánchez C, Guzmán M. Anticancer mechanisms of cannabinoids. Current Oncology. 2016;**23**:S23-S32. DOI: 10.3747/co.23.3080

[47] Ladin DA, Soliman E, Griffin L, Van Dross R. Preclinical and clinical assessment of cannabinoids as anti-cancer agents. Frontiers in Pharmacology. 2016;**7**:361 DOI:10.3389/fphar.2016.00361

[48] McConville P, Elliott WL, Kreger A, Lister R, Moody JB, Trachet E, Urban F, Leopold WR. Preclinical models of tumor growth and response. In: Shields AF, Price P, editors. In Vivo Imaging of Cancer Therapy. Totowa, New Jersey: Humana Press; 2007. pp. 13-32. DOI: 10.1007/978-1-59745-341-7

[49] Borrelli F, Pagano E, Romano B, Panzera S, Maiello F, Coppola D, De Petrocellis L, Buono L, Orlando P, Izzo AA. Colon carcinogenesis is inhibited by the TRPM8 antagonist cannabigerol, a cannabis-derived non-psychotropic cannabinoid. Carcinogenesis. 2014;**35**:2787-2797. DOI: 10.1093/carcin/bgu205

[50] Gallily R, Even-Chen T, Katzavian G, Lehmann D, Dagan A, Mechoulam R. γ-irradiation enhances apoptosis induced by cannabidiol, a non-psychotropic cannabinoid, in cultured HL-60 myeloblastic leukemia cells. Leukemia & Lymphoma. 2003;**44**:1767-1773. DOI: 10.1080/1042819031000103917

[51] Scott KA, Dalgleish AG, Liu WM. The combination of cannabidiol and Δ9-tetrahydrocannabinol enhances the anticancer effects of radiation in an orthotopic murine glioma model. Molecular Cancer Therapeutics. 2014;**13**:2955-2967 DOI: 10.1158/1535-7163.MCT-14-0402

[52] Torres S, Lorente M, Rodríguez-Fornés F, Hernández-Tiedra S, Salazar M, García-Taboada E, Barcia J, Guzmán M, Velasco G. A combined preclinical therapy of cannabinoids and temozolomide against glioma. Molecular Cancer Therapeutics. 2011;**10**:90-103. DOI: 10.1158/1535-7163.MCT-10-0688

[53] De Petrocellis L, Ligresti A, Schiano Moriello A, Iappelli M, Verde R, Stott CG, Cristino L, Orlando P, Di Marzo V. Non-THC cannabinoids inhibit prostate carcinoma growth *in vitro* and *in vivo*: pro-apoptotic effects and underlying mechanisms. British Journal of Pharmacology. 2013;**168**:79-102. DOI: 10.1111/j.1476-5381.2012.02027.x

[54] Galanti G, Fisher T, Kventsel I, Shoham J, Gallily R, Mechoulam R, Lavie G, Amariglio N, Rechavi G, Toren A. Δ9-Tetrahydrocannabinol inhibits cell cycle progression by downregulation of E2F1 in human glioblastoma multiforme cells. Acta Oncologica. 2008;**47**:1062-1070. DOI: 10.1080/02841860701678787

[55] Blázquez C, Carracedo A, Salazar M, Lorente M, Egia A, González-Feria L, Haro A, Velasco G, Guzmán M. Down-regulation of tissue inhibitor of metalloproteinases-1 in gliomas: A new marker of cannabinoid antitumoral activity? Neuropharmacology. 2008;**54**:235-243. DOI: 10.1016/j.neuropharm.2007.06.021

[56] Blázquez C, Salazar M, Carracedo A, Lorente M, Egia A, González-Feria L, Haro A, Velasco G, Guzmán M. Cannabinoids inhibit glioma cell invasion by down-regulating matrix metalloproteinase-2 expression. Cancer Research. 2008;**68**:1945-1952. DOI: 10.1158/0008-5472.CAN-07-5176

[57] Salazar M, Carracedo A, Salanueva ÍJ, Hernández-Tiedra S, Lorente M, Egia A, Vázquez P, Blázquez C, Torres S, García S, Nowak J, Fimia GM, Piacentini M, Cecconi F, Pandolfi PP, González-Feria L, Iovanna JL, Guzmán M, Boya P, Velasco G. Cannabinoid action induces autophagy-mediated cell death through stimulation of ER stress in human glioma cells. The Journal of Clinical Investigation. 2009;**119**:1359-1372. DOI: 10.1172/JCI37948

[58] Preet A, Ganju RK, Groopman JE. Δ^9-Tetrahydrocannabinol inhibits epithelial growth factor-induced lung cancer cell migration *in vitro* as well as its growth and metastasis *in vivo*. Oncogene. 2007;**27**:339-346. DOI: 10.1038/sj.onc.1210641

[59] Martín-Banderas L, Muñoz-Rubio I, Prados J, Álvarez-Fuentes J, Calderón-Montaño JM, López-Lázaro M, Arias JL, Leiva MC, Holgado MA, Fernández-Arévalo M. *In vitro* and *in vivo* evaluation of Δ^9-tetrahidrocannabinol/PLGA nanoparticles for cancer chemotherapy. International Journal of Pharmaceutics. 2015;**487**:205-212. DOI: 10.1016/j.ijpharm.2015.04.054

[60] Vara D, Salazar M, Olea-Herrero N, Guzmán M, Velasco G, Díaz-Laviada I. Anti-tumoral action of cannabinoids on hepatocellular carcinoma: Role of AMPK-dependent activation of autophagy. Cell Death and Differentiation. 2011;**18**:1099-1111. DOI: 10.1038/cdd.2011.32

[61] Vara D, Morell C, Rodríguez-Henche N, Diaz-Laviada I. Involvement of PPARγ in the antitumoral action of cannabinoids on hepatocellular carcinoma. Cell Death & Disease. 2013;**4**:e618. DOI: 10.1038/cddis.2013.141

[62] Carracedo A, Gironella M, Lorente M, Garcia S, Guzmán M, Velasco G, Iovanna JL. Cannabinoids induce apoptosis of pancreatic tumor cells via endoplasmic reticulum stress-related genes. Cancer Research. 2006;**66**:6748-6755. DOI: 10.1158/0008-5472.CAN-06-0169

[63] Caffarel MM, Sarrió D, Palacios J, Guzmán M, Sánchez C. Δ^9-tetrahydrocannabinol inhibits cell cycle progression in human breast cancer cells through Cdc2 regulation. Cancer Research. 2006;**66**:6615-6621. DOI: 10.1158/0008-5472.CAN-05-4566

[64] Caffarel MM, Andradas C, Mira E, Pérez-Gómez E, Cerutti C, Moreno-Bueno G, Flores JM, García-Real I, Palacios J, Mañes S, Guzmán M, Sánchez C. Cannabinoids reduce ErbB2-driven breast cancer progression through Akt inhibition. Molecular Cancer. 2010;**9**:196. DOI: 10.1186/1476-4598-9-196

[65] Armstrong JL, Hill DS, McKee CS, Hernandez-Tiedra S, Lorente M, Lopez-Valero I, Eleni Anagnostou M, Babatunde F, Corazzari M, Redfern CP, Velasco G, Lovat PE. Exploiting cannabinoid-induced cytotoxic autophagy to drive melanoma cell death. Journal of Investigative Dermatology. 2015;**135**:1629-1637. DOI: 10.1038/jid.2015.45

[66] Glodde N, Jakobs M, Bald T, Tüting T, Gaffal E. Differential role of cannabinoids in the pathogenesis of skin cancer. Life Sciences. 2015;**138**:35-40. DOI: 10.1016/j.lfs.2015.04.003

[67] Massi P, Vaccani A, Bianchessi S, Costa B, Macchi P, Parolaro D. The non-psychoactive cannabidiol triggers caspase activation and oxidative stress in human glioma cells. Cellular and Molecular Life Sciences. 2006;**63**:2057-2066. DOI: 10.1007/s00018-006-6156-x

[68] Massi P, Valenti M, Vaccani A, Gasperi V, Perletti G, Marras E, Fezza F, Maccarrone M, Parolaro D. 5-Lipoxygenase and anandamide hydrolase (FAAH) mediate the antitumor activity of cannabidiol, a non-psychoactive cannabinoid. Journal of Neurochemistry. 2008;**104**:1091-1100. DOI: 10.1111/j.1471-4159.2007.05073.x

[69] Soroceanu L, Murase R, Limbad C, Singer E, Allison J, Adrados I, Kawamura R, Pakdel A, Fukuyo Y, Nguyen D, Khan S, Arauz R, Yount GL, Moore DH, Desprez PY, McAllister SD. Id-1 is a key transcriptional regulator of glioblastoma aggressiveness and a novel therapeutic target. Cancer Research. 2013;**73**:1559-1569. DOI: 10.1158/0008-5472.CAN-12-1943

[70] Singer E, Judkins J, Salomonis N, Matlaf L, Soteropoulos P, McAllister S, Soroceanu L. Reactive oxygen species-mediated therapeutic response and resistance in glioblastoma. Cell Death & Disease. 2015;**6**:e1601. DOI: 10.1038/cddis.2014.566

[71] Fisher T, Golan H, Schiby G, PriChen S, Smoum R, Moshe I, Peshes-Yaloz N, Castiel A, Waldman D, Gallily R, Mechoulam R, Toren A. *In vitro* and *in vivo* efficacy of non-psychoactive cannabidiol in neuroblastoma. Current Oncology. 2016;**23**:15-22. DOI: 10.3747/co.23.2893

[72] Haustein M, Ramer R, Linnebacher M, Manda K, Hinz B. Cannabinoids increase lung cancer cell lysis by lymphokine-activated killer cells via upregulation of ICAM-1. Biochemical Pharmacology. 2014;**92**:312-325. DOI: 10.1016/j.bcp.2014.07.014

[73] Ramer R, Rohde A, Merkord J, Rohde H, Hinz B. Decrease of plasminogen activator inhibitor-1 may contribute to the anti-invasive action of cannabidiol on human lung cancer cells. Pharmaceutical Research. 2010;**27**:2162-2174. DOI: 10.1007/s11095-010-0219-2

[74] Ramer R, Merkord J, Rohde H, Hinz B. Cannabidiol inhibits cancer cell invasion via upregulation of tissue inhibitor of matrix metalloproteinases-1. Biochemical Pharmacology. 2010;**79**:955-966. DOI: 10.1016/j.bcp.2009.11.007

[75] Ramer R, Bublitz K, Freimuth N, Merkord J, Rohde H, Haustein M, Borchert P, Schmuhl E, Linnebacher M, Hinz B. Cannabidiol inhibits lung cancer cell invasion and metastasis via intercellular adhesion molecule-1. FASEB Journal. 2012;**26**:1535-1548. DOI: 10.1096/fj.11-198184

[76] Ramer R, Heinemann K, Merkord J, Rohde H, Salamon A, Linnebacher M, Hinz B. COX-2 and PPAR-γ confer cannabidiol-induced apoptosis of human lung cancer cells. Molecular Cancer Therapeutics. 2013;**12**:69-82. DOI: 10.1158/1535-7163.MCT-12-0335

[77] Aviello G, Romano B, Borrelli F, Capasso R, Gallo L, Piscitelli F, Di Marzo V, Izzo AA. Chemopreventive effect of the non-psychotropic phytocannabinoid cannabidiol on experimental colon cancer. Journal of Molecular Medicine. 2012;**90**:925-934. DOI: 10.1007/s00109-011-0856-x

[78] Sreevalsan S, Joseph S, Jutooru I, Chadalapaka G, Safe SH. Induction of apoptosis by cannabinoids in prostate and colon cancer cells is phosphatase dependent. Anticancer Research. 2011;**31**:3799-3807

[79] Ligresti A, Moriello AS, Starowicz K, Matias I, Pisanti S, De Petrocellis L, Laezza C, Portella G, Bifulco M, Di Marzo V. Antitumor activity of plant cannabinoids with emphasis on the effect of cannabidiol on human breast carcinoma. Journal of Pharmacology and Experimental Therapeutics. 2006;**318**:1375-1387. DOI: 10.1124/jpet.106.105247

[80] McAllister SD, Murase R, Christian RT, Lau D, Zielinski AJ, Allison J, Almanza C, Pakdel A, Lee J, Limbad C, Liu Y, Debs RJ, Moore DH, Desprez PY. Pathways mediating the effects of cannabidiol on the reduction of breast cancer cell proliferation, invasion, and metastasis. Breast Cancer Research and Treatment. 2011;**129**:37-47. DOI: 10.1007/s10549-010-1177-4

[81] Shrivastava A, Kuzontkoski PM, Groopman JE, Prasad A. Cannabidiol induces programmed cell death in breast cancer cells by coordinating the cross-talk between apoptosis and autophagy. Molecular Cancer Therapeutics. 2011;**10**:1161-1172. DOI: 10.1158/1535-7163.MCT-10-1100

[82] Elbaz M, Nasser MW, Ravi J, Wani NA, Ahirwar DK, Zhao H, Oghumu S, Satoskar AR, Shilo K, Carson WE, Ganju RK. Modulation of the tumor microenvironment and inhibition of EGF/EGFR pathway: novel anti-tumor mechanisms of cannabidiol in breast cancer. Molecular Oncology. 2015;**9**:906-919. DOI: 10.1016/j.molonc.2014.12.010

[83] Murase R, Kawamura R, Singer E, Pakdel A, Sarma P, Judkins J, Elwakeel E, Dayal S, Martinez-Martinez E, Amere M, Gujjar R, Mahadevan A, Desprez PY, McAllister SD. Targeting multiple cannabinoid anti-tumour pathways with a resorcinol derivative leads to inhibition of advanced stages of breast cancer. British Journal of Pharmacology. 2014;**171**:4464-4477. DOI: 10.1111/bph.12803

[84] Guzmán M, Duarte MJ, Blázquez C, Ravina J, Rosa MC, Galve-Roperh I, Sánchez C, Velasco G, González-Feria L. A pilot clinical study of Δ^9-tetrahydrocannabinol in patients with recurrent glioblastoma multiforme. British Journal of Cancer. 2006;**95**:197-203. DOI: 10.1038/sj.bjc.6603236

[85] https://clinicaltrials.gov/ct2/results?term=cannabis+And+cancer&Search=Search [Accessed: 2016-12-15]

[86] Walsh D, Nelson KA, Mahmoud FA. Established and potential therapeutic applications of cannabinoids in oncology. Support Care Cancer. 2003;**11**:137-143. DOI: 10.1007/s00520-002-0387-7

[87] Ben Amar M. Cannabinoids in medicine: A review of their therapeutic potential. Journal of Ethnopharmacology. 2006;**105**:1-25. DOI: 10.1016/j.jep.2006.02.001

[88] Machado Rocha FC, Stéfano SC, De Cássia Haiek R, Rosa Oliveira LMQ, Da Silveira DX. Therapeutic use of *Cannabis sativa* on chemotherapy-induced nausea and vomiting among cancer patients: systematic review and meta-analysis. European Journal of Cancer Care. 2008;**17**:431-443. DOI: 10.1111/j.1365-2354.2008.00917.x

[89] May BM, Glode AE. Dronabinol for chemotherapy-induced nausea and vomiting unresponsive to antiemetics. Cancer Management and Research. 2016;**8**:49-55. DOI: 10.2147/CMAR.S81425

[90] Meiri E, Jhangiani H, Vredenburgh JJ, Barbato LM, Carter FJ, Yang HM, Baranowski V. Efficacy of dronabinol alone and in combination with ondansetron versus ondansetron alone for delayed chemotherapy-induced nausea and vomiting. Current Medical Research and Opinion. 2007;**23**:533-543. DOI: 10.1185/030079907X167525

[91] Duran M, Pérez E, Abanades S, Vidal X, Saura C, Majem M, Arriola E, Rabanal M, Pastor A, Farré M, Rams N, Laporte JR, Capellà D. Preliminary efficacy and safety of an oromucosal standardized cannabis extract in chemotherapy-induced nausea and vomiting. British Journal of Clinical Pharmacology. 2010;**70**:656-663. DOI: 10.1111/j.1365-2125.2010.03743.x

[92] Abrams DI. Integrating cannabis into clinical cancer care. Current Oncology. 2016;**23**: 8-14. DOI: 10.3747/co.23.3099

[93] Thielmann A, Daeninck PJ. Medical marijuana in cancer: harmful or harm reduction? Clinical Practice. 2013;**10**:371-381. DOI: 10.2217/CPR.13.15

[94] Musty RE, Rossi R. Effects of smoked cannabis and oral Δ^9-tetrahydrocannabinol on nausea and emesis after cancer chemotherapy: A review of State clinical trials. Journal of Cannabis Therapeutics. 2001;**1**:29-42 DOI: 10.1300/J175v01n01_03

[95] Hernandez SL, Sheyner I, Stover KT, Stewart JT. Dronabinol treatment of refractory nausea and vomiting related to peritoneal carcinomatosis. American Journal of Hospice & Palliative Medicine. 2015;**32**:5-7. DOI: 10.1177/1049909113504240

[96] Grotenhermen F. Cannabinoids in cancer pain. Cannabinoids. 2010;**5**:1-3

[97] Cravatt BF, Lichtman AH. The endogenous cannabinoid system and its role in nociceptive behavior. Journal of neurobiology. 2004;**61**:149-160. DOI: 10.1002/neu.20080

[98] Johnson JR, Burnell-Nugent M, Lossignol D, Ganae-Motan ED, Potts R,Fallon MT. Multicenter, double-blind, randomized, placebo-controlled, parallel-group study of the efficacy, safety, and tolerability of THC: CBD extract and THC extract in patients with intractable cancer-related pain. Journal of Pain and Symptom Management. 2010;**39**:167-179. DOI: 10.1016/j.jpainsymman.2009.06.008

[99] Johnson JR, Lossignol D, Burnell-Nugent M, Fallon MT. An open-label extension study to investigate the long-term safety and tolerability of THC/CBD oromucosal spray and oromucosal THC spray in patients with terminal cancer-related pain refractory to strong opioid analgesics. Journal of Pain and Symptom Management. 2013;**46**:207-212. DOI: 10.1016/j.jpainsymman.2012.07.014

[100] Portenoy RK, Ganae-Motan ED, Allende S, Yanagihara R, Shaiova L,Weinstein S, McQuade R, Wright S, Fallon MT. Nabiximols for opioid-treated cancer patients with poor-controlled chronic pain: a randomized, placebo-controlled, graded-dose trial. The Journal of Pain. 2012;**13**:438-449. DOI: 10.1016/j.pain.2012.01.003

[101] Quasthoff S, Hartung HP. Chemotherapy-induced peripheral neuropathy. Journal of Neurology. 2002;**249**:9-17. DOI: 10.1007/PL00007853

[102] Lynch ME, Cesar-Rittenberg P, Hohmann AG. A double-blind, placebo-controlled, crossover pilot trial with extension using an oral mucosal cannabinoid extract for treatment of chemotherapy-induced neuropathic pain. Journal of Pain and Symptom Management. 2014;**47**:166-173. DOI: 10.1016/j.jpainsymman.2013.02.018

[103] Aoyagi T, Terracina KP, Raza A, Matsubara H, Takabe K. Cancer cachexia, mechanism and treatment. World Journal of Gastrointestinal Oncology. 2015;**7**:17-29. DOI: 10.4251/wjgo.v7.i4.17

[104] Kirkham TC, Williams CM. Endogenous cannabinoids and appetite. Nutrition Research Reviews. 2001;**14**:65-86. DOI: 10.1079/NRR200118

[105] Nelson K. A phase II study of delta-9-tetrahydrocannabinol for appetite stimulation in cancer-associated anorexia. Journal of Palliative Care. 1994;**10**:14-18.

[106] Strasser F, Luftner D, Possinger, Gernot Ernst G, Ruhstaller T, Meissner W, Ko YD, Schnelle M, Reif M, Cerny T. Comparison of orally administered cannabis extract and delta-9-tetrahydrocannabinol in treating patients with cancer-related anorexia-cachexia syndrome: a multicenter, phase III, randomized, double-blind, placebo-controlled clinical trial from the Cannabis-In-Cachexia-Study-Group. Journal of Oncology. 2006;**24**:3394-3400. DOI: 10.1200/JCO.2005.05.1847

[107] Maccio A, Madeddu C, Mantovani G. Current pharmacotherapy options for cancer anorexia and cachexia. Expert Opinion on Pharmacotherapy. 2012;**13**:2453-2472. DOI: 10.1517/14656566.2012.734297

[108] Reuter SE, Martin JH. Pharmacokinetics of cannabis in cancer cachexia-anorexia syndrome. Clinical Pharmacokinetics. 2016;**55**:807-812. DOI: 10.1007/s40262-015-0363-2

[109] Brisbois TD, De Kock IH, Watanabe SM, Mirhosseini M, Lamoureux DC, Chasen M, MacDonald N, Baracos VE, Wismer WV. Delta-9-tetrahydrocannabinol may palliate altered chemosensory perception in cancer patients: Results of a randomized, double-blind, placebo-controlled pilot trial. Annals of Oncology. 2011;**22**:2086-2093. DOI: 10.1093/annonc/mdq727

Chapter 7

Endophytic Fungi as Alternative and Reliable Sources for Potent Anticancer Agents

Edwin O. Omeje, Joy E. Ahomafor,
Theophilus U. Onyekaba, Philip O. Monioro,
Ibekwe Nneka, Sunday Onyeloni,
Charles Chime and Jonathan C. Eboka

Additional information is available at the end of the chapter

http://dx.doi.org/10.5772/67797

Abstract

In comparison with other natural sources like plants, highly diverse microorganisms are narrowly explored, especially with respect to their limitless potentials as repositories of exceptionally bioactive natural products. Of these organisms, fungi inhabiting tissues of plant in a noninvasive relationship (endophytic fungi) have proven undeniably useful and unmatchable as sources of potent bioactive molecules against several diseases such as cancer and related ailments. In general terms, endophytic fungi are highly prevalent organisms found in the tissue (intracellular or intercellular) of plants and at least for reasonable portion of their lives. It has been proven that virtually every plant, irrespective of habitat and climate, plays host to wide varieties of endophytes. Endophytic fungi produce metabolites produced by different biosynthetic pathways to that of the host plant, and this robustness equips them to synthesize unlimited structural entities and scaffolds of diverse classes. Interestingly too, the cohabitation/culture of these fungi with certain bacteria offers even stronger hopes for anticancer drug discovery. The endless need for potent drugs has necessitated the search of bioactive molecules from several sources, and endophytic fungi appear to be a recipe. This chapter is an attempt to present the current trend of research with these very promising organisms.

Keywords: microorganism, plants, sources, endophytes, fungi, anticancer, drug discovery

1. Introduction: the emergence of interest in endophytic fungi as sources of bioactive metabolites

Despite the fact that plant natural products (secondary metabolites) have been recognized as the most successful source of potential drug leads [1, 2], their recent implementation in drug discovery and development efforts have somewhat demonstrated a decline in interest [1]. Consequently, the need for new compounds to provide mitigation and relief in diverse human clinical conditions is ever-growing. In addition, the challenges of bacterial drug resistance, the emergence of highly virulent viruses and bacteria with organ transplant-associated complications demand very drastic drug discovery approaches in order to address them [3]. From the earliest times, when man directly tested plant materials for their potentials as medicines or foods to today when structured research approach has led to advancements in the discovery of bioactive natural product, it is evident that so much has been achieved in terms of the number of such agents that have great clinical importance. Notwithstanding, less than 10% of the world's biodiversity has been evaluated for potential biological activity, and therefore, many more useful natural lead compounds await discovery with the challenge being how to access this natural chemical diversity [4]. The search for bioactive natural products with potentials of addressing these identified challenges is as old as man's existence and has always relied heavily on the study of whole plant tissues (morphological parts) such as the roots (bark and inner tissues), leaves, stem (bark and inner tissues) and animal sources [5]. Unfortunately, the use of whole plant or animal tissues for the isolation of bioactive natural products has not been without its serious challenges. Fundamentally, the process leads to destruction of whole plant over time as the tissues are repeatedly collected without replenishment; most times, the existence of these plant species becomes threatened (**endangered**) and they are even lost after some years. Closely associated with this remarkable challenge are the problems of environmental degradation, land spoilage and the usually limited yield of the identified bioactive natural products. Secondly, the use of whole plant tissues in search of bioactive natural products has comparatively witnessed great wastage of research resources as a result of dereplication. Dereplication, which describes the process of fastly identifying or re-isolating already established biomolecules, is not only time and resources wasting but also discourages research zeal and excitement (reduction in interest). As at today, the probability of finding a novel bioactive molecule or chemical scaffold from whole tissues has further reduced because of dereplication. There are usually cross-family interactions among plant species in different biotopes complicated by most times poorly identified plant species, and as such, dereplication becomes a common challenge. Besides, the plant material has fixed biogenetic pathways which are tightly controlled by nature to produce predetermined secondary metabolites. As such and apart from the herculean plant tissue technology, man has little or no control over what a natural plant material produces as secondary metabolites. These identified problems led to loss of popularity in the natural product research efforts and, consequently, the development of combinatorial chemistry. Despite the great chemistry and huge investments witnessed in this era, not much breakthroughs have been recorded and, besides, combinatorial chemistry should act as a compliment to the natural product chemistry [6]. At this point, there arose a dire need for paradigm shift in the search for bioactive natural products. Accordingly, over a decade ago and based on accumulated successful drug discovery story, it appeared that the search for novel secondary metabolites should be refocused and research efforts consequently centered on the organisms that inhabit unique biotopes [1]. Of these organisms, endophytes were quickly recognized as veritable sources of novel bioactive natural products. Endophytes have been viewed as outstanding sources of novel products because there are so many of them occupying literally millions of unique biological niches (higher plant) growing in so many unusual environments. In all these, the endophytic fungi have been shown to be exceptionally useful in the drug discovery process, especially in the western world. An intensive literature search revealed that endophytic populations of the plants in rain forests of the African continent have not been significantly explored. Regrettably, sketchy research data have largely been documented on few usually unharnessed and abridged studies with whole plant tissues. This apparent low interest in researches with microbes as sources of antimetabolites is much more worrisome in trans-Saharan Africa. The reasons are not farfetched, mainly owed to weak infrastructural framework and systems. In Nigeria, for example, which is the acclaimed most populous black nation in Africa (approximately 160 million people—2006 National Population Census data), there are large rainforest zones in strategic locations of the country. Unfortunately, despite this robust biodiversity in Nigeria, bioprospecting for active molecules from these interesting microbes has remained largely unharnessed, and even the few research efforts have relied heavily on the direct plant tissues, with little work on the potentialities of fungal endophytes as veritable sources of novel bioactive compounds. This is a serious aberration and a major affront against any meaningful drug discovery effort of not only in Nigeria but also in several other African Countries. Consequently, there is need to awaken and boost research interest in the use of these specialized microbes (endophytes) for the discovery of potent bioactive molecules against the ever-increasing disease burden globally. In addition, given the rapidly increasing population of Nigeria and accompanying demand for drugs, it is critically important to identify and develop renewable sources of pharmaceuticals and their precursors. It is in line with this thought that we proposed this book chapter on endophytes as alternative and reliable sources of potent anticancer agents. It is our modest expectation that, through concerted research efforts in this promising area of drug discovery process, several strongly potent and safe molecules will be identified, isolated, assayed, characterized and hopefully progress into the several stages of clinical trial program as potential part of the armamentarium against cancer and associated conditions.

2. Endophytic fungi and search for active metabolites

The use of microbial biotopes as reliable sources of bioactive natural products has received significant attention so far [7, 8]. Current available data reveal that more than 40% of novel potent bioactive molecules obtained in a period of nearly two and half decades and half were microorganism-derived. Furthermore, over 60% of the anticancer and 70% of the antimicrobial drugs currently in clinical use are natural products or natural product derivatives. This is not surprising in the light of their evolution over millions of years in diverse ecological niches and natural habitats. The avalanche of microbial diversity with exciting metabolic complexes in plant tissues has been established in the last two decades and is continuing [8]. It is expedient to emphasize that the discovery of an endophytic fungus, from *Taxus brevifolia*, which produces highly selling anticancer agent called ***taxol***, precipitated a surge in interest to researches with endophytes [9]. Accordingly, about a decade ago, it appeared that the search for novel secondary metabolites should be refocused and research efforts consequently centered on the organisms that inhabit unique biotopes [1]. Of these organisms, endophytes were recognized as veritable sources of novel bioactive natural products. Endophytes have been viewed as outstanding sources of novel products because there are so many of them occupying literally millions of unique biological niches (higher plant) growing in so many unusual environment. One very interesting feature of the endophytic fungi is that they are renewable, readily available and environmentally friendly sources of biologically active natural products. An intensive literature search revealed that endophytic populations of the plant in rain forests of the African continent have not been studied apart from few unharnessed studies with whole plant tissues. Despite this ugly and unacceptable picture, it is heartening to note that this trend is gradually changing as current research scholars of African origin, especially those from Nigeria and Cameroun with thrust in natural product chemistry focus more on endophytic fungi nowadays as compared to the use of whole plant tissues. In summary, the inadequacy of systematic exploitation of ecosystems for the discovery of novel microbial compounds had resulted in random sampling and has missed the true potential of many regions [10]. Numerous bioactive molecules have been isolated from endophytic fungi since this ground-breaking discovery [11–13]. It is known that these endophytic fungi are embedded within plant for a substantial part of their life cycle and, as well earlier stated, they are devoid of any established potential to cause diseases in the host [14, 15]. This attribute makes this class of microbes a unique resource base for the discovery and development of potent anticancer molecules without having to destroy whole plant tissues. Additionally, they have been found to be more active when compared to other types of fungi somewhat existing outside the host in terms of metabolic virility [6, 16]. It was previously thought that metabolic products are transferred between host plant and the endophyte, the theory of horizontal transfer from the host plant to its microbial symbiont [9, 11, 17, 18]. This belief has been disproved following the successful sequencing of the *taxadiene synthase* gene from the taxol-producing endophyte which established that the metabolic pathways of both the hosts and the endophytes are independent of each other. The implication of this is that there are ample opportunities available for the manipulation of the endophyte biosynthetic pathways [19] to yield wide varieties of molecules and scaffolds for drug discovery process. 'Endophytism' is, thus, a unique cost–benefit plant microbe association defined by 'location' (not 'function') that is transiently symptomless, unobstructive, and established entirely inside the living host plant tissues [20, 21]. Evidence of plant-associated microorganisms found in the fossilized tissues has revealed that endophyte-plant associations may have evolved from the time higher plants first appeared on the earth surface [22]. The existence of fungi inside the organs of asymptomatic plants has been known since the end of the nineteenth century [23], and the term, 'endophyte' was first proposed in 1866 [24]. Since their discovery and description, they have been isolated from various organs of different plant species, from aboveground tissues of liverworts, hornworts, mosses, lycophytes, equisetopsides, ferns and spermatophytes from the tropics to the arctic, and from the wild to agricultural ecosystems [25]. Interestingly, all plant species studied till date have been found to harbor at least one endophyte. The most frequently encountered endophytes are fungi or bacteria (including actinomycetes), but future projections suggest that there could be revelation of nonendophytic microorganisms [3]. Endophytic fungi are a very diverse polyphyletic group of microorganisms; they can thrive asymptomatically in the tissues of plants aboveground as well as belowground, including stems, leaves and/or roots [26]. Many endophytes have the potential to synthesize various bioactive metabolites that may directly or indirectly be used as therapeutic agents against numerous diseases [3, 19, 21, 27–29]. Occasionally and usually hitting major buck, endophytes that produce host plant secondary metabolites with therapeutic value or potentials have been discovered; some examples include paciltaxel (also known as taxol) [9] and podophyllotoxin [17, 30]. The production of bioactive compounds by endophytes, especially those exclusive to their host plant, is not only important from an ecological perspective but also from a biochemical and molecular standpoint. In contrast to the direct bioprospecting with known medicinal plants (the common problem being that of dereplication), exciting possibilities exist for exploiting endophytic fungi for the production of a plethora of known and novel biologically active secondary metabolites. The potential of microorganisms is further limited by the presence of orphan biosynthetic pathways that remain unexpressed under general laboratory conditions [31]. However, the vast choice of techniques pertaining to the growth and manipulation of microorganisms such as media engineering, coculture, chemical induction, epigenetic modulation and metabolite remodeling, coupled with the fermentation technology for scale-up, make them suitable for production of useful natural products, both known and novel [16]. Of the myriads of ecosystems on earth, those having the greatest biodiversity seem to be ones also having endophytes with the greatest number and the most biodiverse microorganisms. Tropical and temperate rain forests are the most biologically diverse terrestrial ecosystems on earth. As such, one would expect that areas of high plant endemicity also possess specific endophytes that may have evolved with the endemic plant species. Ultimately, biological biodiversity implies chemical biodiversity because of constant chemical innovation that exists in ecosystems where the evolutionary race to survive is most active. Comparatively, tropical rainforests are a remarkable example of this type of environment because competition is great; resources are limited, and selection pressure is at its peak. This gives rise to a high probability that rainforests are excellent source of novel molecular structures and biologically active compounds [32]. Early researches in endophyte bioprospecting showed that a significantly higher number of tropical endophytes produced a larger number of active secondary metabolites than did fungi from temperate endophytes or other tropical substrata [33].

3. Isolation process and characterization of bioactive metabolites from endophytic fungi

The choice of plants for the explorative study of endophytes in search of potent bioactive molecules is a very crucial issue that requires the right information. Since the biochemical pathways of both endophytes and their host are strongly correlated, it is expedient that medicinally useful plants in different cultures are selected for bioprospecting of endophytes. The isolation of endophytic fungi is carried out using the most probable morphological part of the properly identified and document host plant, most times the leaves. The wholesome leaves of the selected plant are collected in sterile plastic bags from designated area with the aid of the geographic position system (GPS) and stored at refrigeration temperature (4°C) in preparation for the isolation of endophytic fungi. There are times during which samples might have to be transported over long distances, and it is required that contingent transport and sterile cold chain arrangements should be made to ensure the integrity of the plant part on arrival. In all the processes, it is required that strict sterility is maintained so as to ensure that no external organisms are introduced as contaminants to the culture. The following procedures are then followed:

(i) The leaves or any other morphological part of interest is washed under flowing tap water for a minimum time of 10 min and dried under sterile dry air.

(ii) With the aid of a sterilized scalpel (use of Bunsen flame) or other techniques, pieces of the leaves are cut out and sterilized further using these agents; 95% ethanol (1–2 min), 3.5% (v/v) sodium hypochlorite (3–4 min), 70% (v/v) ethanol (30–40 s) in that order.

(iii) The sterilized samples will be washed trice in sterile distilled water and allowed to dry on filter papers under aseptic conditions. Subsequently, the samples are placed on the appropriate culture media of interest supplemented with an antibiotic concentration to prevent the growth of bacteria and depending on the substrate that will act as the primary carbon source in the medium. Some of the natural carbon sources include maltose, rice, beans, etc. The plating is usually done in replicates and inside air laminar flow hood of appropriate level of biosafety.

(iv) The plates will then be incubated at room temperature (30–37°C). The fungal mycelium growing out from leaf discs were subsequently transferred to fresh MEA plates by hyphal tip transfers and incubated further at room temperature for 1–2 weeks. The purity of isolated endophytic fungi was checked and their antimicrobial and anticancer activity was determined. The endophytic fungal isolates were maintained in MEA for future studies. This is referred to as the primary culture. When the pure fungal species is identified and fully characterized (after affirmation of interesting activities in this instance, anticancer property using different robust *in vitro* techniques), large-scale production of the fungi will then involve the use of secondary culture technique in larger vessels for the harvest of larger quantity in preparation for isolation of the fungal metabolites. Sometimes, selected bacteria are cocultured with the fungi as a way of stimulating and manipulating and exploiting the metabolic pathways of these organisms. Modifications of these procedures vary from laboratory to laboratory.

4. Identification of endophytic fungal isolates

Essentially, isolated endophytic fungi are identified based on both their macroscopic and microscopic structures [34]. Further identification sequel to establishment of satisfactory biological activities involves the use of biotechnological procedures. There are several taxonomical classification guides available such as found in these references [35–38]. The nonspores are termed and classified as mycelia isolates. The fungal isolates with very interesting biological activity spectrum are further identified based on the analysis of nucleotide sequences of the internal transcribed spacer (ITS) regions of rDNA following the method described by earlier authors [39]. The confirmation of similarity of gene properties of the synthesized nucleotide rDNA sequence of ITS is usually compared with sequences from available GenBank using BLAST program of the National Institutes of Health, United States of America.

5. Large-scale endophytic fungal cultivation and extraction

The large-scale cultivation of the endophytic fungi is also carried out on the selected media as described above and then transferred (inoculated) into a 500-ml or larger Erlenmeyer flasks containing appropriate nutrients depending on target. The setup will be incubated at room temperature for one month standard conditions. The broth is then filtered and extracted with an appropriate solvent such as ethyl acetate. The extract was dried over anhydrous sodium sulfate and then evaporated under vacuum in a rotary evaporator, to yield ethyl acetate extracts. The dried extract will be partitioned into several solvent fractions and recovered for further testing of biological activities. Subsequently, the fractions are subjected to several processes of chromatography and purifications steps to isolate pure metabolites which are tested and fully characterized using physicochemical and spectroscopic methods. In order to maximize the unlimited potentials of the endophytic fungi as reliable repository for anticancer bioactive metabolites and other drug discovery, modern research should target the selection and isolation of samples from diverse ecosystems, manipulating microbial physiology to activate microbial natural-product biosynthetic machinery, and genetically modifying strains for production of unnatural microbial natural products. By manipulating all three of these approaches, the diversity of an extract collection can be maximized, and in doing so, the chance of finding a 'hit' can be increased.

6. An overview of anticancer agents from endophytic fungi

Although some battles have been won since the declaration of the 'war on cancer' in 1971 in the United Sates, the war is ongoing [40]. Furthermore, the much expected breakthrough in anticancer chemotherapy has been seriously challenged. Malignant tumors are one of the most serious diseases that damage human health in the modern world and the second largest deadly disease just after heart diseases [41], and as such, the search for newer anticancer agents remains endless. This search has, in recent times, shifted to the endophytic fungi. Interesting secondary metabolites are derived from endophytes which make them unmatchable synthesizers of very useful complex chemical scaffolds inside their hosts [42, 43]. In comparison, most of these metabolites have been engaged in the fight against diverse diseases of man and animal [44]. Since the advent of taxol from an endophytic fungus, efforts have relied on the manipulation and optimization of the culture conditions and this approach has produced several chemical constituents and novel analogues with quite unique biochemistry [3]. For the purpose of this chapter, we limited our discussion to few selected important categories of bioactive metabolites produced by fungal endophytes of medicinal plants (**Figure 1**). Several authors in the past have reported excellent reviews on endophytes as potential sources of bioactive metabolites. One of such interesting reviews was published by Sanjana et al. [45] in 2012, covering their unmatched potentials as sources for anticancer, antioxidant, immunomodulatory, antiparasitic, antitubercular and insecticidal agents. In the current review, we attempt to present an updated chapter on endophytes as reliable sources of anticancer metabolites. Following the discovery of the multimillion dollar anticancer agent, taxol from the endophytic fungus *Taxomyces andreanae* [9], several others have been studied as potential repositories of anticancer agents. Taxol (paclitaxel) belongs to the diterpenoid class of natural products and is an exceptionally potent anticancer agent. Before, being isolated from the endophytic fungus *Taxomyces andreanae*, it was isolated for the first time, from the bark of *Taxus brevifolia*, commonly called yew plant from the South American pacific. The drug was subsequently approved by the Food and Drug Administration (FDA), USA, for the treatment of selected cancers [46]. The diverse sources of taxol from endophytic fungi are shown in **Table 1**. Lee et al. [47] reported the isolation of a dimeric quinone Torreyanic acid from the endophytic fungus, *Pestalotiopsis microsporum* growing in the plant *Torreya taxifolia*. This compound was shown to possess potent cytotoxic activity through apoptotic mechanisms [47]. Camptothecin, a potent antineoplastic agent from endophytic *Entrophospora infrequens* isolated from the host plant, *Nothapodytes foetida*, was also reported by Puri et al. [48], as having pronounced activity against lung cancer and ovarian cancer cell lines. Several authors attempted the derivatization of analogues of Campothecin, and a successful effort led to the discovery of two clinically useful anticancer drugs: topotecan and irinotecan. These potent anticancer compounds were extracted from the endophytic Fusariumsolani inhabiting *Camptotheca acuminata* [18]. Podophyllotoxin, a nonalkaloid lignin and its analogues are clinically relevant mainly due to their antiviral and anticancer activities; further, they are the precursors of many other useful anticancer drugs including etoposide, Teniposide and etopophos phosphate [49]. Podophyllotoxin and other related aryl tetralin lignans have also been reported to be produced by another novel endophytic fungus, Trametes hirsute with anticancer potential [17]. The different strains of endophytic fungi producing Podophyllotoxin are represented in **Table 2**. Various novel microbial sources of podophyllotoxin include *Aspergillus fumigatus* isolated from *Juniperus communis* [50], *Phialocephala fortinii* isolated from *Podophyllum peltatum* [30] and *Fusarium oxysporum* isolated from *Juniperus recurva* [49]. Ergoflavin, a novel anticancer agent, was isolated from the leaf endophytes of an Indian medicinal plant *Mimusops elengi*, belonging to family Sapotaceae. Ergoflavin is a dimeric xanthene linked at position-2, belonging to the ergochrome class of compounds [51]. Another compound from ergochrome class, i.e., secalonic acid D, a mycotoxin, isolated from the mangrove endophytic fungus also exhibits a good cytotoxic activity on HL60 and K562 cells by inducing leukemia cell apoptosis [52]. Wagenaar et al. [53] studied Rhinocladiella sp. inhabiting *Tripterygium wilfordii* and reported three novel cytochalasins: cytochalasin H, cytochalasin J and epoxycytochalasin H along with a known compound cytochalasin E. These compounds have been identified as 22-oxa-12-cytochalasins and have antitumor activity.

http://dx.doi.org/10.5772/67797

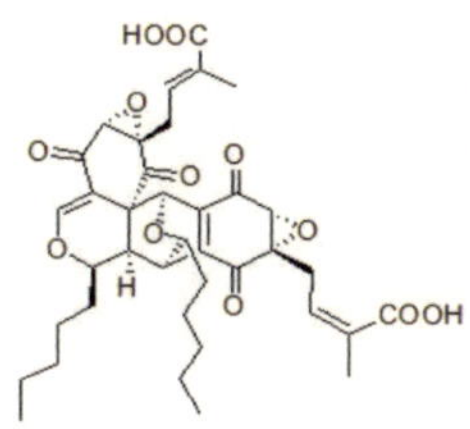

Torreyanic acid

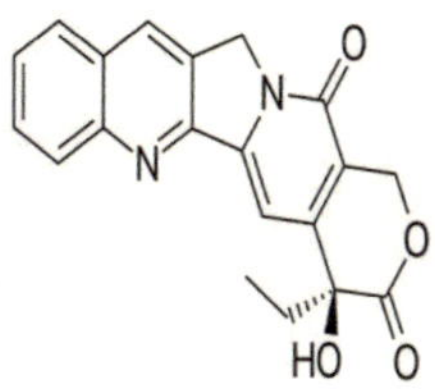

Camptothecin

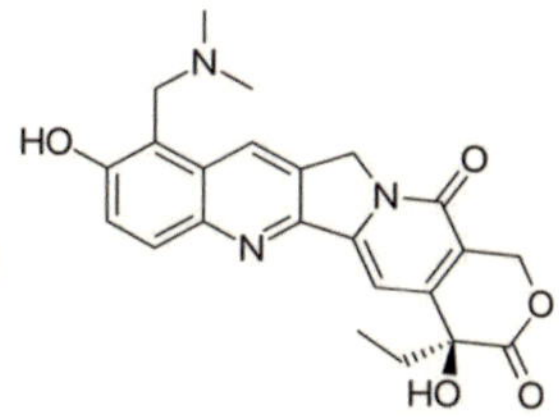

Topothecan

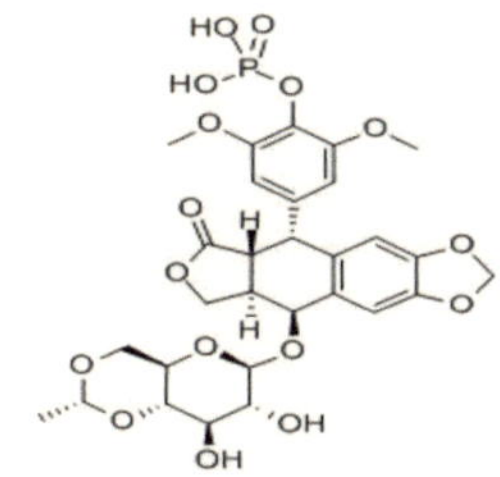

Etopophos

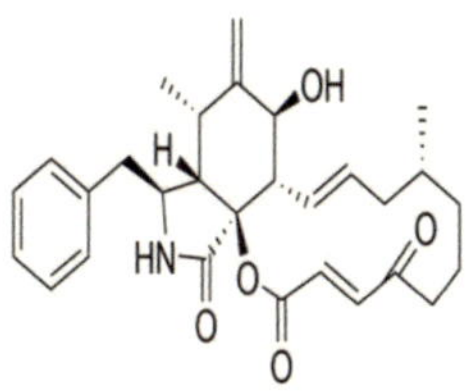

Cytochalasin A

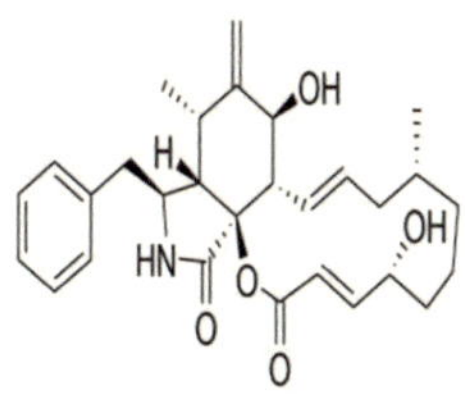

Cytochalasin **B**

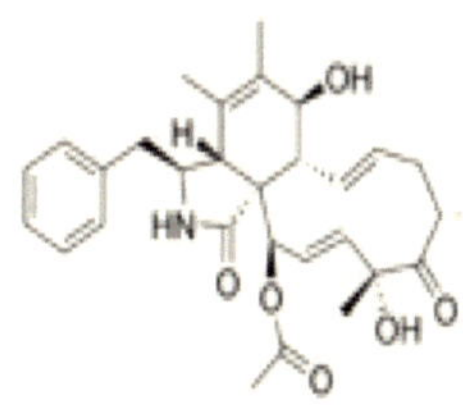

Cytochalasin C

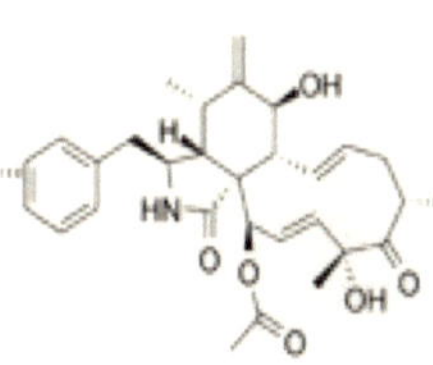

Cytochalasin D

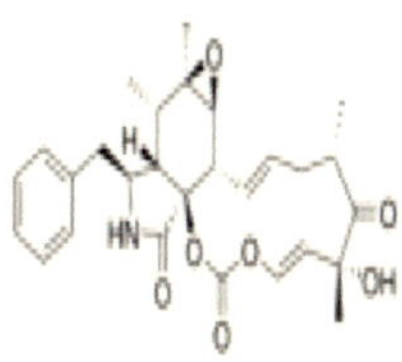

Cytochalasin E

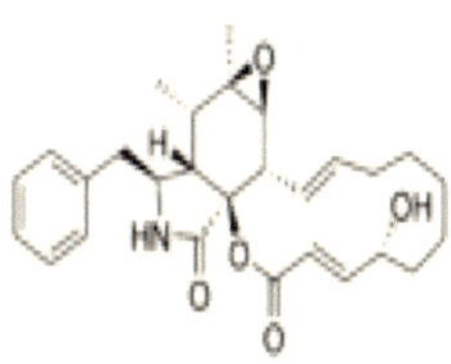

Cytochalasin F

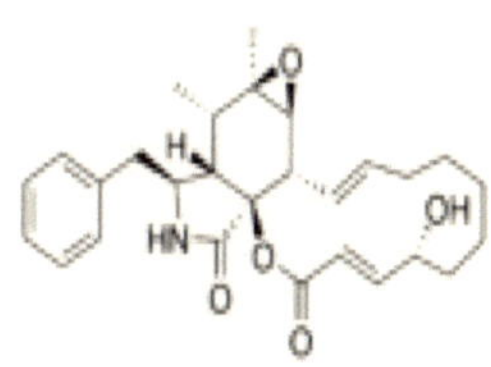

Cytochalasin H

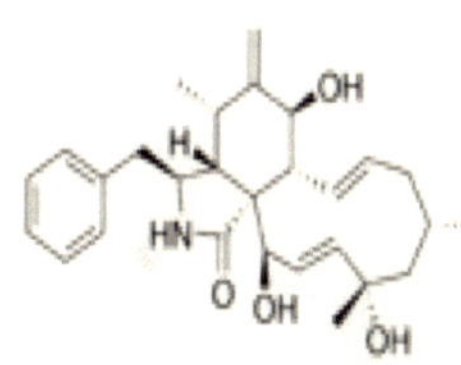

Cytochalasin J

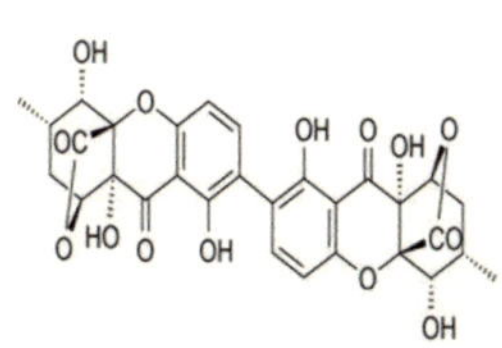

Ergoflavin

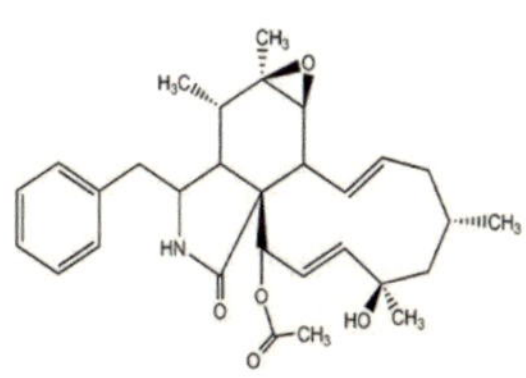

Epoxycytochalasin H

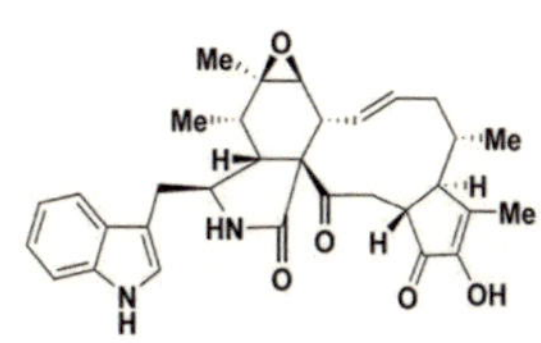

Chaetoglobosin U

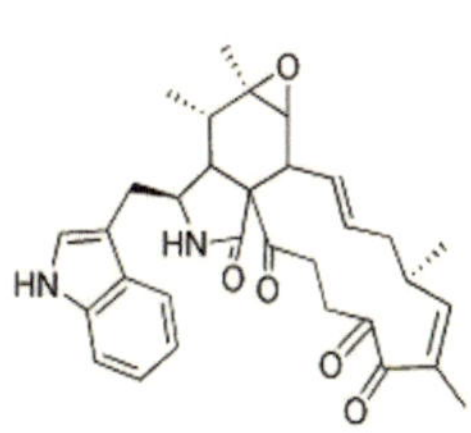

Chaetoglobosin C

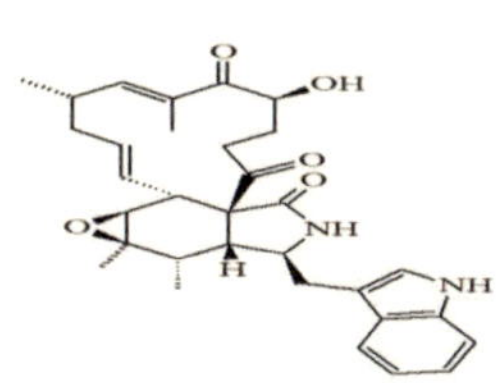

Chaetoglobosin F

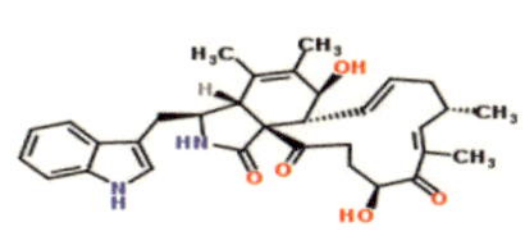

Chaetoglobosin E

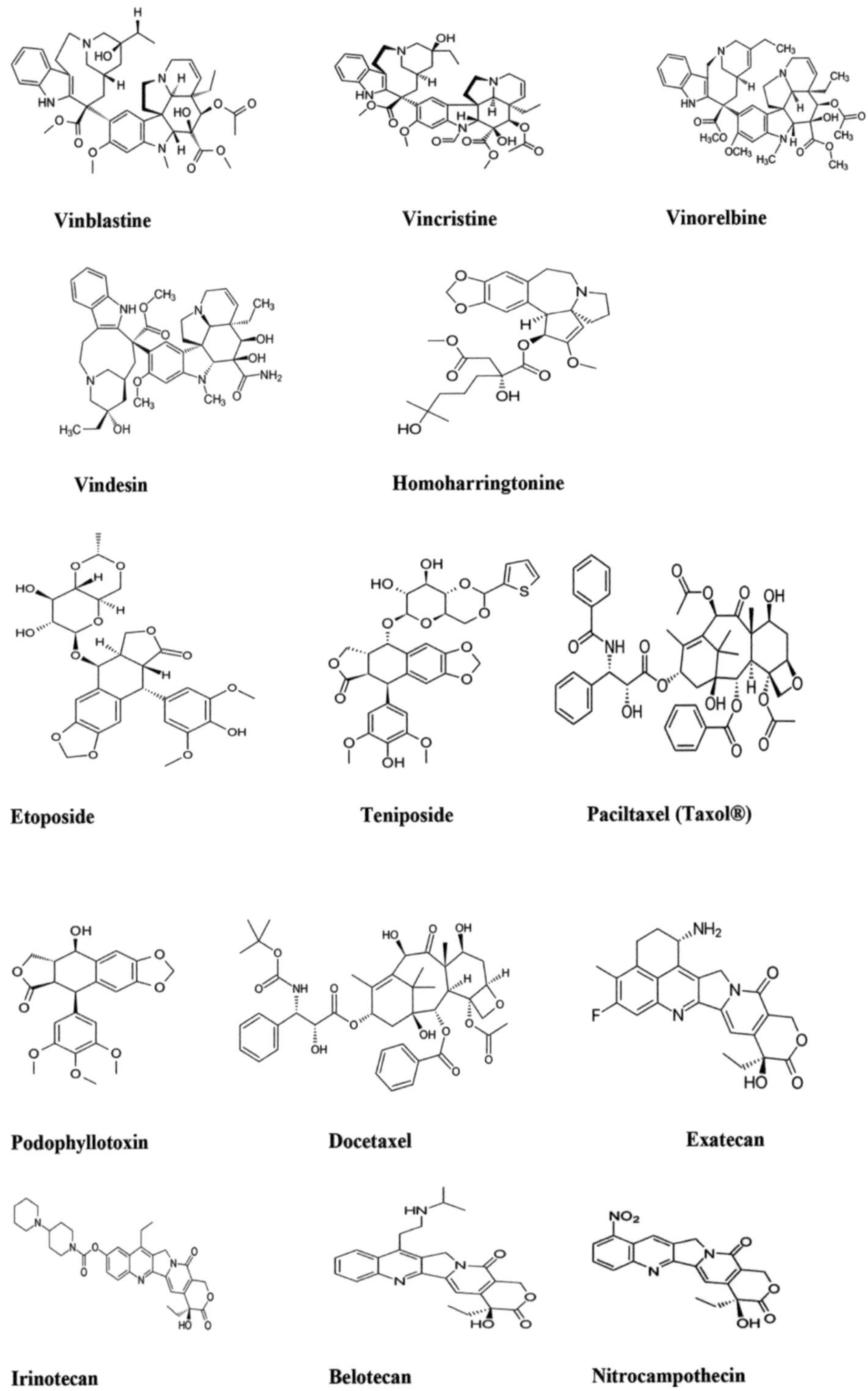

Figure 1. Selected structures of anticancer metabolites from endophytic fungi.

Endophytic fungus	Fungal strain	Host plant	Paclitaxel yield (μg/L)
Alternaria sp.	Ja-69	*Taxus cuspidata*	0.16
Alternaria sp.	–	*Ginkgo biloba*	0.12–0.26
Alternaria alternata	TPF6	*Taxus chinensis* var. *mairei*	84.5
Aspergillus fumigatus	EPTP-1	*Podocarpus* sp.	557.8
Aspergillus niger var. *taxi*	HD86-9	*Taxus cuspidata*	273.6
Botryodiplodia theobromae	BT115	*Taxus baccata*	280.5
Botrytis sp.	XT2	*Taxus chinensis* var. *mairei*	161.24
Botrytis sp.	HD181-23	*Taxus cuspidata*	206.34
Cladosporium cladosporioides	MD2	*Taxus media*	800
Ectostroma sp.	XT5	*Taxus chinensis* var. *mairei*	276.75
Fusarium arthrosporioides	F-40	*Taxus cuspidate*	131
Fusarium lateritium	Tbp-9	*Taxus baccata*	0.13
Fusarium mairei	Y1117	*Taxus chinensis* var. *mairei*	2.7
Fusarium mairei	UH23	*Taxus chinensis* var. *mairei*	286.4
Fusarium solani	–	*Taxus celebica*	1.6
Fusarium solani	Tax-3	*Taxus chinensis*	163.35
Metarhizium anisopliae	H-27	*Taxus chinensis*	846.1
Monochaetia sp.	Tbp-2	*Taxus baccata*	0.10
Mucor rouxianus	DA10	*Taxus chinensis*	–
Ozonium sp.	BT2	*Taxus chinensis* var. *mairei*	4–18
Papulaspora sp.	XT17	*Taxus chinensis* var. *mairei*	10.25
Periconia sp.	No. 2026	*Torreya grandifolia*	0.03–0.83
Pestalotia bicilia	Tbx-2	*Taxus baccata*	1.08
Pestalotiopsis guepinii	W-1f-2	*Wollemia nobilis*	0.49
Pestalotiopsis microspora	Ja-73	*Taxus cuspidata*	0.27
Pestalotiopsis microspora	Ne-32	*Taxus wallachiana*	0.5
Pestalotiopsis microspora	No. 1040	*Taxus wallachiana*	0.06–0.07
Pestalotiopsis microspora	Cp-4	*Taxodium distichum*	0.05–1.49
Pestalotiopsis microspora	Ne 32	*Taxus wallichiana*	0.34–1.83

Adapted from Zhao et al. (2010), *Endophytic* fungi for producing bioactive compounds originally from their host plants [62].

Table 1. Paclitaxel-producing endophytic fungi and their host plants.

A novel cytotoxic cytochalasan-based alkaloid chaetoglobosin U along with four known analogues, chaetoglobosin C, chaetoglobosin F, chaetoglobosin E and ponochalasin A, have been

Endophytic fungus	Fungal strain	Host plant	Podophyllotoxin content or yield
Alternaria sp.	–	*Sinopodophyllum hexandrum* (=*Podophyllum hexandrum*)	–
Alternaria neesex	Ty	*Sinopodophyllum hexandrum*	2.4 μg/L
Fusarium oxysporum	JRE1	*Sabina recurva* (=*Juniperus recurva*)	28 μg/g
Monilia sp.	–	*Dysosma veitchii*	–
Penicillium sp.	–	*Sinopodophyllum hexandrum*	–
Penicillium sp.	–	*Diphylleia sinensis*	–
Penicillium sp.	–	*Dysosma veitchii*	–
Penicillium implicatum	SJ21	*Diphylleia sinensis*	–
Penicillium implication	2BNO1	*Dysosma veitchii*	–
Phialocephala fortinii	PPE5, PPE7	*Sinopodophyllum peltatum*	0.5–189 μg/L
Trametes hirsuta	–	*Sinopodophyllum hexandrum*	30 μg/g

Adapted from Zhao et al. (2010), Endophytic fungi for producing bioactive compounds originally from their host plants.

Table 2. Podophyllotoxin-producing endophytic fungi and their host plants.

produced by the fungal endophyte *Chaetomium globosum* IFB-E019 isolated from *Imperata cylindrica*. Cheatoglobosin U exhibits cytotoxic activity against nasopharyngeal epidermoid tumor KB cell [54]. Chen et al. [55] reported Gliocladicillins A and B as effective antitumor agents in vitro and in vivo. They induced tumor cell apoptosis and also showed a significant inhibition on proliferation of melanoma B16 cells implanted into immunodeficient mice. Vincristine, an alkaloid with cytotoxic activity, was isolated from the endophytic mycelia sterilia inhabiting *Catharanthus roseus* [56]. This drug is mainly used as a chemotherapy regimen in acute lymphoblastic leukemia and nephroblastoma. Likewise, there are large numbers of anticancer agents produced by fungal endophytes inhabiting different medicinal plants. Several of such molecules are presently at different levels of clinical trials, and there are putative hopes that some of them will be approved for use in no distant time. Furthermore, the list of metabolites obtained diverse endophytic fungi with proven potent activity against several cancers is endless, thus indicating that these organisms hold the future in the attempt to conquer cancer therapeutically.

7. Conclusion

No doubt, endophytes remain an unmatchable biodiversity and repository for novel natural compounds with useful biological activities and form simple to complex scaffolds for the generation of more potent of compound. Because of the diversity of potential of advantages including the application of modern biotechnological techniques, metabolic technology and microbial fermentation process, we can better understand and manipulate this important

http://dx.doi.org/10.5772/67797

microorganism resource and make it more beneficial for the mankind [33, 57–60]. We can conclude that the endophytic fungi are a novel and important microbial resource for producing bioactive compounds and have attracted attention of many researchers on their theoretical study as well as their potential applications [61]. The future of discovering anticancer agents from endophytic fungi is undoubtedly bright.

Author details

Edwin O. Omeje[1,2]*, Joy E. Ahomafor[2], Theophilus U. Onyekaba[2,3], Philip O. Monioro[2], Ibekwe Nneka[4], Sunday Onyeloni[2], Charles Chime[5] and Jonathan C. Eboka[2,6]

*Address all correspondence to: edwin.omeje@unn.edu.ng

1 Department of Pharmaceutical and Medicinal Chemistry, Faculty of Pharmaceutical Sciences, University of Nigeria, Nsukka, Nigeria

2 Department of Pharmaceutical Chemistry, Faculty of Pharmacy Sciences, Delta State University, Abraka, Nigeria

3 Department of Pharmaceutical Chemistry, Faculty of Pharmacy, Madonna University, Elele, River State, Nigeria

4 Department of Medicinal Chemistry, National Institute for Pharmaceutical Research and Development (NIPRD), Idu, Abuja, Nigeria

5 Department of Industrial Chemistry, Faculty of Applied Natural Sciences, Enugu State University of Science and Technology, Agbani, Enugu, Enugu State, Nigeria

6 Department of Pharmaceutical Chemistry, Faculty of Pharmacy, University of Benin, Benin City, Edo State, Nigeria

References

[1] Mishra BB, Tiwari VK. Natural products: An evolving role in future drug discovery. European Journal of Medicinal Chemistry. 2011;**46**:4769-4807

[2] Rey-Ladino J, Ross AG, Cripps AW, McManus DP, Quinn R. Natural products and the search for novel vaccine adjuvants. Vaccine. 2011;**29**:6464-6471

[3] Strobel G, Daisy B, Castillo U, Harper J. Natural products from endophytic microorganisms. Journal of Natural Products. 2004;**67**:257-268

[4] Cragg GM, Newman DJ. Biodiversity: A continuing source of novel drug leads. Pure and Applied Chemistry. 2005;**77**:7-24

[5] Dias DA, Urban S, Roessner U. A historical overview of natural products in drug discovery. Metabolites. 2012;**2**(2):303-336

[6] Strobel G, Daisy B. Bioprospecting for microbial endophytes and their natural products. Microbiology and Molecular Biology Reviews. 2003;**66**(4):491-502

[7] Qadri M, Johri S, Shah BA, Khajuria A, Sidiq T, Lattoo SK, Abdin MZ, Riyaz-Ul-Hassan S. Identification and bioactive potential of endophytic fungi isolated from selected plants of the Western Himalaya. SpringerPlus. 2013;**2**:8. DOI: 10.1186/2193-1801-2-8

[8] Porras-Alfaro A, Bayman P. Hidden fungi, emergent properties: Endophytes and microbiomes. Annual Review of Phytopathology. 2011;**49**:291-315

[9] Stierle A, Strobel G, Stierle D. Taxol and taxane production by *Taxomyces andreanae*, an endophytic fungus of pacific yew. Science. 1993;**260**:214-216

[10] Czaran TL, Hoekstra RF, Pagie L. Chemical warfare between microbes promotes biodiversity. Proceedings of the National Academy of Sciences of the United States of America. 2002;**99**:786-790

[11] Strobel G. Harnessing endophytes for industrial microbiology. Current Opinion in Microbiology. 2006;**9**(3):240-244

[12] Wang LW, Zhang YL, Lin FC, Hu YZ, Zhang CL. Natural products with antitumor activity from endophytic fungi. Mini-Reviews in Medicinal Chemistry. 2011;**11**:1056-1074

[13] Zhang Y, Han T, Ming Q, Wu L, Rahman K, Qin L. Alkaloids produced by endophytic fungi: A review. Natural Product Communications. 2012;**7**(7):963-968

[14] Bacon CW, White JF. Microbial Endophytes. New York, NY: Marcel Dekker Inc.; 2000

[15] Souvik K, Christian H, Michael S. Chemical ecology of endophytic fungi: Origins of secondary metabolites. Chemistry and Biology. 2012;**19**:792-798

[16] El Amrani M, Debbab A, Aly AH, Wray V, Dobretsov S, Mueller WEG, Lin WH, Lai DW, Proksch P. Farinomalein derivatives from an unidentified endophytic fungus isolated from the mangrove plant *Avicennia marina*. Tetrahedron Letters. 2012;**53**:6721-6724

[17] Puri SC, Nazir A, Chawla R, Arora R, Riyaz-Ul-Hasan S, Amna T, Ahmed B, Verma V, Singh S, Sagar R, et al. The endophytic fungus *Trametes hirsute* as a novel alternative source of podophyllotoxin and related aryl tetralin lignans. Journal of Biotechnology. 2006;**122**:494-510

[18] Kusari S, Zuhlke S, Spiteller M. An endophytic fungus from *Camptotheca acuminata* that produces camptothecin and analogues. Journal of Natural Products. 2009;**72**(1):2-7

[19] Staniek A, Woerdenbag HJ, Kayser O. Endophytes: Exploiting biodiversity for the improvement of natural-based drug discovery. Journal of Plant Interactions. 2008;**3**:75-93

[20] Kusari S, Spiteller M. Campothecin: Recent advances in plant-endophyte research. In: Patro LR, editor. Natural Resources Conservation and Management. New Delhi, India: Manglam Publications; 2012. pp. 1-32

[21] Kusari S, Spiteller M. Metabolomics of endophytic fungi producing associated plant secondary metabolites: Progress, challenges and opportunities. In: Roessner U, editor. Metabolomics. Rijeka, Croatia: In Tech; 2012. pp. 241-266

[22] Redecker D, Kodner R, Graham LE. Glomalean fungi from the Ordovician. Science. 2000;**289**:1920-1921

[23] Guerin P. Sur la presence d'un champignon dans l'ivraie. Journal de Botanique. 1898;**12**: 230-238

[24] De Bary A. Morphologie und physiologie der Pilze, Flechten and myxomyceten. In: Hofmeister's Handbook of Physiological Botany. Vol. II. Leipzig, Germany: Engelmann; 1866. pp. 1-335

[25] Arnold AE. Understanding the diversity of foliar endophytic fungi: Progress, challenges and frontiers. Fungal Biology Reviews. 2007;**21**:51-66

[26] Selim KA, El-Beih AA, Abd El-Rahman TM, El-Diwany AI. Biology of endophytic fungi. Current Research in Environmental & Applied Mycology. 2012;**2**(1):31-82. DOI: 10.5943/cream/2/1/3

[27] Aly AH, Debbab A, Edrada-Ebel RA, Müller WEG, Kubbutat MHG, Wray V, Ebel R, Proksch P. Protein kinase inhibitors and other cytotoxic metabolites from the fungal endophyte *Stemphylium botryosum* isolated from *Chenopodium album*. Mycosphere. 2010;**1**:153-162

[28] Khawar RN, Mishra A, Gond SK, Stierle A, Stierle D. Anti-cancer compounds derived from fungal endophytes: Their importance and future challenges. Natural Product Reports. 2011;**28**:1208-1228

[29] Debbab A, Aly AH, Edrada-Ebel RA, Wray V, Müller WEG, Totzke F, Zirrgiebel U, Schächtele C, Kubbutat MHG, Lin WH, Mosaddak M, Hakiki A, Proksch P, Ebel R. Bioactive metabolites from endophytic fungus *Stemphylium globuliferum* isolated from *Mentha pulegium*. Journal of Natural Products. 2009;**72**:626-631

[30] Eyberger AL, Dondapati R, Porter JR. Endophyte fungal isolates from *Podophyllum peltatum*. Journal of Natural Products. 2006;**69**:1121-1124

[31] Hertweck C. Hidden biosynthetic treasures brought to light. Nature Chemical Biology. 2009;**5**:450-452

[32] Redell P, Gordon V. Lessons from nature: Can ecology provide new leads in the search for novel bioactive chemicals from rainforest? In: Wrigley SK, Hayes MA, Thomas R, Chrystal EJT, Nicholson N, editors. Biodiversity: New Leads for Pharmaceutical and Agrochemical Industries. Cambridge, United Kingdom: The Royal Society of Chemistry; 2000. pp. 205-212

[33] Bill G, Dombrowski A, Pelaez F, Polishook J, An Z. Recent and future discoveries of pharmacologically active metabolites from tropical fungi. In: Watling R, Frankland JC, Ainsworth AM, Isaac S, Robinson CH, editors. Tropical Mycology: Mycromycetes. Vol. 2. New York, NY: CABI Publishing; 2002. pp. 165-194

[34] Thirawatthana P, Tanapat P, Jittra P, Anthony JSW, Prakitsin S. Antimicrobial and anticancer activities of endophytic fungi from *Mitrajyna javanica* Koord and Val. African Journal of Microbiology Research. 2013;**7**(49):5565-5572. DOI: 10.5897/AJMR12.2352

[35] Ainsworth GC, Sparrow FK, Sussman AS. The Fungi: An Advanced Treatise. Vol. 4A. New York, USA: Academic Press; 1973

[36] Ellis MB. More Dematiaceous Hyphomycetes. Kew, Surrey, England: Common Wealth Mycological Institute; 1976

[37] von Arx JA. The Genera of Fungi Sporulating in Pure Culture. Vaduz, Liechtenstein: A.R. Gantner Verlag KG; 1978

[38] Barnett HL, Hunter BB. Illustrated Genera of Imperfect Fungi. 4th ed. St. Paul, MN: APS Press; 1998

[39] Rogers SO, Bendich AJ. Extraction of total cellular DNA from plants, algae and fungi. Plant Molecular Biology Manual. 1994;**D1**:1-8

[40] Michelakis ED, Webster L, Mackey JR. Dichloroacetate (DCA) as a potential metabolic-targeting therapy for cancer. British Journal of Cancer. 2008;**99**(7):989-994. DOI: 0.1038/sj.bjc.6604554

[41] Tu J-T, Sun H-X, Ye Y-P. Immunomodulatory and antitumour activity of triterpenoid fractions from the rhizomes of *Astilbe chinensis*. Journal of Ethnopharmacology. 2008;**119**:266-271

[42] Owen NL, Hundley N. Endophytes—The chemical synthesizers inside plants. Science Progress. 2004;**87**:79-99

[43] Tan RX, Zou WX. Endophytes: A rich source of functional metabolites. Natural Product Reports. 2001;**18**:448-459

[44] Tejesvi MV, Mahesh B, Nalini MS, Prakash HS, Kini KR, Subbiah V, Shetty HS. Endophytic fungal assemblages from inner bark and twig of *Terminalia arjuna* W. and A. (Combretaceae). World Journal of Microbiology and Biotechnology. 2005;**21**:1535-1540

[45] Sanjana K, Suruchi G, Maroof A, Manoj KD. Endophytic fungi from medicinal plants: A treasure hunt for bioactive metabolites. Phytochemistry Reviews. 2012. DOI: 10.1007/s11101-012-9260-6

[46] Cremasco MA, Hritzko BJ, Linda Wang NH. Experimental purification of paclitaxel from a complex mixture of taxanes using a simulated moving bed. Brazilian Journal of Chemical Engineering. 2009;**26**(1):207-218

[47] Lee JC, Strobel GA, Lobkovsky E, Clardy J. Torreyanic acid: A selectively cytotoxic quinone dimer from the endophytic fungus *Pestalotiopsis microspora*. Journal of Organic Chemistry. 1996;**61**(10):3232-3233

[48] Puri SC, Verma V, Amna T, Qazi GN, Spiteller M. An endophytic fungus from *Nothapodytes foetida* that produces camptothecin. Journal of Natural Products. 2005;**68**:1717-1719

[49] Kour AS, Shawl S, Rehman S, Sultan P, Qazi PH, Suden P, Khajuria RK, Verma V. Isolation and identification of an endophytic strain of *Fusarium oxysporum* producing podophyllotoxin from *Juniperus recurva*. World Journal of Microbiology and Biotechnology. 2008;**24**:1115-1121

[50] Kusari S, Lamshoft M, Spiteller M. *Aspergillus fumigates* Fresenius, an endophytic fungus from *Juniperus communis* L. Horstmann as a novel source of the anticancer pro-drug deoxypodophyllotoxin. Journal of Applied Microbiology. 2009;**107**(3):1019-1030

[51] Deshmukh SK, Mishra PD, Kulkarni-Almeida A, et al. Anti-inflammatory and anticancer activity of ergoflavin isolated from an endophytic fungus. Chemistry & Biodiversity. 2009;**6**(5):784-789

[52] Zhang JY, Tao LY, Liang YJ, et al. Secalonic acid D induced leukemia cell apoptosis and cell cycle arrest of G1 with involvement of GSK-3b/b-catenin/c-Myc pathway. Cell Cycle. 2009;**8**(15):2444-2450

[53] Wagenaar MM, Corwin J, Strobel G, Clardy J. Three new cytochalasins produced by an endophytic fungus in the genus Rhinocladiella. Journal of Natural Products. 2000;**63**(12):1692-1695

[54] Ding G, Song YC, Chen JR, Xu C, Ge HM, Wang XT, Tan RX. Chaetoglobosin U, a cytochalasin alkaloid from endophytic *Chaetomium globosum* IFB-E019. Journal of Natural Products. 2006;**69**(2):302-304

[55] Chen Y, Guo H, Du Z, Liu XZ, Che Y, Ye X. Ecology-based screen identifies new metabolites from a Cordyceps-colonizing fungus as cancer cell proliferation inhibitors and apoptosis inducers. Cell Proliferation. 2009;**42**:838-884

[56] Yang X, Zhang L, Guo B, Guo S. Preliminary study of vincristine-producing endophytic fungus isolated from leaves of *Catharanthus roseus*. Chinese Traditional and Herbal Drugs. 2004;**35**:79-81

[57] Aly AH, Debbab A, Kjer J, Proksch P. Fungal endophytes from higher plants: A prolific source of phytochemicals and other bioactive natural products. Fungal Diversity. 2010;**41**:1-6

[58] Bara R, Aly AH, Pretsch A, Wray V, Wang BG, Proksch P, Debbab A. Antibiotically active metabolites from *Talaromyces wortmannii*, an endophyte of Aloe vera. The Journal of Antibiotics. 2013;**66**(8):491-493. DOI: 10.1038/ja.2013.28

[59] Bara R, Aly AH, Wray V, Lin WH, Proksch P, Debbab A. Talaromins A and B, new cyclic peptides from the endophytic fungus *Talaromyces wortmannii*. Tetrahedron Letters. 2013;**54**:1686-1689

[60] Colegate SM, Molyneux RJ. Bioactive Natural Products: Detection, Isolation and Structure Determination. Boca Raton, FL, USA: CRC Press; 2008. pp. 421-437

[61] Dias DA, Urban S, Roessner U. A historical overview of natural products in drug discovery. Metabolites. 2012;**2**:303-336

[62] Zhao J, Zhou L, Wang J, Shan T, Zhong L , Liu X, Gao X. A. Mendez Vilas (Ed). Endophytic fungi for producing bioactive compounds originally from their host plants. 2010. Current Research Technology and Education Topics in Applied Microbiology and Microbial Biotechnology, pp. 567-576

Section 4

Phytotherapy and Modern Formulations for Treatment of Skin Cancer

Chapter 8

Flavonoids: Promising Natural Products for Treatment of Skin Cancer (Melanoma)

Raimundo Gonçalves de Oliveira Júnior,
Christiane Adrielly Alves Ferraz,
Mariana Gama e Silva, Érica Martins de Lavor,
Larissa Araújo Rolim, Julianeli Tolentino de Lima,
Audrey Fleury, Laurent Picot,
Jullyana de Souza Siqueira Quintans,
Lucindo José Quintans Júnior and
Jackson Roberto Guedes da Silva Almeida

Additional information is available at the end of the chapter

http://dx.doi.org/10.5772/67573

Abstract

Melanoma, which is the most malignant skin cancer type, has got one of the fastest increasing incidence rates of all cancer types in the world. When belatedly diagnosed, melanoma is extremely invasive and metastatic. Although there are effective drugs used to treat melanoma, some cell lines have proven resistant to chemotherapy. In this context, several research groups on natural products have investigated the anticancer effect of new natural molecules in the treatment of melanoma. Flavonoids have shown to play an important role in chemoprevention and inhibition of the proliferation, migration, and invasion of melanoma cells. In this chapter, we present a systematic review performed through a literature search over a period of 20 years, using specialized databases. Analysis of all selected manuscripts demonstrated that at least 97 flavonoids have already been investigated for the treatment of melanoma using *in vitro* or *in vivo* models. Most of the bioactive flavonoids belong to the classes of flavones (38.0%), flavonols (17.5%), or isoflavonoids (17.5%). Apigenin, diosmin, fisetin, luteolin, and quercetin were considered as the most studied flavonoids for melanoma treatment. In general, flavonoids have shown to be a promising source of molecules with great potential for the treatment of melanoma.

Keywords: cancer, melanoma treatment, herbal medicines, medicinal plants, flavonoids

---

1. Introduction

Natural products have contributed significantly to new drugs discovery. Historically, natural products derived from plants, microorganisms, and animals have been a promising source of medicinal preparations and molecules with therapeutic potential, for various diseases, including cancer treatment. The study of natural products also contributed to the provision of unique chemical structures, which were chemically modified, resulting in the development of new drugs [1–3].

An analysis of the new medicines approved by the US Food and Drug Administration (FDA) between 1981 and 2010 revealed that 34% of those drugs were based on small molecules from natural compounds or derivatives of natural compounds (semisynthetic products). This includes drugs such as statins, tubulin-binding anticancer, and immunosuppressant drugs. In this context, it is evident the contribution of natural products for drug discovery [3–5].

In the search for new anticancer drugs, natural products have provided many structural models with different mechanisms of action, for the treatment of melanoma regional or distant metastatic melanoma. Vinblastine from *Vinca rosea* and paclitaxel, which originates from a Chinese plant, is an example of anticancer agent obtained from natural sources. The therapy also includes drugs with different mechanisms of action, such as immunomodulatory agents, BRAF, and MEK inhibitors, and most recently, use of vaccines [6, 7]. However, even with recent advances in anticancer therapy, there is still a demand to develop new effective anticancer drugs for the melanoma treatment [8].

Despite the diversity of treatments for melanoma, the high resistance of tumor cells to conventional therapies drives the search for new anticancer agents that have less toxic effects, and greater effectiveness, incentive to develop new therapies that can be used individually or in combination with other drugs bringing therapeutic benefits for the patient. The polyphenolic compounds like flavonoids possess a large spectrum of pharmacological activity, including anticancer activity. These secondary metabolites have molecular mechanisms of action in tumor cells already understood, acting in enzymes and receptors associated and signal transduction pathways relating to cellular proliferation, differentiation, apoptosis, inflammation, angiogenesis, and metastasis [9–11].

2. Pathological aspects of skin cancer (melanoma)

2.1. Definition

Melanomas are malignant skin tumors deriving from melanocytes, the melanin-producing cells, that typically occur in the skin but may rarely occur in mucous membranes (vulva, vagina, and rectum), or uvea, the pigmented layer of the eye, lying beneath the sclera and cornea, and comprising the iris, choroid, and ciliary body. Melanomas account for less than 2% of skin cancers but are responsible for 80% of the mortality of patients with skin cancer [12]. They are classified in several subtypes, according to their tissue origin, tumor form, spreading and infiltrating behavior, metastatic potential, etc. These includes (a) superficial spreading melanoma, that tend to start growing outwards rather than downwards into the skin, (b) nodular melanoma, that tends to grow downwards, deeper into the skin, (c) lentigo maligna melanoma, that develops from very slow growing pigmented areas of skin called lentigo maligna or Hutchinson's melanotic freckle, (d) acral lentiginous melanoma, most commonly found on the palms of the hands and soles of the feet or around the big toenail, and (e) amelanotic melanoma, that usually have no, or very little color, occasionally are pink or red, or have light brown or gray around the edges [13].

2.2. Etiology

The precise etiology of melanoma depends on several individual factors and is probably multifactorial in most cases [12]. Sun exposure (particularly UVB radiation) and genetic susceptibility (including faulty DNA repair) have been reported as major environmental and genetic factors associated with the risk of melanoma initiation and promotion [14, 15]. Precursor lesions, particularly dysplastic nevi/atypical moles, probably play a critical role in melanoma initiation [16]. Moreover, the distribution of melanoma among various work forces suggests that occupational risk factors could play an important role in the etiology of this cancer. For example, melanoma incidence is significantly higher in populations working in printing and press, petrochemical, and telecommunications industries [17].

2.3. Progression

The development of a melanoma tumor is considered a multistage process that involves various genetic and epigenetic alterations. From a histopathological point of view, the following steps can be considered: (a) common acquired nevi and dysplastic nevi, (b) radial growth phase melanoma, in which melanocytes undergo changes that enable them to survive and proliferate (c) vertical growth phase melanoma, in which tumor cells deeply invade into the dermis/hypodermis, and (d) malignant metastatic melanoma, in which the cells may eventually invade the endothelium and migrate to distant tissues [18–20]. When diagnosed in the early stages, melanoma can be easily treated by surgical excision of the primary tumor [21]. However, when the disease is at an advanced stage the treatment is very difficult because the cancer cells have a high capacity to cause metastases (including brain metastases) and acquire resistance to conventional therapy [22, 23]. The progression of cutaneous melanoma in the skin can be classified using the Clark method [18, 19] (**Figure 1**).

This classification is not very used, contrary to the TNM one, which is regularly revised by the American Joint Committee on Cancer (AJCC) [24, 25]. The TNM classification is based on the thickness of the primary tumor (T, also known as Breslow's index), presence of metastatic cells in the neighboring lymph nodes (N), and localization of metastasis in the body (M) (**Table 1**). The T criterion is subdivided into four categories from T1 to T4 discriminating melanomas from 1 –4 mm thick. Each category is subdivided into two subgroups that report the presence (a) or not (b) of ulceration of the primary tumor. The survival rate decreases with an increase in

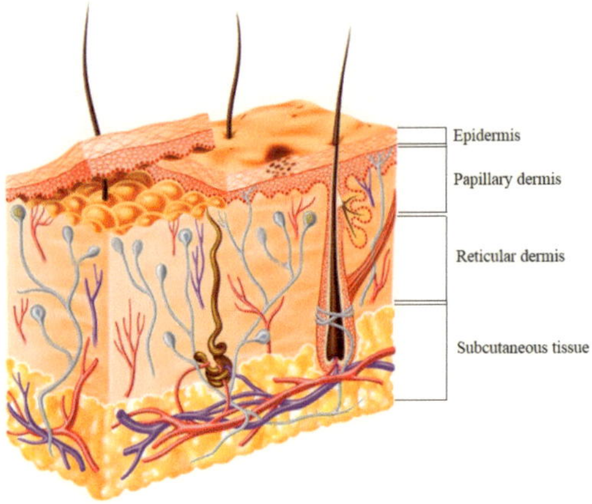

Stages and description

I. Melanoma is found exclusively in epidermidis

II. Melanoma penetrates the upper part of the dermis (papillary dermis)

III. Melanoma penetrates to the junction of papillary dermis with the reticular dermis

IV. Melanoma penetrates the reticular dermis

V. Melanoma penetrates the subcutaneous tissue

Figure 1. Progression stages of the cutaneous melanoma, according to the Clark skin infiltration classification [18, 19].

T classification	**Tumor thickness**	**Ulceration-mitosis**
T1	≤1.0 mm	a. Without ulceration and mitosis < 1/mm^2 b. With ulceration or mitosis ≥ 1/mm^2
T2	1.01–2.0 mm	a. Without ulceration b. With ulceration
T3	2.01–4.0 mm	a. Without ulceration b. With ulceration
T4	>4.0 mm	a. Without ulceration b. With ulceration
N classification	**Metastatic lymph nodes**	**Size of metastatic lymph nodes**
N0	0	–
N1	1	a. Micrometastasis b. Macrometastasis
N2	2–3	a. Micrometastasis b. Macrometastasis c. In transit without metastatic nodule
N3	≥4	–
M classification	**Site**	**Seric LDH**
M0	0	–
M1a	Subcutaneous tissue and/or metastatic lymph nodes	Normal
M1b	Lung metastasis viscera metastasis	Normal
M1c	Distant metastasis	High

Table 1. The TNM classification of melanoma progression (adapted from Ref. [26]).

the thickness of the tumor, which may, however, be smaller in the presence of ulceration. The classification N evaluates the number of neighboring lymph nodes containing metastatic melanoma cells. This criterion is subdivided into four categories from N0 to N3, as well as three subgroups according to the presence of small metastases detected after biopsy (a), large metastasis detected after clinical examination (b) and metastases in transit (c) (melanoma cells located between the primary tumor and the lymph node region in lymph channels). The classification M, with four categories from M0 to M1c, evaluates the localization of metastases in the organism, as well as the increase in serum lactate dehydrogenase concentration [24].

According to the TNM parameters, four melanoma progression stages can be defined (**Table 2**).

The only efficient treatment is the early surgical resection of the primary melanoma, when tumor cells have not already spread to nearby lymph nodes (stages I and II). Advanced and metastatic melanoma (stages III and IV) has very poor prognosis as most chemotherapeutical agents used to treat cancers are ineffective in killing melanoma cells, which are constitutively or adaptively resistant to proapoptotic drugs [22]. Melanoma is also resistant to radiotherapy [27, 28]. The overall positive responses to melanoma monotherapy using conventional anticancer drugs are weak and range from 4 to 26% [22]. Additionally, melanoma tumor displays pronounced neoangiogenesis [29] and a high ability to escape immune cell that explain why the 5-year survival rate for metastatic melanoma ranges from 5 to 10%, with a median survival of less than 8 months [30, 31]. Brain metastasis is present in 75% of stage IV melanoma patients, and constitutes a major cause of mortality because of the low permeability of the blood-brain barrier to chemotherapeutic drugs [30].

2.4. Epidemiology

Since 2005, World Health Organization (WHO) has identified the cutaneous melanoma as a priority public health concern as 132,000 new cases are registered every year in the world [32]. Since the early 1970s, the incidence of malignant melanoma has increased significantly, for example an average 4% every year in the United States [12, 14, 33]. The melanoma death rate in

Stage		T	N	M
I	IA	T1a	N0	M0
	IB	T1b-T2a	N0	M0
II	IIa	T2b/T3a	N0	M0
	IIb	T3b-T4a	N0	M0
	IIc	T4b	N0	M0
III	IIIa	T1 to T4b	N1a-N2a	M0
	IIIb	T1 to T4a	N1b-N2b-N2c	M0
	IIIc	T1 to T4b	N3	M0
IV	-	T1 to T4b	N1 to N3	M1

Table 2. Melanoma progression stages based on the TNM classification (adapted from Ref. [26]).

2012 was the highest in Australia and New Zealand (3.5/100,000) and Europe (2.3 per 100,000 people). In 2014, 76,100 new cases were diagnosed in the United States and 9710 patients with cutaneous melanoma died, according to the American Cancer Society. The wide disparity in melanoma incidence throughout the world depends upon the variation of early sun-exposure behaviors, recreational and vacation histories, nevus phenotypes and skin phototypes, distribution of melanoma risk genotypes, and discrepancies in epidemiological registrations between countries [34]. According to the WHO, a large number of atypical nevi (moles) are the strongest risk factor for malignant melanoma in fair-skinned populations. Malignant melanoma is more common among people with a pale complexion, blue eyes, and red or fair hair. It is over 20 times more frequent in White people compared to African-Americans and the risk increases with the age, although it also affects young adults, especially women. High, intermittent exposure to solar UV appears to be a significant risk factor for the development of malignant melanoma [14, 35], particularly for White people living in tropical regions [36, 37]. The incidence of malignant melanoma in White populations generally increases with decreasing latitude, with the highest recorded incidence occurring in Australia, where the annual rates are 10 and over 20 times the rates in Europe for women and men, respectively. Several epidemiological studies support a positive association with history of sunburn, particularly sunburn at an early age [34]. The role of cumulative sun exposure in the development of malignant melanoma is equivocal. However, malignant melanoma risk is higher in people with a history of nonmelanoma skin cancers and solar keratoses, both of which are indicators of cumulative UV exposure [38].

2.5. Immunity and immunotherapy of melanomas

Activation of genes in transformed melanocytes leads to the expression or overexpression of tumour-associated antigens. Several melanoma-associated antigens (MAA) have been identified and classified according to their tissue expression and structure [39, 40]. These include proteic antigens that can be recognized as MHC-I—peptide complexes by cytolytic T lymphocytes, membrane gangliosides, and conformational antigens inducing strong humoral responses by B-lymphocytes. MAGE-1, −2, −3 and −4 antigens are expressed by metastatic melanoma while their expression is absent in melanocytes and weak in primary melanoma tumors, indicating that the corresponding genes are activated during malignant transformation and progression [41]. Other MAA such as Melan-A/melanoma antigen recognized by T-cells (MART-1), tyrosinase, Pme117/gp100, gp75/tyrosine-related protein (TRP)-1 and AIM-2 are expressed in normally differentiated melanocytes and melanoma cells but absent in other tumor cells, suggesting the possibility to target them for a specific destruction of melanoma tumors [42, 43]. The expression of various gangliosides present in the membranes of melanocytes and melanoma cells (GM3, GD3, GM2, GD2 and *O*-acetyl GD3) is also significantly increased during malignant transformation [44]. Given that malignant melanoma is one of the most immunogenic tumor and that melanomas are highly resistant to chemotherapy and radiotherapy, immunotherapy appears as one of the most promising and relevant strategies to destroy melanoma tumors and metastatic cells.

Promising results have been reported using *ex-vivo* stimulation of tumor-infiltrating lymphocytes by cytokines and MAA, potentiation of T-cell cytotoxic activity by blocking CTL-A4

http://dx.doi.org/10.5772/67573

co-inhibitory receptor (using monoclonal antibodies), CAR-T strategies, and combination of immunotherapy with chemotherapeutics (e.g., dacarbazine/CTL-A4 blockade) [22, 31, 45–49]. Interferon-α and interleukin-2 monotherapeutic treatments give an overall positive response in 13–25% patients, and constitute a first-line therapy for nonmetastatic patients. Ipilimumab, an anti-CTLA-4 monoclonal antibody, targeting a T-cell receptor decreasing T-cell activation and cytotoxicity, allows a long-term survival benefit in one-third of metastatic melanoma patients, and a complete remission in patients [50]. As a consequence, a high research effort is dedicated to the development of new antibodies activating antitumoral immunity and to the discovery of new natural drugs with cytostatic, antimetastatic, and/or antiangiogenic activity that could stimulate the immune system and be used in chemoimmunotherapy protocols to synergize with chemotherapeutic drugs and immune effectors.

In this view, only a few natural molecules have proved their efficacy to limit tumor growth and inhibit the invasiveness of highly aggressive melanoma cells in *in vitro* and *in vivo* models. The efficacy of such molecules is related to their antiangiogenic activity (e.g., resveratrol [51], curcumin [52]), to their capacity to induce melanoma cell death regardless of their apoptosis-sensitivity (e.g., narciclasine [53], carotenoids [54–59]), to their ability to target components of apoptotic pathways to overcome melanoma cells resistance to anticancer drugs (e.g., epigallocatechin gallate [60–62]), or to their strong stimulatory effect on antitumoral immunity (e.g. *Lentinula edodes* polysaccharides [63]). Considering the clinical efficacy of melanoma immunotherapy, combined to the high potential of natural compounds to limit melanoma growth and restore melanoma sensitivity to apoptosis inducers without impairing antitumoral immunity, an important research effort should be undertaken to assess the efficacy of original natural cytostatic compounds, highlight the molecular and cellular mechanisms involved in their pharmacological action, and study if these molecules favor *in vivo* melanoma rejection via their immune regulatory properties. Considering the fast growth of melanoma and failure of current treatments, the identification and clinical development of such efficient molecules will obviously have a significant impact on patient survival rate and duration.

3. Molecular and cellular pathways involved in melanoma biogenesis and progression

3.1. Implication of the MAPK pathway

The receptor tyrosine kinase MAPK pathway triggers a signaling cascade that regulates cell growth, proliferation, differentiation, and survival in response to a wide variety of extracellular stimuli including hormones, cytokines, and growth factors through the activation of tyrosine kinase receptors. As mutations of components of the MAPK pathway are associated with increased activity of ERK1/2 proteins [64], deregulation of this pathway contribute to both development and progression of melanoma. In particular, mutations in B-RAF, a member of the RAF kinase family, have been identified in up to 70% of malignant melanoma [65].

Binding of a ligand to the membrane bound tyrosine kinases receptors (RTKs) or integrins adhesion to extracellular matrix triggers the activation of the RAS GTPases which further lead to activation/transduction of the MAPK signaling pathway. Ras GTPases are small proteins bound to the cytoplasmic membrane. The RAS gene encodes three isoforms with tissue-specific pattern: HRAS, KRAS, and NRAS [64]. Downstream targets of RAS proteins are the PI3K/Akt pathway and the serine threonine kinase RAF proteins [66, 67]. Activated B-RAF then leads to the activation of the MEK/ERKs kinases, which targets a variety of signaling pathways such as cell growth, proliferation, protein synthesis, and apoptosis.

The RAF kinase family consists of three cytoplasmic proteins (A-RAF, B-RAF, and C-RAF) which participate in the MAPK transduction pathway. Unlike, c-RAF and A-RAF, mutations in B-RAF have been identified in up to 70% of malignant melanoma [68, 65]. Most frequent activating somatic mutations in B-RAF occur at the V599E where a valine replaces a glutamic acid [68]. Identification of such activating mutations in B-RAF proteins leads to the development of new drugs, such as B-RAF inhibitors, as anticancer strategies [69].

These oncogenic B-RAF proteins are able to transform fibroblastic cell line and lead to hyperactivation of the ERK proteins [68]. Constitutive ERK leads to increased proliferation apoptosis resistance in melanoma cells [69]. Interestingly, suppression of the tumor suppressor PTEN and activating mutations in B-RAF are both necessary in melanoma development highlighting the importance of the PI3K/Akt pathway upregulation in melanoma growth and apoptosis resistance [70].

Indeed, the tumor suppressor PTEN is downregulated in melanoma and this is associated with PI3K/Akt hyperactivation [71]. Apoptosis resistance could be mediated through activation of the NF-KB pathway, target of hyperactive ERK proteins [72]. Oncogenic B-RAF also leads to inhibition of the LKB1-AMPK pathway, a central signaling pathway at a crossroad between metabolism and proliferation regulation through, in particular, inhibition of the mTOR pathway. This study highlights a new pathway in tumor growth regulation [73]. Finally, expression of MCL-1, a member of the Bcl-2 pathway, whose alternative splicing leads to proteins with either pro- and antiapoptotic activities, is increased in melanoma metastasis associated with oncogenic B-RAF [74]. Oncogenic B-RAF may also trigger the antiapoptosis pathway through inhibition of the proapoptotic Bim proteins [75].

Besides, downregulation of a downstream target of the MAPK pathway, MITF (microphthalmia-associated transcription factor), the master regulator of melanocyte development, survival, and function, is associated with poor diagnosis and melanoma progression [76]. Finally, cKIT, a tyrosine kinase receptor, might trigger proliferation signals in melanoma through activation of the MAPK pathway [77].

Others signaling pathways contribute to melanoma progression and metastasis such as the noncanonical Wnt signaling [78] and deregulation of the cyclin-dependent kinase inhibitor 2A (CDKN2A) pathway involved proliferation and apoptosis control [23].

3.2. Implication of extracellular vesicles (EV) in melanoma biogenesis and progression

Extracellular vesicles (EVs) are small vesicles released by most cell types in the extracellular environment, and as a consequence can be retrieved from various body fluids, especially plasma. EV might split into apoptotic bodies (>1 μm), microparticles (100 nm to 1 μm) released after membrane blebbing and exosomes (<100 nm), vesicles with an endosomal origin release after multivesicular bodies fuse with the plasma membrane [79]. EVs are biological vectors that convey lipids, different classes of proteins (cytoskeleton, adhesion, raft associated proteins, histones, chaperones [80], glycoproteins, and chemokines [81] or even morphogens such as Hedgehog proteins [82]. EVs also harbor nucleic acids [83] able to modulate the differentiation of the target cells [84]. EVs communicate with their target cells via receptor-ligand interaction, through transfer of membrane proteins [85, 86], can fuse with the plasma membrane [87], or transfer their components into target cells via phagocytosis [88] or endocytosis [89]. The ability of EVs released from antigen presenting cells to convey MHC class II proteins [90] highlights their immunomodulatory properties and their potential as therapeutic agents in anticancer strategies [91]. Moreover, as they carry tumor antigens via MCH class I proteins, EVs can initiate antitumor response *in vitro* [92] and *in vivo* [93]. Nevertheless, the composition of EVs and the message they convey depend both on the cells they originate from and the conditions triggering their release. Indeed, EVs from dendritic cells can also suppress immune response in inflammatory diseases models such as DTH (delayed-type hypersensitivity) mice [94]. This ability to attenuate immune response might be associated with the capacity of EV to induce expression of molecules able to inactivate T-cells or suppress immune response [95].

In addition to their immunomodulatory properties, the role of EVs in inflammation, angiogenesis, and proliferation has been widely demonstrated [96–98]. This suggests an implication for EVs in tumor survival and progression. In this study, exosomal markers, such as CD63, could be found also on a wide range of subpopulations of EVs, and as long as there is no determination of the cellular origin of vesicles, we chose to use the term EV to refer to both exosomes and microparticles.

3.3. Role of circulating EV in melanoma biogenesis and progression

Circulating EV can trigger inflammatory pathways in target cells [96], stimulate angiogenesis [82, 99, 100], protect against apoptosis [101], or stimulate proliferation [102].

Plasma levels of EV harboring CD63 in melanoma-engrafted SCID mice correlate to tumor size, suggesting a role of the tumor in EV secretion [103]. However, other suggests that circulating rates of EV do not differ between melanoma and healthy patients [104–106] but instead, EV protein composition might differ. In particular, plasmatic EVs from melanoma patients are enriched in platelet-derived EV involved in neovascularization (CD42a harboring EV) and antitumour immune responses (CD8 harboring EV) [105]. Furthermore, circulating endothelial and platelet derived-EV (EEV) and procoagulant EV are significantly higher in melanoma patients [107]. Such procoagulant EVs stimulate proinflammatory cytokines secretion by macrophages and drive melanoma metastasis *in vivo* [108] reinforcing the implication of EV in melanoma progression.

3.4. A role of EV in melanoma metastasis

EV release is exacerbated in human malignant [109] and murine [110] melanoma cell lines. Furthermore, in comparison with murine melanocyte cell line, metastastic melanoma cell lines secrete highly procoagulant EV harboring phosphatidylserine and enriched in tissue factor proteins suggesting that melanocyte transformation into cancer cells is associated with the secretion of such EVs [110]. Besides, Wnt5a, a noncanonical Wnt signaling ligand in involved melanoma progression [78] induces the release of melanoma exosomes enriched in proangiogenic proteins and pro-inflammatory cytokines [111].

Proteomic analysis of human malignant melanoma cell lines A375 reveals an enrichment in proteins involved in angiogenesis and matrix remodeling such as annexin A1 and hyaluronan and proteoglycan link protein 1 (HAPLN1) [109]. Analysis of EV microRNA content reveals enrichment in miRNA involved in cell growth, proliferation, and apoptosis. Uptake of such EV promotes the invasion ability of normal melanocytes [109]. Furthermore, tumor-derived EV harbor FAS ligand involved in antitumor response through lymphocytes apoptosis [112]. Finally, human (SK-Mel28/-202/-265/-35) and mouse (B16-F10) cell line–derived exosomes are enriched in TYRP2 (tyrosinase-related protein-2), VLA-4 and Hsp90 proteins. Indeed, B16F10-derived exosomes are enriched in prooncogenic proteins such as the oncogene MET which has been described a role in cell transformation, proliferation, survival, invasion, and metastasis [113–115]. BM cell treatment with such exosomes led to an increase in tumor size compared to nontreated mice. Compared to EV derived from B16F1, a poor metastatic cell line, injection of B16F10 EV led to increased metastatic lesions and a wider tissue distribution (brain, bone) [106]. This is in agreement with previous studies suggesting that highly metastasis cells are enriched in oncogene Met72 and are more deleterious than B16F1-derived EV [116]. These data strongly suggest that EV from melanoma cells is able to suppress antitumor response and stimulate tumor progression but also their ability to trigger melanoma invasion and metastasis. However, different populations of EV have distinct procoagulant properties [117]. Thus, it is therefore necessary to identify the cell origin of EV in order to determine their role in cancer progression.

3.5. Role of microRNAs in melanoma progression

MicroRNAs are noncoding small RNAs able to bind target mRNAs, through their 3′UTRs leading to their degradation. Binding of microRNAs to their targets allows regulating a wide variety of cellular mechanisms such as proliferation, angiogenesis, inflammation, and survival.

A role for microRNAs in melanoma progression was first demonstrated through different miRNA expression signatures associated with the developmental lineage and differentiation state of solid tumors [118]. Furthermore, a microarray analysis demonstrates a specific targeting between A375 cell line and the A375 cells-derived EV of 28 miRNAs involved in cellular growth, development, and proliferation [109]. Relevance of microRNAs implication in melanoma development was illustrated by the fact that miRNAS loci are retrieved in genomic regions altered in melanoma [119]. MITF (microphthalmia-associated transcription factor) the master regulator of melanocyte development, survival, and function, which is often dysregulated in melanoma is a target of miR-137 [120] and miR-182 [121]. Finally, a number of microRNAs such as miR-214 [122] and miR-223 [123], but also miR-137, miR-182, miR-221/222, and miR-34a, have been involved in melanoma progression (for a review see [124]). In particular, miR-221 and miR-222 are involved in tumor proliferation and an increased in invasion and migration abilities through targeting of p27Kip1/CDKN1B (cyclin-dependent kinase inhibitor 1B) and the tyrosine kinase receptor c-KIT receptor [124, 125].

However, five members of the Let-7 family are downregulated in primary melanoma suggesting that these microRNAs might trigger anticancer responses. In particular, Let7b which targets cyclins exerts antitumoral responses through inhibition of cancer cycle progression [126].

http://dx.doi.org/10.5772/67573

MicroRNAs can also be transported via EV and regulate the pathway in distant target cells. In particular, circulating EV from metastatic melanoma patients harbors a specific miRNA signature. Indeed, those EVs are enriched in oncogenics miRNAs mir17 and miR19a suggesting a role for miRNAs-associated EV in tumor progression and metastasis [127]. On the other hand, circulating EV in advanced melanoma patients shows a decrease in miR-125b which downregulation has been described in melanoma progression [128].

Finally, deep-RNA sequencing allows identifying an enrichment of 23 specific microRNAs in small EV including miR-199a-3p, miR-150-5p, miR-142-3p, and miR-486-5p known to be involved in melanoma progression or identified in melanoma metastasis or patient blood samples [129]. In particular, miR-214 has been associated with melanoma metastasis [122]. Interestingly, *in silico* analysis reveals that some of these miRNAs could target the BRAF pathway which is often deregulated in melanoma [129]. Metastatic cell lines secrete EV enriched in the oncogenic miR-222. Furthermore, miR-222 associated with EV can be transferred into target cells and promote tumorigenesis through activation the Akt/PI3K pathway [130].

3.6. Identification of new markers for melanoma diagnosis and prognosis

Circulating concentrations of lactate dehydrogenase [79], S100 and MIA (Melanoma Inhibitory Activity), two small proteins expressed by melanoma cells, are significantly higher in melanoma patients [131] and thus are widely used a proteins markers in order to monitor melanoma progression. LDH concentrations might be a better prognosis factor to classify advanced melanoma [132, 133].

Other circulating factors such as circulating nucleic acids or EV could be used in melanoma detection as a prognosis factor in advanced stages of diseases. Indeed, circulating EVs from stage III to stage IV are enriched TYRP2 (tyrosinase-related protein-2), a specific melanoma protein, VLA-4 (very late antigen 4) and HSP90. Furthermore, these enriched EVs correlated with poor survival prognosis [106]. These authors identified a specific exosomes protein signature that could be used as a prognosis marker in stages III and IV melanoma patients [106].

Besides, circulating EV carries melanoma markers such as S100B and MIA proteins. Concentrations of EV-S100B and EV-MIA are higher in stage IV melanoma patients and such EV was associated to poor prognosis in patients [104]. Detection of such EV could be used as an additional diagnosis and prognosis marker of melanoma patients. In contrast, these authors did not find an increase in TYRP2 containing exosomes in plasma of melanoma patients. This discrepancy could be due to difference in EV isolation, or EV concentrations/number analysis (NTA analysis vs. EV-protein concentration determination). Finally, circulating EV enriched in oncogenes miRNAs mir17 and miR19a could be used as predictive markers in melanoma patients [127].

In addition, some microRNAs detected in patient metastasis such as miR-150, miR-342-3p, miR-455-3p, miR-145, miR-155, and miR-497 could be used as a specific signature to predict postsurvival recurrence with a high expression of miR-145, miR-155 in metastatic tissue associated with longer survival [134]. Finally, identification of a specific signature of 16 differentially expressed microRNAs in patient blood samples represents a new noninvasive tool in diagnosis applications [135]. Finally, other authors suggest that microRNAs from blood patients could be used to monitor melanoma recurrence [136, 137].

4. Current melanoma treatment

The treatment options for regional or distant metastatic melanoma have expanded in recent years and are directly influenced by disease stage at diagnosis and the extent of metastases. The therapy used includes several drugs with different mechanisms of action, including chemotherapies, immunomodulatory agents, the serine/threonine protein kinase BRAF, mitogen-activated protein kinase (MEK) inhibitors, and most recently, use of vaccines [6, 7]. The primary treatment of this cancer type is surgical excision, sentinel lymph node dissection, radical lymph node dissection, and isolated limb perfusion [138, 139].

Chemotherapy may now be considered a second or third line in patients with resistance to immunotherapy and targeted therapy [140]. Tumor cells may evade the immune attack by some mechanisms, such as impaired antigen presentation, expression of factors with immunosuppressive properties, such as transforming growth factor-beta (TGF-β), vascular endothelial growth factor (VEGF), interleukin-2 (IL-2), and induction of resistance to apoptosis. In addition, melanoma cells further express receptors on the cell surface which function as checkpoints to the immune system response, as the cytotoxic T-lymphocyte-associated protein 4 (CTLA-4) and programmed cell death protein 1 (PD-1). The ipilimumab is an anti-CTLA-4 monoclonal antibody and the nivolumab and pembrolizumab are also monoclonal antibodies directed against the PD-1 receptor, that blocking the inhibitory ligand's suppression of immune response. Thus, the main objectives of immunotherapy are to activate an immune response through the immunostimulation of IL-2, the upregulation of tumor-inhibitory T cells, and the inhibition of the immune control points [141, 142].

In addition to the immunological approach, targeted therapies have also been employed in the treatment of melanoma, such as BRAF and MEK inhibitors. The BRAF gene is responsible for encoding the B-raf protein that participates in the regulation of the mitogen-activated protein kinase/extracellular signal-regulated kinase (MAPK/ERK) signaling pathway, which regulates cell proliferation, differentiation, and cell cycle progression [142]. The discovery that BRAF was mutated in about 50% of melanomas led to the development of BRAF kinase inhibitors as vemurafenib and dabrafenib. However, most patients acquire resistance mechanisms to BRAF kinase inhibition [141, 143]. In view of the development of resistance to single BRAF blockade, several combination schemes have been developed, as the combination therapy with MEK inhibitors trametinib and cobimetinib [144–146].

Despite these advances, about 80% of patients develop resistance to the current standard of treatment with the combination of a selective BRAF and MEK inhibitors, which stimulates research for new treatment alternatives. The use of triple combining therapy has also been the subject of investigations and demonstrated prolonged responses [147]. Preclinical assays performed with the triple combination of BRAF and MEK inhibitors and anti-PD-1 demonstrated high antitumor activity and phase I/II clinical studies have shown promise in BRAFV600-mutated melanoma [148]. Moreover, vaccines have also been investigated and in 2015 the Food and Drug Administration (FDA) approved the Talimogene laherparepvec (T-VEC), an oncolytic virus derived from herpes simplex type 1, which can selectively replicate within tumors and produce granulocyte macrophage colony stimulating factor (GM-CSF) which promotes increased antitumor immune response [149].

http://dx.doi.org/10.5772/67573

5. Chemical and biological aspects of flavonoids

Flavonoids are phenolic constituents commonly found in a variety of fruits, vegetables, and medicinal plants. They add color, flavor, and aroma to plants, and play an important role in protection mechanisms against pathogens, ultraviolet radiation, and herbivores. Flavonoids comprise an important class of secondary metabolites, with numerous possibilities of chemical structures [150, 151].

Flavonoids have a basic phenylbenzopyrone skeleton (C_6-C_3-C_6), admitting several substitution possibilities. In accordance with the substitution pattern of A, B, and C rings of the basic structure, flavonoids can be classified as chalcones, aurones, flavones, flavonols, flavanols, flavanones, isoflavones, flavanonols, among others [10]. The most common classes of flavonoids are shown in **Figure 2**.

Flavonoids may include the polyhydroxylated or polymethoxylated form. There are more than 8000 flavonoids identified, some of the most abundant are quercetin, catechin, and kaempferol, which are often combined with glycosidic units (commonly glucose, galactose, and rhamnose) through C-C or C-O-C bonds [152, 153]. The structural diversity of flavonoids directly influences their chemical, physical and pharmacological properties.

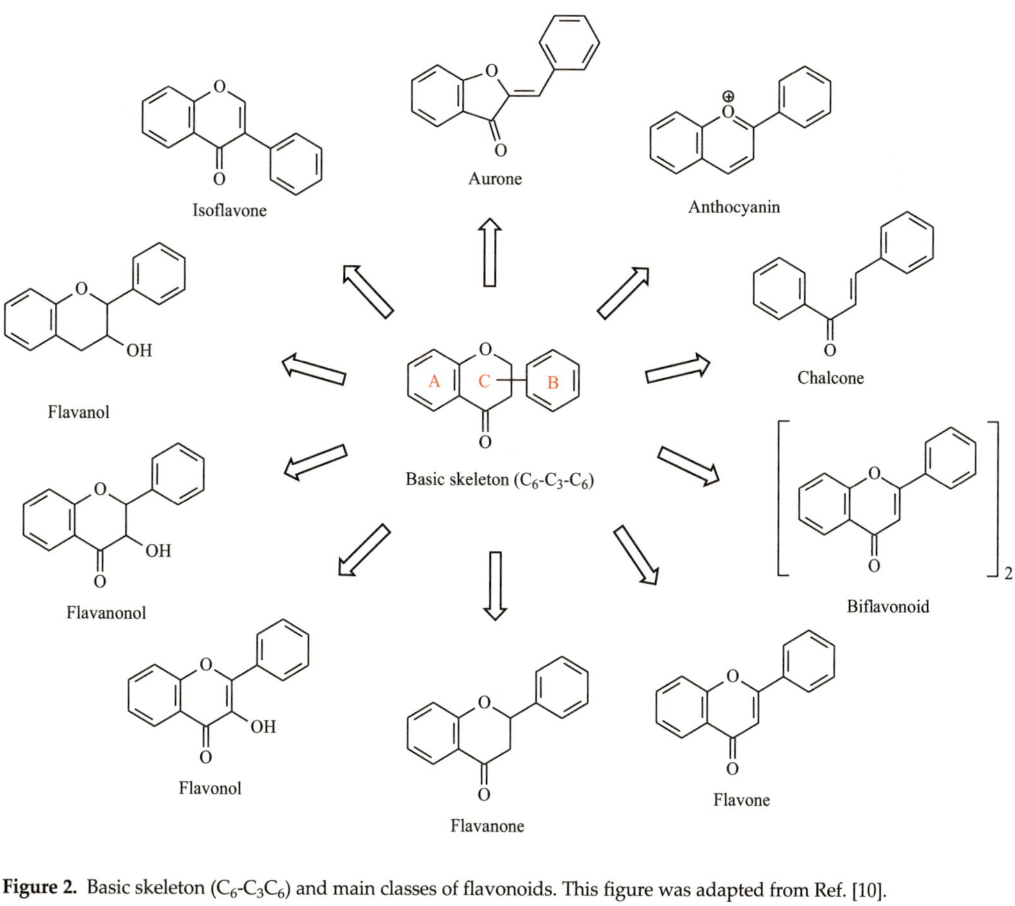

Figure 2. Basic skeleton (C_6-C_3C_6) and main classes of flavonoids. This figure was adapted from Ref. [10].

Several studies have demonstrated the therapeutic properties of flavonoids obtained from plants or through synthesis. In fact, the structural diversity of flavonoids contributes to the diverse pharmacological activities reported for these compounds. *In vitro* and *in vivo* assays have shown the antioxidant, anti-inflammatory, antinociceptive, cardioprotective, photoprotective, antidepressant, antimicrobial, and cytotoxic effects of flavonoids [154, 155].

Recently, flavonoids have been shown to be potent antitumor agents. These compounds showed promising effect against different tumor cell lines, including human melanoma cells [156, 157]. In addition, flavonoids typically exhibit low toxicity in biological systems, which make them an alternative therapy compared with traditional anticancer drugs [158–161].

6. Bioactivity of flavonoids on melanoma

In this section, the authors present a systematic review performed through a literature search over a period of 20 years (January 1996–December 2016). This literature search was performed through specialized databases (PUBMED, LILACS, SCIELO, Science Direct, and Web of Science) using different combinations of the following keywords: flavonoid, flavonoid derivative, melanoma, skin cancer, treatment, and anticancer therapy. We did not contact investigators and we did not attempt to identify unpublished data.

Manuscripts were selected based on the inclusion criteria: articles published in English, Portuguese, Spanish, or French and articles with keywords in the title, abstract, or keywords, as well as studies involving anticancer activity of natural flavonoids necessarily against melanoma in *in vitro* or *in vivo* models. Other review articles, meta-analysis, abstracts, conferences, editorial/letters, case reports, conference proceedings, or articles that did not meet the inclusion criteria were excluded from this systematic review.

For the selection of the manuscripts, two independent investigators (RGOJ and CAAF) first selected the articles according to the title, then to the abstract, and finally through an analysis of the full-text publication. A consensus between the investigators was reached as a clarification for in order to clarify all disagreements. The selected articles were manually reviewed with the purpose of identifying and excluding the works that did not fit the criteria described above.

The primary search identified 164 articles. However, among these, 39 manuscripts were indexed in two or more databases and were considered only once, resulting in 125 articles. After an initial screening of titles, abstracts, full text, and time of publication, 43 articles were selected, while the remainder did not meet the inclusion criteria (n = 82). Although many articles presented promising anticancer activity for plant extracts rich in flavonoids, we considered only articles that showed anticancer activity of the isolated flavonoids on melanoma cell lines. Investigations involving synthetic flavonoids were also excluded from this review. A flowchart illustrating the progressive study selection and numbers at each stage is shown in **Figure 3**.

Analysis of all selected manuscripts demonstrated that at least 97 flavonoids have already been investigated for the treatment of melanoma using *in vitro* or *in vivo* models. Most of the bioactive flavonoids belong to the classes of flavones (38%), flavonols (17.5%), or isoflavonoids

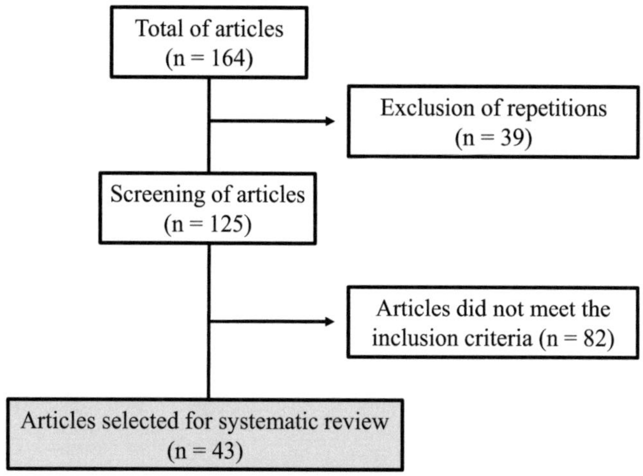

Figure 3. Flowchart of included studies for the systematic review.

(17.5%), which has aroused the interest of several research groups in natural and synthetic products in the world. All information about these flavonoids for the treatment of melanoma was reported in **Box 1**. Next, we highlight the anticancer properties of the main tested flavonoids on melanoma cells (apigenin, diosmin, fisetin, luteolin, and quercetin).

6.1. Bioactivity of apigenin on melanoma

Apigenin (4′,5,7,-trihydroxyflavone) is a nonmutagenic and low-toxicity dietary flavonoid commonly present in many fruits, vegetables, and medicinal plants. This flavone has a broad spectrum of antiproliferative activities against many types of cancer cells, including melanoma. Recent studies have demonstrated that apigenin inhibits cell growth through cell cycle arrest and apoptosis in malignant human melanoma cell lines. Hasnat et al. [169] showed that treatment with 50 μM apigenin significantly reduced viable cell percentages in A375 and A2058 human melanoma cells. Treatment with apigenin for 24 h also decreased human melanoma cell numbers in a dose-dependent manner. A similar result was observed by Spoerlein et al. [170], who evaluated the cytotoxic potential and the effect of apigenin on the cell cycle of 518A2 human melanoma cells. Apigenin also caused a dose-dependent decrease in the percentage of transwell-migrated cells, and ~90 and ~70% inhibitions of cell migration were recorded upon treatment with 20 μM of apigenin, respectively, for A2058 and A375 cells [169].

The cytotoxic effects of apigenin were related to its ability to reduce integrin protein levels and inhibit the phosphorylation of focal adhesion kinase (FAK) and extracellular signal-regulated kinase (ERK1/2). Furthermore, apigenin treatment increased apoptotic factors such as caspase-3 and cleaved poly(ADP-ribose) polymerase in a dose-dependent manner. Cao et al. [172] have also demonstrated that apigenin suppressed STAT3 phosphorylation, decreased STAT3 nuclear localization, and inhibited STAT3 transcriptional activity. Apigenin also downregulated STAT3 target genes MMP-2, MMP-9, VEGF, and Twist1, which are involved in cell migration and invasion. In this same investigation, it was determined the *in vivo* antimetastatic effect of

Flavonoid	Model	Cell line	Concentration or dose	Effectiveness	Possible mechanisms of action	Reference
Aurones						
2,6-Dihydroxy-2-[(4-hydroxyphenyl)methyl]-3-benzofuranone	*In vitro*	B16-BL6 (MM)	ND	Preliminary test determined $IC_{50} > 100$ μM.	NE	[162]
Anthocyanins						
Cyanidin-3-*O*-β-glucopyranoside (C-3-G)	*In vitro*	M14 (HM)	5 or 10 μM	A treatment with a single dose of C-3-G decreased cell proliferation without affecting cell viability and without inducing apoptosis or necrosis. C-3-G treatment also induced increase of cAMP levels and upregulation of tyrosinase expression and activity resulting in an enhanced melanin synthesis and melanosome maturation.	Upregulation of the melanoma differentiation antigen Melan-A/MART-1 in treated cells respect to the untreated control was recorded.	[163]
Biflavonoids						
Pteridium III	*In vitro*	A375 (HM)	ND	Preliminary test determined IC_{50} equal to 106.7 μM.	NE	[164]
Chalcones						
2′,4′-Dihydroxychalcone	*In vitro*	B16-BL6 (MM)	ND	Preliminary test determined IC_{50} equal to 44.3 μM.	NE	[162]
4,4′-Dihydroxy-2′-methoxychalcone	*In vitro*	B16-BL6 (MM)	ND	Preliminary test determined IC_{50} equal to 56.3 μM.	NE	[162]
Isoliquiritigenin (ISL)	*In vitro*	B16-BL6 (MM)	ND	Preliminary test determined IC_{50} equal to 80.5 μM.	NE	[162]
	In vitro and *in vivo* (mice)	B16F0 (MM)	5–25 μg/ml	A significant concentration- and time-dependent reduction in cell proliferation was observed. The cell inhibition rate ranged from 18 to 79% and 35 to 91% after 24 and 48 h of ISL treatment (5, 10, 15, 20, and 25 μg/mL), respectively. ISL	ISL increased reactive oxygen species (ROS) formation during B16F0 cell differentiation, but no specific target was evaluated.	[165]

Flavonoid	Model	Cell line	Concentration or dose	Effectiveness	Possible mechanisms of action	Reference
				did not show significant activity in the *in vivo* model.		
Phloretin	*In vitro*	M14 (HM)	1–40 μM	Cell viability was 31.6% in M14 cells exposed to 40 μM of this compound. Phloretin induced apoptosis in a concentration dependent manner with significant effect at 20 μM after 48 h of treatment.	NE	[166]
α,2′,4,4′-tetrahydroxydihydrochalcone	*In vitro*	B16-BL6 (MM)	ND	Preliminary test determined $IC_{50} > 100$ μM.	NE	[162]
Flavones						
5,3′,4′-Trihydroxy-6,7,5′-trimethoxyflavone	*In vitro*	B16F10 (MM)	ND	Preliminary test determined IC_{50} equal to 14 μM.	NE	[167]
5,4′-Dihydroxy-6,7,3′,5′-tetramethoxyflavone	*In vitro*	B16F10 (MM)	ND	Preliminary test determined IC_{50} equal to 241 μM.	NE	[167]
5,6,3′-Trihydroxy-7,4′-Dimethoxyflavone	*In vitro*	B16F10 (MM)	ND	Preliminary test determined IC_{50} equal to 18 μM.	NE	[167]
5,6,4′-Trihydroxy-7,3′,5′-trimethoxyflavone	*In vitro*	B16F10 (MM)	ND	Preliminary test determined IC_{50} equal to 39 μM.	NE	[167]
5,6,7-Trihydroxybaicalein	*In vitro*	B16F10 (MM)	ND	Preliminary test determined IC_{50} equal to 11 μM.	NE	[167]
5,6-Dihydroxy-7,3′,4′-trimethoxyflavone	*In vitro*	B16F10 (MM)	ND	Preliminary test determined IC_{50} equal to 29 μM.	NE	[167]
5,7-Dihydroxy-6-methoxyhispidulin	*In vitro*	B16F10 (MM)	ND	Preliminary test determined IC_{50} equal to 67 μM.	NE	[167]
5,7-Dihydroxy-7-methoxyflavone	*In vitro*	B16F10 (MM)	ND	Preliminary test determined IC_{50} equal to 119 μM.	NE	[167]
6-Hydroxyluteolin	*In vitro*	B16F10 (MM)	ND	Preliminary test determined IC_{50} equal to 13 μM.	NE	[167]
6-Methoxyflavone	*In vitro*	B16F10 (MM)	ND	Preliminary test determined IC_{50} equal to 398 μM.	NE	[167]

Flavonoid	Model	Cell line	Concentration or dose	Effectiveness	Possible mechanisms of action	Reference
6-Prenylapigenin	*In vitro*	B16 (MM)	ND	Preliminary test determined IC_{50} equal to 32.5 μM.	NE	[168]
Albanin	*In vitro*	B16 (MM)	ND	Preliminary test determined IC_{50} equal to 84.7 μM.	NE	[168]
Apigenin	*In vitro*	B16F10 (MM)	ND	Preliminary test determined IC_{50} equal to 26 μM.	NE	[167]
	In vitro	A375 and A2058 (HM)	0–50 μM	Treatment with 50 μM apigenin significantly reduced viable cell percentages in both types of melanoma cells. Apigenin exhibited dose-dependent inhibition of melanoma cell migration, unlike untreated controls.	Apigenin reduced integrin protein levels and inhibited the phosphorylation of focal adhesion kinase (FAK) and extracellular signal regulated kinase (ERK1/2). Furthermore, apigenin treatment increased apoptotic factors such as caspase-3 and cleaved poly (ADP-ribose) polymerase in a dose dependent manner.	[169]
	In vitro	518A2 (HM)	ND	Preliminary test determined $IC_{50} > 50$ μM. The flavonoid also reduced cell migration.	Apigenin induced an arrest of the cell cycle of 518A2 melanoma cells at the G2/M transition and also attenuated the expression and secretion of the metastasis relevant matrix metalloproteinases MMP-2 and MMP-9.	[170]
	In vitro	MDA-MB-435 (HM)	1–50 μM	Preliminary test determined $IC_{50} > 50$ μM.	NE	[171]
	In vitro and *in vivo* (mice)	B16F10 (MM), A375 and G361 (HM)	0–40 μM (in vitro tests) and 150 mg/kg (*in vivo* tests)	Apigenin (5 and 10 μM) also dose-dependently inhibited B16F10, A375 G361 cell migration and invasion. Apigenin-treated mice had significant fewer metastatic nodules.	Apigenin suppressed STAT3 phosphorylation, decreased STAT3 nuclear localization and inhibited STAT3 transcriptional activity. Apigenin also downregulated STAT3 target genes MMP-2, MMP-9, VEGF and Twist1, which are involved in cell migration and invasion.	[172]

Flavonoid	Model	Cell line	Concentration or dose	Effectiveness	Possible mechanisms of action	Reference
Artocarpin	*In vitro*	B16 (MM)	ND	Preliminary test determined IC_{50} equal to 10.3 μM.	NE	[168]
Baicalein	*In vitro*	B16F10 (MM)	0–200 μM	Treatment with 40 μM baicalein resulted in approximately 87% inhibition of cell growth. Baicalein also inhibited the migration and invasion of B16F10 cells.	Baicalein reduced the expression of MMPs and tightening TJ through the suppression of claudin expression, possibly in association with a suppression of the phosphoinositide 3-kinase/ Akt signaling pathway.	[173]
	In vitro	B16F10 (MM)	3.156–50 μM	Preliminary test determined IC_{50} equal to 50 μM.	NE	[174]
Brosimone I	*In vitro*	B16 (MM)	ND	Preliminary test determined IC_{50} equal to 10.7 μM.	NE	[168]
Chrysin	*In vitro*	518A2 (HM)	ND	Preliminary test determined IC_{50} > 50 μM. The flavonoid also reduced cell migration.	Apigenin induced an arrest of the cell cycle of 518A2 melanoma cells at the G2/M transition and also attenuated the expression and secretion of the metastasisrelevant matrix metalloproteinases MMP-2 and MMP-9.	[170]
	In vitro	B16BL6 (MM)	ND	Preliminary test determined IC_{50} equal to 20.5 μM.	NE	[175]
	In vitro	B16F10 (MM)	ND	Preliminary test determined IC_{50} equal to 51 μM.	NE	[167]
Cirsilineol	*In vitro*	B16F10 (MM)	ND	Preliminary test determined IC_{50} equal to 73 μM.	NE	[167]
Cirsiliol	*In vitro*	B16F10 (MM)	ND	Preliminary test determined IC_{50} equal to 9 μM.	NE	[167]
Cudraflavone B	*In vitro*	B16 (MM)	ND	Preliminary test determined IC_{50} equal to 12.5 μM.	NE	[168]
Cudraflavone C	*In vitro*	B16 (MM)	ND	Preliminary test determined IC_{50} equal to 9.2 μM.	NE	[168]

Flavonoid	Model	Cell line	Concentration or dose	Effectiveness	Possible mechanisms of action	Reference
Desmethoxylcentaureidin	*In vitro*	B16F10 (MM)	ND	Preliminary test determined IC_{50} equal to 64 μM.	NE	[167]
Diosmin	*In vivo* (mice)	B16F10 (MM)	0.2% solution (*ad libitum* as drink)	Animals treated with diosmin presented a reduction in the number of subpleural mestases in comparison to the negative control group.	NE	[176]
	In vivo (mice)	B16F10 (MM)	551 mg/kg/day Diosmin alone or combined with different doses of IFN-α	IFN-α showed a dose-dependent antiinvasive and antiproliferative activity in our study, while diosmin showed an antiinvasive activity similar to the lower dose of IFN-α used. Combination of diosmin and IFN-α have shown synergistic effect.	NE	[177]
	In vivo (mice)	B16F10 (MM)	0.2% solution (*ad libitum* as drink)	Group treated with diosmin showed the greatest reduction (52%) in the number of metastatic nodules.	NE	[178]
	In vivo (mice)	B16F10 (MM)	20 mg/day	Diosmin decreased the number of metastatic nodules (52%), implantation (79%), growth (67%) and invasion (45%) index.	NE	[179]
Eupafolin	*In vitro*	B16F10 (MM)	ND	Preliminary test determined IC_{50} equal to 16 μM.	NE	[167]
Eupatilin	*In vitro*	B16F10 (MM)	ND	Preliminary test determined IC_{50} equal to 58 μM.	NE	[167]
	In vitro	B16F10 (MM)	10^{-4}–10^{-8} M	Preliminary test determined IC_{50} from 33 to 85 μM.	NE	[180]
Eupatorin	*In vitro*	B16F10 (MM)	ND	Preliminary test determined IC_{50} equal to 44 μM.	NE	[167]
Isolinariin A	*In vitro*	C32 (HM)	ND	Preliminary test determined IC_{50} equal to 11.76 μM.	NE	[181]

Flavonoid	Model	Cell line	Concentration or dose	Effectiveness	Possible mechanisms of action	Reference
Isolinariin B	*In vitro*	C32 (HM)	ND	Preliminary test determined IC_{50} equal to 21.47 μM.	NE	[181]
Jaceosidin	*In vitro*	B16F10 (MM)	ND	Preliminary test determined IC_{50} equal to 27 μM.	NE	[167]
	In vitro	B16F10 (MM)	10^{-4} to 10^{-8} M	Preliminary test determined IC_{50} from 32 to 49 μM.	NE	[180]
Kuwanon C	*In vitro*	B16 (MM)	ND	Preliminary test determined IC_{50} equal to 14.2 μM.	NE	[168]
Linariin	*In vitro*	C32 (HM)	ND	Preliminary test determined IC_{50} equal to 12.6 μM.	NE	[181]
Luteolin	*In vitro*	B16F10 (MM)	ND	Preliminary test determined IC_{50} equal to 21 μM.	NE	[167]
	In vitro	MDA-MB-435 (HM)	1–50 μM	Preliminary test determined IC_{50} equal to 30.3 μM.	NE	[171]
	In vitro	A375 (HM)	0–80 μM	Preliminary test determined IC_{50} equal to 115.1 μM. Luteolin also inhibited colony formation and induced apoptosis in a dose and time-dependent manner by disturbing cellular integrity as evident from morphological evaluation.	Accumulation of cells in G0/G1 (60.4-72.6%) phase for A375 cells after 24 h treatment indicated cell cycle arresting potential of this flavonoid, but no specific target was investigated.	[182]
	In vitro	B16F10 (MM)	3.156–50 μM	Preliminary test determined $IC_{50} > 50$ μM.	NE	[174]
	In vitro	A2058 (HM)	0–80 μg/ml	Luteolin inhibited cell proliferation ($IC_{50} = 35$ μg/ml) and increased apoptotic body formation. Luteolin induces apoptosis by Endoplasmic Reticulum (ER) stress via increasing Reactive Oxygen Species (ROS) levels.	Luteolin increased expression of the ER stress-related proteins; protein kinase RNA-like ER kinase, phosphor eukaryotic translation initiation factor 2α, activating transcription factor (ATF) 6, CCAAT/enhancer-binding protein-homologous protein (CHOP), and cleaved caspase 12. Furthermore, luteolin	[183]

Flavonoid	Model	Cell line	Concentration or dose	Effectiveness	Possible mechanisms of action	Reference
					increased the level of intracellular ROS, leading to ROS mediated apoptosis and ER stress.	
	In vitro and *in vivo* (mice)	B16F10	5–50 μM (in vitro tests) and 10–20 mg (*in vivo* tests)	Luteolin suppressed the hypoxia-induced changes in the cells in a dose-dependent manner. In experimental metastasis model mice, treatment with luteolin reduced metastatic colonization in the lungs by 50%.	Luteolin inhibited the hypoxia-induced epithelial-mesenchymal transition in malignant melanoma cells both *in vitro* and *in vivo* via the regulation of β3 integrin.	[184]
Morin	*In vitro*	B16 (MM)	ND	Preliminary test determined IC_{50} equal to 170 μM.	NE	[168]
Norartocarpin	*In vitro*	B16 (MM)	ND	Preliminary test determined IC_{50} equal to 7.8 μM.	NE	[168]
Pectolinarigenin	*In vitro*	B16F10 (MM)	ND	Preliminary test determined IC_{50} equal to 64 μM.	NE	[167]
Pectolinarin	*In vitro*	C32 (HM)	ND	Preliminary test determined IC_{50} equal to 7.17 μM.	NE	[181]
Tangeretin	*In vivo* (mice)	B16F10 (MM)	20 mg/day	Tangeretin decreased the number of metastatic nodules, implantation, growth and invasion index.	NE	[179]
Flavanones						
3,7-Dihydroxy-6-methoxyflavanone	*In vitro*	B16-BL16 (MM)	ND	Preliminary test determined $IC_{50} > 100$ μM.	NE	[162]
3,7-Dihydroxyflavanone	*In vitro*	B16-BL16 (MM)	ND	Preliminary test determined $IC_{50} > 100$ μM.	NE	[162]
7-Hydroxy-6-methoxyflavanone	*In vitro*	B16-BL16 (MM)	ND	Preliminary test determined IC_{50} equal to 6.7 μM.	NE	[162]
7-Hydroxyflavanone	*In vitro*	B16-BL16 (MM)	ND	Preliminary test determined IC_{50} equal to 99.9 μM.	NE	[162]
Alnustinol	*In vitro*	B16-BL16 (MM)	ND	Preliminary test determined $IC_{50} > 100$ μM.	NE	[162]

Flavonoid	Model	Cell line	Concentration or dose	Effectiveness	Possible mechanisms of action	Reference
Artocarpanone	*In vitro*	B16 (MM)	ND	Preliminary test determined IC_{50} equal to 122.2 μM.	NE	[168]
Dihydrobaicalein	*In vitro*	B16-BL16 (MM)	ND	Preliminary test determined $IC_{50} > 100$ μM.	NE	[162]
Dihydrooroxylin A	*In vitro*	B16-BL16 (MM)	ND	Preliminary test determined IC_{50} equal to 72.6 μM.	NE	[162]
Eriodictyol	*In vitro*	B16F10 (MM)	3.156–50 μM	Preliminary test determined $IC_{50} > 50$ μM.	NE	[174]
Garbanzol	*In vitro*	B16-BL16 (MM)	ND	Preliminary test determined $IC_{50} > 100$ μM.	NE	[162]
Isoxanthohumol (IXN)	*In vitro*	B16 (MM) and A375 (HM)	0–100 μM	The treatment of both celllines with IXN resulted in dose-dependent decrease of cell viability (IC_{50} 21.88–24.18 μM).	PI3K/Akt and MEK-ERK signaling pathways between B16 and A375 cells were involved.	[185]
Liquiritigenin	*In vitro*	B16-BL16 (MM)	ND	Preliminary test determined IC_{50} equal to 97.7 μM.	NE	[162]
Naringenin	*In vitro*	C32 and A375 (HM)	ND	Preliminary test determined IC_{50} equal to 0.6 and 13.8 μM for C32 and A375 cells, respectively.	NE	[189]
	In vitro	B16-BL16 (MM)	ND	Preliminary test determined $IC_{50} > 100$ μM.	NE	[162]
Flavonols						
Alnusin	*In vitro*	B16-BL16 (MM)	ND	Preliminary test determined $IC_{50} > 100$ μM.	NE	[162]
Drabanemoroside	*In vitro*	SK-MEL-2 (HM) and B16F1 (MM)	ND	Preliminary test determined IC_{50} equal to 1.9 μg/ml for SK-MEL-2. The compound was not effective against B16F1 cells ($IC_{50} > 40$ μg/ml).	NE	[189]
Fisetin	*In vitro*	A375 (HM)	20–80 μM	Preliminary test determined IC_{50} equal to 38.1 and 20.3 μM at 24 and 48 h after treatment.	Fisetin inhibited mTOR and p70S6K through direct binding while the observed inhibitory	[186]

Flavonoid	Model	Cell line	Concentration or dose	Effectiveness	Possible mechanisms of action	Reference
					effect of fisetin on AKT was mediated indirectly, through targeting interrelated pathways.	
	In vitro and *in vivo* (mice)	A375 (HM)	10 and 20 μM, in combination with sorafenib (2 and 5 μM)	Combination treatment (fisetin + sorafenib) more effectively reduced the migration and invasion of BRAF-mutated melanoma cells both in vitro and in raft cultures compared to individual agents. In addition, fisetin potentiated the antiinvasive and antimetastatic effects of sorafenib *in vivo*.	Combination treatment (fisetin + sorafenib) promoted a decrease in N cadherin, vimentin and fibronectin and an increase in E-cadherin both in vitro and in xenograft tumors. Furthermore, combination therapy effectively inhibited Snail1, Twist1, Slug and ZEB1 protein expression compared to monotherapy. The expression of MMP-2 and MMP-9 in xenograft tumors was further reduced in combination treatment compared to individual agents.	[187]
	In vitro and *in vivo* (mice)	451Lu (HM)	20–100 μM (in vitro tests) and 1 and 2 mg/kg (*in vivo* tests)	IC_{50} was estimated to be 80, 37.2, and 17.5 μM at 24, 48, and 72 hours of treatment, respectively. A smaller average tumor volume was consistently observed in mice treated with fisetin. This was more marked in animals receiving 1 mg fisetin than in animals receiving the 2 mg dose, indicating a nonlinear dose response.	Fisetin decreased cell viability with G1-phase arrest and disruption of Wnt/β-catenin signaling.	[188]
	In vitro	451Lu and A375 (HM)	20–80 μM	The efficacy of fisetin in the induction of apoptosis varied with cell type as A375 cells were more susceptible to fisetin treatment compared to 451Lu cells. Results confirm apoptosis as the primary mechanism through which fisetin inhibits melanoma cell growth.	Fisetin treatment induced endoplasmic reticulum (ER) stress in highly aggressive A375 and 451Lu human melanoma cells, as revealed by upregulation of ER stress markers including IRE1a, XBP1s, ATF4 and GRP78. Both extrinsic and intrinsic apoptosis	[189]

http://dx.doi.org/10.5772/67573

Flavonoid	Model	Cell line	Concentration or dose	Effectiveness	Possible mechanisms of action	Reference
					pathways are involved in fisetin cytotoxic effects.	
Galangin	*In vitro*	B16F10 (MM)	0–100 μM	Preliminary test determined IC_{50} equal to 145 μM. Galangin. Microscopical analysis revealed the reduced number of cells and morphological aberrations after a 24 h treatment. The appearance of apoptotic cells such as cell shrinking, rounding and partial detachment was evident at a galangin concentration of 100 μM.	Galangin activated apoptosis signaling cascades by cleavage of procaspase-9, procaspase-3 and PARP in B16F10 cells. Moreover, galangin significantly induced activation of phosphor-p38 MAPK in a time and dose dependent manner.	[190, 192]
	In vitro and *in vivo* (mice)	B16F10 (MM)	0–200 μM (in vitro tests) and 50 mg/kg (*in vivo* tests)	Galangin decreased the proliferation of B16F10 cells in a dose-dependent manner. The cell viabilities were 67.9% at 50 mM group, 54.5% at 100 mM group, and 48.7% at 200 mM group, respectively. A significant reduced number of migrating cells was observed when the cells were treated with galangin for 24 h. *In vivo* models showed that galangin inhibited lung metastasis of B16F10 cells.	Molecular data showed that FAK mRNA level were reduced dose-dependently. Galangin also reduced phosphorylation of FAK (Tyr397) protein and suppressed the transcription of FAK gene, indicating FAK expression is a candidate target of galangin.	[191]
	In vitro	B16 (MM)	10–250 μg/ml	Preliminary test determined IC_{50} equal to 91.65 μg/ml.	Inhibitory effect on melanin production and tyrosinase activity.	[194]
Galangin-7-methyl ether	*In vitro*	B16BL6 (MM)	ND	Preliminary test determined IC_{50} equal to 20.8 μM.	NE	[175]
Icaritin	*In vitro*	A375S, A375R, A2058, and MEWO (all HM)	2.5–80 μM	Preliminary test determined IC_{50} equal to 2.7, 6.9, 14, and 15.6 μM in A375S, A375R, A2058, and MEWO cells, respectively, after 72h of treatment.	Icaritin suppressed p-STAT3 (tyr705) level in parallel with increases of p-STAT3 (ser727), p-ERK and p-AKT. The flavonoid significantly inhibited STAT3 nuclear translocation and reduced	[195]

Flavonoid	Model	Cell line	Concentration or dose	Effectiveness	Possible mechanisms of action	Reference
					the levels of STAT3 -targeted genes. Icaritin also inhibited IGF-1-induced STAT3 activation through downregulation of total IGF-1R level.	
Isorhamnetin	*In vitro*	SK-MEL-2 (HM) and B16F1 (MM)	ND	Preliminary test determined $IC_{50} > 40$ μg/ml for both cell lines.	NE	[189]
Isorhamnetin-3-*O*-β-D-glucoside	*In vitro*	SK-MEL-2 (HM) and B16F1 (MM)	ND	Preliminary test determined $IC_{50} > 40$ μg/ml for both cell lines.	NE	[189]
Kaempferol	*In vitro*	MDA-MB-435 (HM)	1–50 μM	Preliminary test determined IC_{50} equal to 1.5 μM.	NE	[171]
	In vitro	SK-MEL-2 (HM)	ND	Preliminary test determined IC_{50} equal to 6.9 μM.	NE	[196]
Kaempferol-3-*O*-rhamnoside	*In vitro*	SK-MEL-2 (HM)	ND	Preliminary test determined IC_{50} equal to 33.9 μM.	NE	[196]
Myricetin	*In vitro*	B16F10 (MM)	3.156–50 μM	Preliminary test determined IC_{50} equal to μM.	NE	[174]
Quercetin	*In vitro*	B16F10 (MM)	3.156–50 μM	Preliminary test determined $IC_{50} > 50$ μM.	NE	[174]
	In vitro and *in vivo* (mice)	B16F10 (MM)	25–50 μM (in vitro tests) and 7.5–15 mg/kg (*in vivo* tests), in combination with different doses of sulforaphane.	Quercetin and sulforaphane in combination inhibit the proliferation and migration of melanoma cells more effectively than either compound used alone. These compounds in combination significantly suppressed melanoma growth as compared to their individual use in a mouse model.	This combined effect was predominantly due to a decrease in MMP −9 expression in the mouse tumors.	[197]
	In vitro and	A375, A2058 (HM)	0–60 μM (in vitro tests) and 100 mg/kg (*in vivo* tests)	Exposure to quercetin resulted in inhibition of proliferation of melanoma cells, induction of cell	Quercetin inhibited the activation of STAT3 signaling by interfering with STAT3 phosphorylation, and	[198]

http://dx.doi.org/10.5772/67573

Flavonoid	Model	Cell line	Concentration or dose	Effectiveness	Possible mechanisms of action	Reference
	in vivo (mice)	and B16F10 (MM)		apoptosis, and suppression of migratory and invasive properties. Furthermore, quercetin suppressed A375 tumor growth and STAT3 activities in xenografted mice model, and inhibited murine B16F10 cells lung metastasis in an animal model.	reducing STAT3 nuclear localization.	
	In vitro	A375, A2058, SK-MEL-2 and MeWo (HM)	0–80 μM	Quercetin dose-dependently inhibited HGF-stimulated melanoma cell migration and invasion.	Suppression of the HGF/c-Met signaling pathway contributes to the antimetastatic action of quercetin in melanoma.	[199]
	In vitro	SK-MEL-2 (HM)	ND	Preliminary test determined IC_{50} equal to 4.7 μM.	NE	[194]
	In vitro	SK-MEL-2 (HM) and B16F1 (MM)	ND	Preliminary test determined IC_{50} equal to 21.1 and 8.2 μg/ml for SK-MEL-2 and B16F1 cell lines, respectively.	NE	[189]
Quercetin-3-*O*-rhamnoside	*In vitro*	SK-MEL-2 (HM)	ND	Preliminary test determined IC_{50} equal to 41.5 μM.	NE	[194]
Quercetin-3-*O*-β-D-glucopyranoside	*In vitro*	SK-MEL-2 (HM) and B16F1 (MM)	ND	Preliminary test determined IC_{50} > 40 μg/ml for both cell lines.	NE	[189]
Rhamnetin-3-*O*-rhamnoside	*In vitro*	SK-MEL-2 (HM)	ND	Preliminary test determined IC_{50} > 100 μM.	NE	[194]
Rhamnocitrin-3-*O*-rhamnoside	*In vitro*	SK-MEL-2 (HM)	ND	Preliminary test determined IC_{50} equal to 34.1 μM.	NE	[194]
Rutin	*In vivo* (mice)	B16F10 (MM)	20 mg/day	Rutin decreased the number of metastatic nodules, implantation, growth and invasion index.	NE	[179]

Flavonoid	Model	Cell line	Concentration or dose	Effectiveness	Possible mechanisms of action	Reference
Flavanols						
Epigallocatechin	*In vitro*	CHL-1 and WM266-4 (HM)	0.1–200 μM	Preliminary test determined IC_{50} equal to 10.3 and 51.2 μM for CHL-1 and WM266-4 cells.	Expression of ER stress and apoptosis markers.	[200]
Flavanonols						
Aromadendrin	*In vitro*	M14 (HM)	1–40 μM	The compound was not able to inhibit cell proliferation at 1–40 μM concentrations.	NE	[166]
Pinobanksin	*In vitro*	B16BL6 (MM)	ND	Preliminary test determined IC_{50} > 200 μM.	NE	[175]
Pinobanksin 5-methylether	*In vitro*	B16BL6 (MM)	ND	Preliminary test determined IC_{50} equal to 187 μM.	NE	[175]
Silymarin	*In vitro*	A375-S2 (HM)	1×10^{-5} to 1×10^{-4} M	It was assessed the effect of silymarin on anti-Fas agonistic antibody CH11 treated human malignant melanoma, A375-S2 cells. Pretreatment with silymarin significantly induced cell apoptosis in CH11-treated A375-S2 cells.	Caspase-8, −9, −3 and pan caspase inhibitors partially reversed silymarin induced apoptosis of CH11-treated cells. The expression of Fas-associated proteins with death domain (FADD), procaspase-8 and −3 was increased by silymarin pretreatment.	[201]
Isoflavonoids						
2′-Hydroxybiochanin A	*In vitro*	B16-BL6 (MM)	ND	Preliminary test determined IC_{50} >100 μM.	NE	[162]
4′-Methoxy-2′,3,7-trihydroxyisoflavanone	*In vitro*	B16-BL6 (MM)	ND	Preliminary test determined IC_{50} >100 μM.	NE	[162]
7-*O*-Methylvestitol	*In vitro*	B16-BL6 (MM)	ND	Preliminary test determined IC_{50} equal to 24.1 μM.	NE	[162]
Biochanin A	*In vitro*	B16-BL6 (MM)	ND	Preliminary test determined IC_{50} >100 μM.	NE	[162]
Calycosin	*In vitro*	B16-BL6 (MM)	ND	Preliminary test determined IC_{50} >100 μM.	NE	[162]

Flavonoid	Model	Cell line	Concentration or dose	Effectiveness	Possible mechanisms of action	Reference
Daidzein	*In vitro*	B16-BL6 (MM)	ND	Preliminary test determined IC_{50} >100 μM.	NE	[162]
Ferreirin	*In vitro*	B16-BL6 (MM)	ND	Preliminary test determined IC_{50} >100 μM.	NE	[162]
Formononetin	*In vitro*	B16-BL6 (MM)	ND	Preliminary test determined IC_{50} >100 μM.	NE	[162]
Genistein	*In vitro*	518A2 (HM)	ND	Preliminary test determined IC_{50} > 50 μM. The flavonoid also reduced cell migration.	Apigenin induced an arrest of the cell cycle of 518A2 melanoma cells at the G2/M transition and also attenuated the expression and secretion of the metastasisrelevant matrix metalloproteinases MMP-2 and MMP-9.	[170]
	In vitro	M14 (HM)	12–100 μM	Genistin reduced cell proliferation in 40.9% at 100 μM dose.	Cytotoxic activity of genistin was related to its antioxidant effect, but no specific target was investigated.	[202]
Isoangustone A (IAA)	*In vitro* and *in vivo* (mice)	SK-MEL-28 and SK MEL-5 (HM)	0–20 μM (in vitro tests) and 2–10 mg/kg (*in vivo* tests)	Treatment with 20 μM of IAA inhibited the growth of SK-MEL-28 cells up to 67% as compared with untreated control cells. Moreover, in a xenograft mouse model, IAA significantly decreased tumor growth, volume, and weight of SK-MEL-28 xenografts.	IAA significantly blocked cell-cycle progression at the G1-phase and inhibited the expression of G1-phase regulatory proteins, including cyclins D1 and E in the SK-MEL-28 cell line. IAA suppressed the phosphorylation of Akt, GSK-3b, and JNK1/2. IAA also bound to phosphoinositide 3-kinase (PI3K), MKK4, and MKK7, strongly inhibiting their kinase activities in an ATP-competitive manner.	[203]
Isovestitol	*In vitro*	B16-BL6 (MM)	ND	Preliminary test determined IC_{50} equal to 33.6 μM.	NE	[162]
Mucronulatol	*In vitro*	B16-BL6 (MM)	ND	Preliminary test determined IC_{50} equal to 30.4 μM.	NE	[162]

Flavonoid	Model	Cell line	Concentration or dose	Effectiveness	Possible mechanisms of action	Reference
Pratensein	*In vitro*	B16-BL6 (MM)	ND	Preliminary test determined IC_{50} >100 μM.	NE	[162]
Vestitol	*In vitro*	B16-BL6 (MM)	ND	Preliminary test determined IC_{50} equal to 57.4 μM.	NE	[162]
Vestitone	*In vitro*	B16-BL6 (MM)	ND	Preliminary test determined IC_{50} >100 μM.	NE	[162]
Violanone	*In vitro*	B16-BL6 (MM)	ND	Preliminary test determined IC_{50} >100 μM.	NE	[162]
Xenognosin B	*In vitro*	B16-BL6 (MM)	ND	Preliminary test determined IC_{50} equal to 34.1 μM.	NE	[162]

ND: not described; NE: not evaluated; HM: human melanoma cell line; MM: murine melanoma cell line.

Box 1. Anticancer activity of flavonoids on melanoma cell lines.

apigenin in an experimental lung metastasis model. Apigenin-treated mice had significant fewer metastatic nodules when compared to the vehicle control group, suggesting apigenin inhibits the metastasis potential of B16F10 melanoma cells *in vivo* mouse model (**Figure 4**).

6.2. Bioactivity of diosmin on melanoma

Diosmin is a glycosylated flavonoid commonly used as an active constituent of several pharmaceutical products, mainly for cardiovascular diseases treatment. Diosmin is used in the treatment of venous insufficiency, because of its vasoprotector and venotonic properties. In addition, it acts as an antioxidant, anti-inflammatory, and antimutagenic molecule, regulating the activity of several enzymes, including cyclooxygenases and cytochrome P450 proteins [177, 179]. Interestingly, the anticancer effects of diosmin have also been studied [176, 178], suggesting that this flavonoid presents a broad spectrum of pharmacological activities.

Conesa et al. [179] performed a comparative study with three different flavonoids (tangeretin, rutin, and diosmin) using an experimental model of B16F10 melanoma cell-induced pulmonary metastasis. The greatest reduction in the number of metastatic nodules (52%) was obtained with diosmin treatment. Similarly, diosmin presented a relevant decreasing in implantation, growth, and invasion index (79.40, 67.44, and 45.23%, respectively). These results were confirmed by another study developed by Martínez et al. [178], suggesting diosmin is an effective agent against metastatic stages of melanoma.

The antimetastatic effect of diosmin has also been evaluated in combination with IFN-α [176, 177], an important cytokine that has shown the significant effect in the treatment of metastatic melanoma in high doses. In both investigations, it was verified that synergistic antiproliferative and antimetastatic effects shown by the combination of the flavonoid and the lowest dose of IFN-α, which was similar to that produced by the highest dose of the cytokine alone. These results suggest that diosmin may be used in combination with IFN-α in an attempt to reduce its therapeutic dose, thereby reducing the side effects promoted by continued cytokine use.

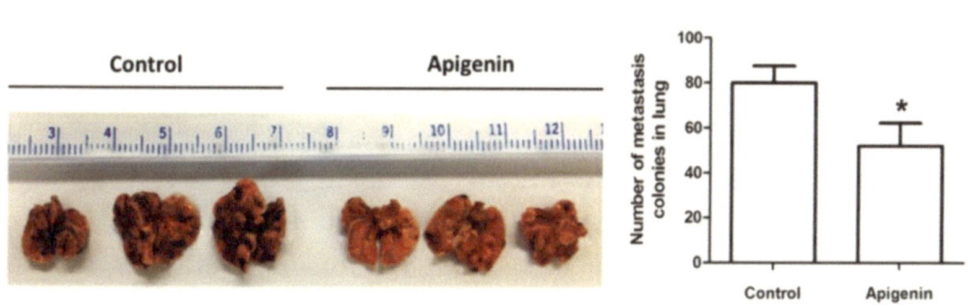

Figure 4. Apigenin inhibited murine melanoma B16F10 cell lung metastasis. B16F10 melanoma cells were injected into the tail vein of the C57BL/6 mice. These mice then received intragastric administration of vehicle or apigenin (150 mg/kg/day) for 24 consecutive days. Lung metastasis of B16F10 melanoma cells in the mouse model (upper) and the metastasis nodules number in the lungs (bottom) were shown. Data were mean ± SD, $n = 8$, $*p < 0.05$. This figure was taken from Ref. [172].

6.3. Bioactivity of fisetin on melanoma

Fisetin (3,7,3′,4′-tetrahydroxyflavone) is a flavonol also found in many fruits and vegetables, such as strawberries, apples, persimmons, kiwi, onions, and cucumbers. This flavonoid has shown a relevant neuroprotective effect, aiding in memory and cognition processes, as well as reducing behavioral deficits. Recently, the effect of fisetin on anticancer therapy has also been studied [186].

Investigation conducted by Syed et al. [188] determined an IC_{50} value of 38.1 and 20.3 μM against A375 human melanoma cell line, at 24 and 48 h after treatment. In a subsequent study, Syed et al. [191] have demonstrated that fisetin induces apoptosis in melanoma cells. The efficacy of fisetin in the induction of apoptosis varied with cell type and preliminary results confirmed apoptosis as the primary mechanism through which fisetin inhibits melanoma cell growth. The possible mechanisms involved include upregulation of ER stress markers such as IRE1a, XBP1s, ATF4, and GRP78. In addition, both extrinsic and intrinsic apoptosis pathways are involved in fisetin cytotoxic effects.

The effect of fisetin was also evaluated on the growth of metastatic 451Lu human melanoma cells, which exhibit constitutive Wnt signaling in addition to harboring a mutation in the B-Raf gene. The IC_{50} value was estimated to be 17.5 μM at 72 h of treatment in the MTT assay. In an *in vivo* model, a smaller average tumor volume was consistently observed in mice treated with fisetin. This was more marked in animals receiving 1 mg fisetin than in animals receiving the 2 mg dose, indicating a nonlinear dose response. The authors attributed this effect to a decreasing of cell viability with G1-phase arrest and disruption of Wnt/β-catenin signaling mediated by fisetin [186].

A recent report evaluated the effect of fisetin in combination with sorafenib, a multi-kinase inhibitor of mutant and wild-type BRAF and CRAF kinases, on melanoma cell invasion and metastasis. In this study, fisetin potentiated the anti-invasive and antimetastatic effects of sorafenib *in vivo*, suggesting that this flavonoid can be used as an alternative agent in melanoma therapy reducing doses of anticancer drugs used for this purpose [187].

6.4. Bioactivity of luteolin on melanoma

Luteolin is a common flavone that exists in many types of plants including fruits, vegetables, and medicinal herbs. This flavonoid presents potential for cancer prevention and therapy [174]. Concerning to melanoma treatment, George et al. [182] showed that luteolin possesses relevant cytotoxicity against A375 human melanoma cell line, with an IC_{50} value of 115.1 μM in a preliminary test. Luteolin also inhibited colony formation and induced apoptosis in a dose and time-dependent manner by disturbing cellular integrity. Accumulation of cells in the G0/G1 (60.4–72.6%) phase for A375 cells after 24 h treatment indicated cell cycle arresting potential of this flavonoid, suggesting that luteolin inhibits cell proliferation and promotes cell cycle arrest and apoptosis in human melanoma cells. A similar result was demonstrated by Casagrande and Darbon [204], who highlighted the involvement of the regulation of cyclin-dependent kinases CDK2 and CDK1 in the antiproliferative effect of luteolin on OCM-1 human melanoma cells.

In a recent investigation, the inhibitory effect of luteolin on melanoma cell proliferation was related to ER stress induced. In this context, luteolin increased the expression of the ER stress-related proteins, such as protein kinase RNA-like ER kinase, phosphorylation eukaryotic translation initiation factor 2α, activating transcription factor (ATF) 6, CCAAT/enhancer-binding protein-homologous protein (CHOP), and cleaved caspase 12. In addition, luteolin increased the level of intracellular ROS, leading to ROS-mediated apoptosis and ER stress, suggesting that luteolin induces apoptosis by ER stress via increasing ROS levels [183].

Anticancer potential of luteolin has also evaluated *in vivo*. In experimental metastasis model, mice treatment with luteolin (10 or 20 mg/kg) reduced metastatic colonization in the lungs by 50%. This treatment increased E-cadherin expression while reduced the expression of vimentin and β3 integrin in the tumor tissues [184]. These results encourage the use of luteolin as an anticancer chemopreventive and chemotherapeutic agent.

6.5. Bioactivity of quercetin on melanoma

Quercetin is a noncarcinogenic dietary flavonoid with low toxicity, has been shown to exert antioxidant, anti-inflammatory, neuroprotective, and antimelanoma activities [193]. A preliminary study showed that quercetin presents a weak cytotoxic effect on B16F10 murine melanoma cells, with an IC_{50} value > 50 μM [174]. However, Casagrande and Darbon [204] and Kim et al. [196] showed that quercetin presents a considerable antiproliferative effect on OCM-1 and SK-MEL-2 human melanoma cells, with an IC_{50} value between 4.7 and 19 μM. In these investigations, the authors demonstrated that the presence of hydroxyl group at the 3′-position of the ring B in quercetin favors the cytotoxic effect and a G1 cell cycle arrest. The involvement of the regulation of cyclin-dependent kinases CDK2 and CDK1 may also be present in its anticancer effect.

Cao et al. [198] evaluated the involvement of STAT3 signaling in the inhibitory effects of quercetin on melanoma cell growth, migration, and invasion. Quercetin treatment promoted inhibition in proliferation of melanoma cells, induction of cell apoptosis, and suppression of migratory and invasive properties. Furthermore, mechanistic study indicated that quercetin inhibits the activation of STAT3 signaling by interfering with STAT3 phosphorylation, and reducing STAT3 nuclear localization. In an animal model, quercetin inhibited murine B16F10 cells lung metastasis, indicating that quercetin possesses antitumor potential.

7. Brief structure-activity relationship (SAR) considerations

Nagao et al. [167] evaluated the cytotoxic activity of 21 flavones and the effect of the substitution patterns on their anticancer potential, although the authors highlight that the number of compounds examined might not be sufficient to determine the structure-activity relationships. Generally, the data show that the growth inhibitory activity of one flavone against the three different tumor cell lines (including a murine melanoma cell line) is not always the same, suggesting differences in the sensitivity of tumor cells to flavones.

The influences of ring A substituents against B16F10 cells were examined. Comparing the antiproliferative activity of four 3′,4′-di-OH-flavones, the order of contribution was found to be 5-OH-6,7-di-OCH_3 > 5,6,7-tri-OH > 5,7-di-OH-6-OCH_3 > 5,7-di-OH. In contrast, in the

3′-OH-4′-OCH_3-flavones (desmethoxycentaureidin, eupatorin, and 5,6,3′-trihydroxy-7,4′-dimethoxyflavone), the order is 5,6-di-OH-7-OCH_3 > 5-OH-6,7-di-OCH_3 > 5,7-di-OH-6-OCH_3. In the 3′,4′-di-OCH_3-flavones (eupatilin and 5,6-dihydroxy-7,3′,4′-trimethoxyflavone), the order is 5,6-di-OH-7-OCH_3 > 5,7-di-OH-6-OCH_3, and in the 3′-OCH_3-4′-OH-flavones (jaceosidin and cirsilineol), it is 5,7-di-OH-6-OCH_3 > 5-OH-6,7-di-OCH_3. In addition, for ring B substituents, 3′,4′-di-OH and 3′,4′-di-OH-5′-OCH_3 showed a greater effect than the others, but the influence of 3′,5′-di-OCH_3-4′-OH appears to be not relevant [167].

Another investigation evaluated the effects of polyhydroxylated flavonoids on the growth of B16F10 melanoma cells. In general, the results suggest that the presence of a C2–C3 double bond and three adjacent hydroxyl groups in the A- or B-rings confers greater antiproliferative activity [174]. Casagrande and Darbon [204] investigated the effects of a series of flavonoids on cell proliferation and cell cycle distribution in human melanoma cells (OCM-1). Interestingly, the presence of a hydroxyl group at the 3′-position of the ring B in quercetin and luteolin was correlated to a G1 cell cycle arrest while its absence in kaempferol and apigenin was correlated to a G2 block.

The presence of isoprenoid units in the cytotoxic effect of flavonoids has also been evaluated for melanoma cells [168]. The results indicated that isoprenoid substitutions in flavonoids enhance their cytotoxic potential, and that the position of attachment and the number of isoprenoid-substituent moieties per molecule influence flavonoid cytotoxicity. This is probably related to their lipophilicity and affinity properties, which favor penetration into the cell membrane.

Acknowledgements

The authors thank FACEPE (Fundação de Amparo à Ciência e Tecnologia do Estado de Pernambuco) for financial support.

Author details

Raimundo Gonçalves de Oliveira Júnior[1], Christiane Adrielly Alves Ferraz[1], Mariana Gama e Silva[1], Érica Martins de Lavor[1], Larissa Araújo Rolim[1], Julianeli Tolentino de Lima[1], Audrey Fleury[2], Laurent Picot[2], Jullyana de Souza Siqueira Quintans[3], Lucindo José Quintans Júnior[3] and Jackson Roberto Guedes da Silva Almeida[1]*

*Address all correspondence to: jackson.guedes@univasf.edu.br

1 Center for Studies and Research of Medicinal Plants, Federal University of San Francisco Valley, Petrolina, Pernambuco, Brazil

2 Faculty of Science and Technology, University of La Rochelle, La Rochelle, France

3 Department of Physiology, Federal University of Sergipe (DFS/UFS), São Cristóvão, Sergipe, Brazil

References

[1] Cragg GM, Newman DJ. Natural products: a continuing source of novel drug leads. Biochimica et Biophysica Acta. 2013; **1830**: 3670–3695.

[2] Shen B. A new golden age of natural products drug discovery. Cell. 2015; **163**: 1297–1300.

[3] Cragg GM, Newman DJ. Natural products as sources of new drugs from 1981 to 2014. Journal of Natural Products. 2016; **79**: 629–661.

[4] Carter GT. Natural products and pharma 2011: strategic changes spur new opportunities. Natural Product Reports. 2011; **28**: 1783–1789.

[5] Harvey AL, Edrada-Ebel R, Quinn RJ. The re-emergence of natural products for drug discovery in the genomics era. Nature Reviews Drug Discovery. 2015; **14**: 1–19.

[6] Saiag P, Bosquet L, Guillot B. Management of adult patients with cutaneous melanoma without distant metastasis. European Journal of Dermatology. 2007; **17**: 325–31.

[7] Bilir SP, Ma Q, Zhao Z, Wehler E, Munakata J, Barber B. Economic burden of toxicities associated with treating metastatic melanoma in the United States. Health Drug Benefits. 2016; **9**: 203–213.

[8] Kuphal S, Bosserhoff A. Recent progress in understanding the pathology of malignant melanoma. Journal of Pathology. 2009; **219**: 400–409.

[9] Shin SY, Woo Y, Hyun J, Yong Y, Koh D, Lee YL, Lim Y. Relationship between the structures of flavonoids and their NF-κB-dependent transcriptional activities. Bioorganic & Medicinal Chemistry Letters. 2011; **21**: 6036–6041.

[10] Ravishankar D, Rajora AK, Greco F, Osborn HMI. Flavonoids as prospective compounds for anti-cancer therapy. International Journal of Biochemistry & Cell Biology. 2013; **45**: 2821–2831.

[11] Bouzaiene NN, Chaabane F, Sassi A, Chekir-Ghedira L, Ghedira K. Effect of apigenin-7-glucoside, genkwanin and naringenin on tyrosinase activity and melanin synthesis in B16F10 melanoma cells. Life Sciences. 2016; **144**: 80–85.

[12] MacKie RM, Hauschild A, Eggermont AMM. Epidemiology of invasive cutaneous melanoma. Annals of Oncology: Official Journal of the European Society for Medical Oncology/ESMO. 2009; **20**: vi1–7.

[13] Tobias, JS, Hochhauser D. Cancer and its Management. 6th edition, Wiley-Blackwell; 2013.

[14] Armstrong BK, Kricker A. The epidemiology of UV induced skin cancer. Journal of Photochemistry and Photobiology. B, Biology. 2001; **63**(1–3): 8–18.

[15] Kraemer KH, Lee MM, Andrews AD, Lambert WC. The role of sunlight and DNA repair in melanoma and non-melanoma skin cancer. The xeroderma pigmentosum paradigm. Archives of Dermatology. 1994; **130**(8): 1018–21.

[16] Melamed RD, Aydin IT, Rajan GS, Phelps R, Silvers DN, Emmett KJ, Brunner G, Rabadan R, Celebi JT. Genomic characterization of dysplastic nevi unveils implications for diagnosis of melanoma. Journal of Investigative Dermatology, 2016; 24.

[17] Koh HK, Sinks TH, Geller AC, Miller DR, Lew RA. Etiology of melanoma. Cancer Treatment and Research. 1993; **65**: 1–28.

[18] Clark WH, Ainsworth AM, Bernardino EA, Yang CH, Mihm CM, Reed RJ. The developmental biology of primary human malignant melanomas. Seminars in Oncology. 1975; **2**(2): 83–103.

[19] Clark WH, Elder DE, Guerry D, Epstein MN, Greene MH, Van HM. A study of tumor progression: the precursor lesions of superficial spreading and nodular melanoma. Human Pathology. 1984; **15**(12): 1147–65.

[20] Conde-Perez A, Larue L. Human relevance of NRAS/BRAF mouse melanoma models. European Journal of Cell Biology. 2014; **93**(1–2): 82–86.

[21] Liu J, Fukunaga-Kalabis M, Li L, Herlyn M. Developmental pathways activated in melanocytes and melanoma. Archives of Biochemistry and Biophysics. 2014; **563**: 13–21.

[22] Locatelli C, Filippin-Monteiro FB, Creczynski-Pasa TB. Recent Advances in the Biology, Therapy and Management of Melanoma. (L. Davids, Ed.). InTech DTP, Croatia; 2013.

[23] Palmieri, G, Ombra, M, Colombino M, Casula M, Sini M, Manca A, Paliogiannis P, Ascierto PA, Cossu A. Multiple molecular pathways in melanomagenesis: characterization of therapeutic targets. Frontiers in Oncology. 2015; 5: 1–16.

[24] Balch CM, Soong SJ, Gershenwald JE, Thompson JF, Reintgen DS, Cascinelli N, Urist M, McMasters KM, Ross MI, Kirkwood JM, Atkins MB, Thompson JA, Coit DG, Byrd D, Desmond R, Zhang Y, Liu PY, Lyman GH, Morabito A. Prognostic factors analysis of 17,600 melanoma patients: validation of the American Joint Committee on Cancer melanoma staging system. Journal of Clinical Oncology?: Official Journal of the American Society of Clinical Oncology. 2001; **19**(16): 3622–34.

[25] Balch CM, Gershenwald JE, Soong SJ, Thompson JF, Atkins MB, Byrd DR, Buzaid AC, Cochran AJ, Coit DG, Ding S, Eggermont AM, Flaherty KT, Gimotty PA, Kirkwood JM, McMasters KM, Mihm MC Jr, Morton DL, Ross MI, Sober AJ, Sondak VK. Final version of 2009 AJCC melanoma staging and classification. Journal of Clinical Oncology: Official Journal of the American Society of Clinical Oncology. 2009; **27**(36): 6199–206.

[26] Wevers KP. Progression in melanoma: considerations and implications in dissecting nodal fields [thesis]. Netherlands: University of Groningen; 2013.

[27] Pak BJ, Lee J, Thai BL, Fuchs SY, Shaked Y, Ronai Z, Kerbel RS, Ben-David Y. Radiation resistance of human melanoma analysed by retroviral insertional mutagenesis reveals a possible role for dopachrome tautomerase. Oncogene. 2004; **23**(1): 30–38.

[28] Satyamoorthy K, Chehab NH, Waterman MJ, Lien MC, El-Deiry WS, Herlyn M, Halazonetis TD. Aberrant regulation and function of wild-type p53 in radioresistant

melanoma cells. Cell Growth & Differentiation?: The Molecular Biology Journal of the American Association for Cancer Research. 2000; **11**(9): 467–74.

[29] Marneros AG. Tumor angiogenesis in melanoma. Hematology/Oncology Clinics of North America. 2009; **23**(3): 431–446.

[30] Hall WA, Djalilian HR, Nussbaum ES, Cho KH. Long-term survival with metastatic cancer to the brain. Medical Oncology (Northwood, London, England). 2000; **17**(4): 279–86.

[31] Nardin A, Wong WC, Tow C, Molina TJ, Tissier F, Audebourg A, Garcette M, Caignard A, Avril MF, Abastado JP, Prévost-Blondel A. Dacarbazine promotes stromal remodeling and lymphocyte infiltration in cutaneous melanoma lesions. The Journal of Investigative Dermatology. 2001; **131**(9): 1896–905.

[32] WHO. Health Effects of UV Radiation. Accessed in: http://www.who.int/uv/health/en/. 2016.

[33] Grange F. Epidemiology of cutaneous melanoma: descriptive data in France and Europe. Annales de Dermatologie et de Vénéréologie. 2005; **132**: 975–82.

[34] Wu S, Han J, Laden F, Qureshi AA. Long-term ultraviolet flux, other potential risk factors, and skin cancer risk: a cohort study. Cancer Epidemiology and Prevention Biomarkers. 2014; 23(6): 1080–1089.

[35] Holman CD, Armstrong BK. Cutaneous malignant melanoma and indicators of total accumulated exposure to the sun: an analysis separating histogenetic types. Journal of the National Cancer Institute. 1984; **73**(1): 75–82.

[36] Leiter U, Garbe C. Epidemiology of melanoma and nonmelanoma skin cancer—the role of sunlight. Sunlight, Vitamin D and Skin Cancer. 2008; **624**: 89–103.

[37] Sturm RA. Skin colour and skin cancer—MC1R, the genetic link. Melanoma Research. 2002; **12**(5): 405–16.

[38] McGregor JM, Yu CC, Dublin EA, Levison DA, MacDonald DM. Aberrant expression of p53 tumour-suppressor protein in non-melanoma skin cancer. The British Journal of Dermatology. 1992; **127**(5): 463–9.

[39] Forslund KÖ, Nordqvist K. The melanoma antigen genes—any clues to their functions in normal tissues? Experimental Cell Research. 2001; **265**(2): 185–194.

[40] Sang M, Wang L, Ding C, Zhou X, Wang B, Lian Y, Shan B. Melanoma-associated antigen genes – An update. Cancer Letters. 2011; **302**(2): 85–90.

[41] Brasseur F, Rimoldi D, Liénard D, Lethé B, Carrel S, Arienti F, Suter L, Vanwijck R, Bourlond A, Humblet Y. Expression of MAGE genes in primary and metastatic cutaneous melanoma. International Journal of Cancer. 1995; **63**(3): 375–80.

[42] de Vries TJ, Fourkour A, Wobbes T, Verkroost G, Ruiter DJ, van Muijen GN. Heterogeneous expression of immunotherapy candidate proteins gp100, MART-1, and tyrosinase in human melanoma cell lines and in human melanocytic lesions. Cancer Research. 1997; **57**(15): 3223–9.

[43] de Vries TJ, Trancikova D, Ruiter DJ, van Muijen GN. High expression of immunotherapy candidate proteins gp100, MART-1, tyrosinase and TRP-1 in uveal melanoma. British Journal of Cancer. 1998; **78**(9): 1156–61.

[44] Ritter G, Livingston PO. Ganglioside antigens expressed by human cancer cells. Seminars in Cancer Biology. 1991; **2**(6): 401–9.

[45] Cebon J, Gedye C, John T, Davis ID. Immunotherapy of advanced or metastatic melanoma. Clinical Advances in Hematology & Oncology: H&O. 2007; **5**(12): 994–1006.

[46] Itzhaki O, Levy D, Zikich D, Treves AJ,Markel G, Schachter J, BesserMJ. Adoptive T-cell transfer in melanoma. Immunotherapy. 2013; 5(1): 79–90.

[47] Knight DA, Ngiow SF, Li M, Parmenter T, Mok S, Cass A, Haynes NM, Kinross K, Yagita H, Koya RC, Graeber TG, Ribas A, McArthur GA, Smyth MJ. Host immunity contributes to the anti-melanoma activity of BRAF inhibitors. The Journal of Clinical Investigation. 2013; **123**(3): 1371–81.

[48] Menzies AM, Long GV. Recent advances in melanoma systemic therapy. BRAF inhibitors, CTLA4 antibodies and beyond. European Journal of Cancer (Oxford, England: 1990). 2013; **49**(15): 3229–41.

[49] Prickett TD, Crystal JS, Cohen CJ, Pasetto A, Parkhurst MR, Gartner JJ, Yao X, Wang R, Gros A, Li YF, El-Gamil M, Trebska-McGowan K, Rosenberg SA, Robbins PF. Durable complete response from metastatic melanoma after transfer of autologous T cells recognizing 10 mutated tumor antigens. Cancer Immunology Research. 2016; **4**(8): 669–678.

[50] Di Giacomo A, Danielli R, Calabrò L, Guidoboni M, Miracco C. Ipilimumab in the common daily practice: Feasibility, safety, and efficacy in heavily pretreated metastatic melanoma patients. Journal of Clinical Oncology: Official Journal of the American Society of Clinical Oncology. 2009; **27**: 20002.

[51] Wang M, Yu T, Zhu C, Sun H, Qiu Y. Resveratrol triggers protective autophagy through the ceramide/Akt/mTOR pathway in melanoma B16 cells. Nutrition and Cancer. 2014; **66**(3): 435–40.

[52] Gupta SC, Kismali G, Aggarwal BB. Curcumin, a component of turmeric: from farm to pharmacy. BioFactors (Oxford, England). 2013; **39**(1): 2–13.

[53] Van Goietsenoven G, Hutton J, Becker JP, Lallemand B, Robert F. Targeting of eEF1A with Amaryllidaceae isocarbostyrils as a strategy to combat melanomas. FASEB Journal?: Official Publication of the Federation of American Societies for Experimental Biology. 2010; **24**(11): 4575–84.

[54] Baudelet PH, Gagez AL, Bérard JB, Juin C, Bridiau N. Antiproliferative activity of Cyanophora paradoxa pigments in melanoma, breast and lung cancer cells. Marine Drugs. 2013; **11**(11): 4390–406.

[55] Gagez AL, Thiery V, Pasquet V, Cadoret JP, Picot L. Epoxycarotenoids and cancer. Review. Current Bioactive Compounds. 2012; **8**(2): 109–141.

[56] Kumar SR, Hosokawa M, Miyashita K. Fucoxanthin: a marine carotenoid exerting anti-cancer effects by affecting multiple mechanisms. Marine Drugs. 2013; **11**(12): 5130–47.

[57] Mimouni V, Ulmann L, Pasquet V, Mathieu M, Picot L. The potential of microalgae for the production of bioactive molecules of pharmaceutical interest. Current Pharmaceutical Biotechnology. 2012; 13: 2733–2750.

[58] Pasquet V, Morisset P, Ihammouine S, Chepied A, Aumailley L. Antiproliferative activity of violaxanthin isolated from bioguided fractionation of *Dunaliella tertiolecta* extracts. Marine Drugs. 2011; **9**(5): 819–31.

[59] Xu XL, Hu DN, Iacob C, Jordan A, Gandhi S. Effects of Zeaxanthin on growth and invasion of human uveal melanoma in nude mouse model. Journal of Ophthalmology. 2015; **2015**: 392305.

[60] Alqathama A, Prieto JM. Natural products with therapeutic potential in melanoma metastasis. Natural Products Reports, 2015; **32**(8): 1170–1182.

[61] Nihal M, Ahmad N, Mukhtar H, Wood GS. Anti-proliferative and proapoptotic effects of (?)-epigallocatechin-3-gallate on human melanoma: Possible implications for the chemoprevention of melanoma. International Journal of Cancer. 2005; **114**(4): 513–521.

[62] Zhang L, Wei Y, Zhang J. Novel mechanisms of anticancer activities of green tea component epigallocatechin-3-gallate. Anti-Cancer Agents in Medicinal Chemistry. 2014; **14** (6): 779–86.

[63] Tanaka K, Ishikawa S, Matsui Y, Tamesada M, Harashima N, Harada M. Oral ingestion of *Lentinula edodes* mycelia extract inhibits B16 melanoma growth via mitigation of regulatory T cell-mediated immunosuppression. Cancer Science. 2011; **102**(3): 516–21.

[64] Palmieri G, Capone M, Ascierto ML, Gentilcore G, Stroncek DF, Casula M, Sini MC, Palla M, Mozzillo N, Ascierto PA. Main roads to melanoma. Journal of Translational Medicine. 2009; **7**: 86.

[65] Dhomen N, Marais R. New insight into BRAF mutations in cancer. Current Opinion in Genetics & Development. 2007; **17**(1): 31–39.

[66] Campbell PM, Der CJ. Oncogenic Ras and its role in tumor cell invasion and metastasis. Seminars in Cancer Biology. 2004; **14**(2): 105–114.

[67] Giehl K. Oncogenic Ras in tumour progression and metastasis. Biological Chemistry. 2005; **386**(3): 193–205.

[68] Davies H, Bignell GR, Cox C, Stephens P, Edkins S, et al. 2002. Mutations of the BRAF gene in human cancer. Nature, **417**(6892): 949–954.

[69] Karasarides M, Chiloeches A, Hayward R, Niculescu-Duvaz D, Scanlon I, et al. B-RAF is a therapeutic target in melanoma. Oncogene. 2004; **23**(37): 6292–6298.

[70] Dankort D, Curley DP, Cartlidge RA, Nelson B, Karnezis AN, et al. Braf (V600E) cooperates with Pten loss to induce metastatic melanoma. Nature Genetics. 2009; **41**(5): 544–552.

[71] Haluska FG, Tsao H, Wu H, Haluska FS, Lazar A, et al. Genetic alterations in signaling pathways in melanoma. Clinical Cancer Research. 2006; **12**(7): 2301s–2307s.

[72] Dhawan P, Singh AB, Ellis DL, Richmond A. Constitutive Activation of Akt/protein kinase B in melanoma leads to up-regulation of nuclear factor-κB and tumor progression. Cancer Research. 2002; **62**(24): 7335–7342.

[73] Zheng B, Jeong JH, Asara JM, Yuan YY, Granter SR, et al. Oncogenic B-RAF negatively regulates the tumor suppressor LKB1 to promote melanoma cell proliferation. Molecular Cell. 2009; **33**(2): 237–247.

[74] McKee CS, Hill DS, Redfern CPF, Armstrong JL, Lovat PE. Oncogenic BRAF signalling increases Mcl-1 expression in cutaneous metastatic melanoma. Experimental Dermatology. 2013; **22**(11): 767–769.

[75] Cartlidge RA, Thomas GR, Cagnol S, Jong KA, Molton SA, et al. Oncogenic BRAF (V600E) inhibits BIM expression to promote melanoma cell survival. Pigment Cell & Melanoma Research. 2008; **21**(5): 534–544.

[76] Hoek KS, Eichhoff OM, Schlegel NC, Döbbeling U, Kobert N, et al. In vivo switching of human melanoma cells between proliferative and invasive states. Cancer Research. 2008; **68**(3): 650–656.

[77] Smalley KSM, Sondak VK, Weber JS. c-KIT signaling as the driving oncogenic event in sub-groups of melanomas. Histology and Histopathology. 2009; **24**(5): 643–650.

[78] Weeraratna AT, Jiang Y, Hostetter G, Rosenblatt K, Duray P, et al. Wnt5a signaling directly affects cell motility and invasion of metastatic melanoma. Cancer Cell. 2002; **1** (3): 279–288.

[79] Deichmann M, Benner A, Bock M, Jäckel A, Uhl K, et al. S100-Beta, melanoma-inhibiting activity, and lactate dehydrogenase discriminate progressive from nonprogressive American Joint Committee on Cancer stage IV melanoma. Journal of Clinical Oncology: Official Journal of the American Society of Clinical Oncology. 1999; **17**(6): 1891–1896.

[80] Thery C, Boussac M, Veron P, Ricciardi-Castagnoli P, Raposo G, et al. Proteomic analysis of dendritic cell-derived exosomes: a secreted subcellular compartment distinct from apoptotic vesicles. The Journal of Immunology. 2001; **166**(12): 7309–7318.

[81] Garcia BA, Smalley DM, Cho, Shabanowitz J, Ley K, et al. The platelet microparticle proteome. Journal of Proteome Research. 2005; **4**(5): 1516–1521.

[82] Martínez MC, Larbret F, Zobairi F, Coulombe J, Debili N, et al. Transfer of differentiation signal by membrane microvesicles harboring hedgehog morphogens. Blood. 2006; **108** (9): 3012–3020.

[83] Valadi H, Ekström K, Bossios A, Sjöstrand M, Lee JJ, et al. Exosome-mediated transfer of mRNAs and microRNAs is a novel mechanism of genetic exchange between cells. Nature Cell Biology. 2007; **9**(6): 654–659.

[84] Ismail N, Wang Y, Dakhlallah D, Moldovan L, Agarwal K, et al. Macrophage microvesicles induce macrophage differentiation and miR-223 transfer. Blood. 2013; **121**(6): 984–995.

[85] Fritzsching B, Schwer B, Kartenbeck J, Pedal A, Horejsi V, et al. Release and intercellular transfer of cell surface CD81 via microparticles. The Journal of Immunology. 2002; **169** (10): 5531–5537.

[86] Rozmyslowicz T, Majka M, Kijowski J, Murphy S, Conover D, et al. Platelet- and megakaryocyte-derived microparticles transfer CXCR4 receptor to CXCR4-null cells and make them susceptible to infection by X4-HIV. [Miscellaneous Article]. AIDS. 2003; **17**(1): 33–42.

[87] del Conde I. Tissue-factor-bearing microvesicles arise from lipid rafts and fuse with activated platelets to initiate coagulation. Blood. 2005; **106**(5): 1604–1611.

[88] Feng D, Zhao WL, Ye YY, Bai XC, Liu RQ, et al. Cellular internalization of exosomes occurs through phagocytosis. Traffic. 2010. **11**(5): 675–687.

[89] Morelli AE. Endocytosis, intracellular sorting, and processing of exosomes by dendritic cells. Blood. 2004; **104**(10): 3257–3266.

[90] Raposo G, Nijman HW, Stoorvogel W, Liejendekker R, Harding CV, et al. B lymphocytes secrete antigen-presenting vesicles. The Journal of Experimental Medicine. 1996; **183**(3): 1161–1172.

[91] Chaput N, Théry C. Exosomes: immune properties and potential clinical implementations. Seminars in Immunopathology. 2011; **33**(5): 419–440.

[92] Wolfers J, Lozier A, Raposo G, Regnault A, Théry C, et al. Tumor-derived exosomes are a source of shared tumor rejection antigens for CTL cross-priming. Nature Medicine. 2001; **7**(3): 297–303.

[93] Zitvogel L, Regnault A, Lozier A, Wolfers J, Flament C, et al. Eradication of established murine tumors using a novel cell-free vaccine: dendritic cell derived exosomes. Nature Medicine. 1998; **4**(5): 594–600.

[94] Kim SH, Bianco NR, Shufesky WJ, Morelli AE, Robbins PD. Effective treatment of inflammatory disease models with exosomes derived from dendritic cells genetically modified to express IL-4. Journal of Immunology (Baltimore, Md.: 1950). 2007; **179**(4): 2242–2249.

[95] Zhang HG, Grizzle WE. Exosomes and cancer: a newly described pathway of immune suppression. Clinical Cancer Research: An Official Journal of the American Association for Cancer Research. 2011; **17**(5): 959–964.

[96] Andriantsitohaina R, Gaceb A, Vergori L, Martínez MC. Microparticles as Regulators of Cardiovascular Inflammation. Trends in Cardiovascular Medicine. 2012; **22**(4): 88–92.

[97] Hugel B, Martínez MC, Kunzelmann C, Freyssinet JM. Membrane microparticles: two sides of the coin. Physiology. 2005; **20**(1): 22–27.

[98] Yáñez-Mó M, Siljander PRM, Andreu Z, Zavec AB, Borràs FE, et al. Biological properties of extracellular vesicles and their physiological functions. Journal of Extracellular Vesicles. 2015; **4**.

[99] Mackie AR, Klyachko E, Thorne T, Schultz KM, Millay M, et al. Sonic hedgehog-modified human CD34+ cells preserve cardiac function after acute myocardial infarction. Circulation Research. 2012, **111**(3): 312–321.

[100] Paulis L, Fauconnier J, Cazorla O, Thireau J, Soleti R, Vidal B, Ouillé A, Bartholome M, Bideaux P, Roubille F, Guennec JY, Andriantsitohaina R, Martinez MC, Lacampagne A. Activation of Sonic hedgehog signaling in ventricular cardiomyocytes exerts cardioprotection against ischemia reperfusion injuries. Scientific Reports. 2015; 5 (7983): 1–10.

[101] Soleti R, Lauret E, Andriantsitohaina R, Carmen Martínez M. Internalization and induction of antioxidant messages by microvesicles contribute to the antiapoptotic effects on human endothelial cells. Free Radical Biology and Medicine. 2012; **53**(11): 2159–2170.

[102] Baj-Krzyworzeka M, Majka M, Pratico D, Ratajczak J, Vilaire G, Kijowski J, Reca R, Janowska-Wieczorek A, Ratajczak MZ. Platelet-derived microparticles stimulate proliferation, survival, adhesion, and chemotaxis of hematopoietic cells. Experimental Hematology. 2002; **30**(5): 450–459.

[103] Logozzi M, De Milito A, Lugini L, Borghi M, Calabrò L, Spada M, Perdicchio M, Marino ML, Federici C, Iessi E, Brambilla D, Venturi G, Lozupone F, Santinami M, Huber V, Maio M, Rivoltini L, Fais S. High levels of exosomes expressing CD63 and caveolin-1 in plasma of melanoma patients. PLoS One. 2009; 4(4): e5219.

[104] Alegre E, Zubiri L, Perez-Gracia JL, González-Cao M, Soria L Martín-Algarra S, González A. Circulating melanoma exosomes as diagnostic and prognosis biomarkers. Clinica Chimica Acta. 2016; **454**: 28–32.

[105] Koliha N, Heider U, Ozimkowski T, Wiemann M, Bosio A, Wild S. Melanoma affects the composition of blood cell-derived extracellular vesicles. Frontiers in Immunology. 2016; 7(282): 1–12.

[106] Peinado H, Alečković M, Lavotshkin S, Matei I, Costa-Silva B, Moreno-Bueno G, Hergueta-Redondo M, Williams C, García-Santos G, Ghajar C, Nitadori-Hoshino A, Hoffman C, Badal K, Garcia BA, Callahan MK, Yuan J, Martins VR, Skog J, Kaplan RN, Brady MS, Wolchok JD, Chapman PB, Kang Y, Bromberg J, Lyden D. Melanoma exosomes educate bone marrow progenitor cells toward a pro-metastatic phenotype through MET. Nature Medicine. 2012; **18**(6): 883–891.

[107] Laresche C, Pelletier F, Garnache-Ottou F, Lihoreau T, Biichlé S, Mourey G, Saas P, Humbert P, Seilles E, Aubin F. Increased levels of circulating microparticles are associated with increased procoagulant activity in patients with cutaneous malignant melanoma. The Journal of Investigative Dermatology. 2014; **134**(1): 176–182.

[108] Lima LG, Chammas R, Monteiro RQ, Moreira MEC, Barcinski MA. Tumor-derived microvesicles modulate the establishment of metastatic melanoma in a phosphatidylserine-dependent manner. Cancer Letters. 2009; **283**(2): 168–175.

[109] Xiao D, Ohlendorf J, Chen Y, Taylor DD, Rai SN, Waigel S, Zacharias W, Hao H, McMasters KM. Identifying mRNA, microRNA and protein profiles of melanoma exosomes. PLoS One. 2012; **7**(10).

[110] Lima LG, Oliveira AS, Campos LC, Bonamino M, Chammas R, Werneck C, Vicente CP, Barcinski MA, Petersen LC, Monteiro RQ. Malignant transformation in melanocytes is associated with increased production of procoagulant microvesicles. Thrombosis and Haemostasis. 2011; **106**(4): 712–723.

[111] Ekström EJ, Bergenfelz C, von Bülow V, Serifler F, Carlemalm E, Jönsson G, Andersson T, Leandersson K. WNT5A induces release of exosomes containing pro-angiogenic and immunosuppressive factors from malignant melanoma cells. Molecular Cancer. 2014; **13**: 88.

[112] Andreola G, Rivoltini L, Castelli C, Huber V, Perego P, Deho P, Squarcina P, Accornero P, Lozupone F, Lugini L, Stringaro A, Molinari A, Arancia G, Gentile M, Parmiani G, Fais S. Induction of lymphocyte apoptosis by tumor cell secretion of FasL-bearing microvesicles. The Journal of Experimental Medicine. 2002; **195**(10): 1303–1316.

[113] Birchmeier C, Birchmeier W, Gherardi E, Vande Woude GF. Met, metastasis, motility and more. Nature Reviews. Molecular Cell Biology. 2003; **4**(12): 915–925.

[114] Boccaccio C, Comoglio PM. Invasive growth: a MET-driven genetic programme for cancer and stem cells. Nature Reviews. Cancer. 2006; **6**(8): 637–645.

[115] Peruzzi B, Bottaro DP. Targeting the c-Met signaling pathway in cancer. Clinical Cancer Research: An Official Journal of the American Association for Cancer Research. 2006; **12** (12): 3657–3660.

[116] Hao S, Ye Z, Li F, Meng Q, Qureshi M, Yang J, Xiang J. Epigenetic transfer of metastatic activity by uptake of highly metastatic B16 melanoma cell-released exosomes. Experimental Oncology. 2006; **28**(2): 126–131.

[117] Muhsin-Sharafaldine MR, Saunderson SC, Dunn AC, Faed JM, Kleffmann T, McLellan AD. Procoagulant and immunogenic properties of melanoma exosomes, microvesicles and apoptotic vesicles. Oncotarget. 2016; **7**(35): 56279–56294.

[118] Lu J, Getz G, Miska EA, Alvarez-Saavedra E, Lamb J, Peck D, Sweet-Cordero A, Ebert BL, Mak RH, Ferrando AA, Downing JR, Jacks T, Horvitz HR, Golub TR. MicroRNA expression profiles classify human cancers. Nature. 2005; **435**(7043): 834–838.

[119] Zhang L, Huang J, Yang N, Greshock J, Megraw MS, et al. 2006. MicroRNAs exhibit high frequency genomic alterations in human cancer. Proceedings of the National Academy of Sciences of the United States of America, **103**(24): 9136–9141.

[120] Bemis LT, Chen R, Amato CM, Classen EH, Robinson SE, Coffey DG, Erickson PF, Shellman YG, Robinson WA. MicroRNA-137 targets microphthalmia-associated transcription factor in melanoma cell lines. Cancer Research. 2008; **68**(5): 1362–1368.

[121] Segura MF, Hanniford D, Menendez S, Reavie L, Zou X, Alvarez-Diaz S, Zakrzewski J, Blochin E, Rose A, Bogunovic D, Polsky D, Wei J, Lee P, Belitskaya-Levy I, Bhardwaj N, Osman I, Hernando E. Aberrant miR-182 expression promotes melanoma metastasis by repressing FOXO3 and microphthalmia-associated transcription factor. Proceedings of the National Academy of Sciences of the United States of America. 2009; **106**(6): 1814–1819.

[122] Penna E, Orso F, Cimino D, Tenaglia E, Lembo A, Quaglino E, Poliseno L, Haimovic A, Osella-Abate S, De Pittà C, Pinatel E, Stadler MB, Provero P, Bernengo MG, Osman I, Taverna D. MicroRNA-214 contributes to melanoma tumour progression through suppression of TFAP2C. The EMBO Journal. 2011; **30**(10): 1990–2007.

[123] Sand M, Skrygan M, Sand D, Georgas D, Gambichler T, Hahn SA, Altmeyer P, Bechara FG. Comparative microarray analysis of microRNA expression profiles in primary cutaneous malignant melanoma, cutaneous malignant melanoma metastases, and benign melanocytic nevi. Cell and Tissue Research. 2013; **351**(1): 85–98.

[124] Felicetti F, Errico MC, Bottero L, Segnalini P, Stoppacciaro A, Biffoni M, Felli N, Mattia G, Petrini M, Colombo MP, Peschle C, Carè A. The promyelocytic leukemia zinc finger-microRNA-221/-222 pathway controls melanoma progression through multiple oncogenic mechanisms. Cancer Research. 2008; **68**(8): 2745–2754.

[125] Mueller DW, Bosserhoff AK. Role of miRNAs in the progression of malignant melanoma. British Journal of Cancer. 2009; **101**(4): 551–556.

[126] Schultz J, Lorenz P, Gross G, Ibrahim S, Kunz M. MicroRNA let-7b targets important cell cycle molecules in malignant melanoma cells and interferes with anchorage-independent growth. Cell Research. 2008; **18**(5): 549–557.

[127] Pfeffer SR, Grossmann KF, Cassidy PB, Yang CH, Fan M, Kopelovich L, Leachman SA, Pfeffer LM. Detection of exosomal miRNAs in the plasma of melanoma patients. Journal of Clinical Medicine. 2015; **4**(12): 2012–2027.

[128] Alegre E, Sanmamed MF, Rodriguez C, Carranza O, Martín-Algarra S, González A. Study of circulating microRNA-125b levels in serum exosomes in advanced melanoma. Archives of Pathology & Laboratory Medicine. 2014; **138**(6): 828–832.

[129] Lunavat TR, Cheng L, Kim DK, Bhadury J, Jang SC, Lässer C, Sharples RA, López MD, Nilsson J, Gho YS, Hill AF, Lötvall J. Small RNA deep sequencing discriminates subsets of extracellular vesicles released by melanoma cells—evidence of unique microRNA cargos. RNA Biology. 2015; **12**(8): 810–823.

[130] Felicetti F, De Feo A, Coscia C, Puglisi R, Pedini F, Pasquini L, Bellenghi M, Errico MC, Pagani E, Carè A. Exosome-mediated transfer of miR-222 is sufficient to increase tumor malignancy in melanoma. Journal of Translational Medicine. 2016; **14**.

[131] Auge JM, Molina R, Filella X, Bosch E, Gonzalez Cao M, Puig S, Malvehy J, Castel T, Ballesta AM. S-100beta and MIA in advanced melanoma in relation to prognostic factors. Anticancer Research. 2005; **25**(3A): 1779–1782.

[132] Alegre E, Sammamed M, Fernández-Landázuri S, Zubiri L, González Á. Circulating biomarkers in malignant melanoma. Advances in Clinical Chemistry. 2015; **69**: 47–89.

[133] Díaz-Lagares A, Alegre E, Arroyo A, González-Cao M, Zudaire ME, Viteri S, Martín-Algarra S, González A. Evaluation of multiple serum markers in advanced melanoma. Tumour Biology: The Journal of the International Society for Oncodevelopmental Biology and Medicine. 2011; **32**(6): 1155–1161.

[134] Segura MF, Belitskaya-Lévy I, Rose AE, Zakrzewski J, Gaziel A, Hanniford D, Darvishian F, Berman RS, Shapiro RL, Pavlick AC, Osman I, Hernando E. Melanoma microRNA signature predicts post-recurrence survival. Clinical Cancer Research. 2010; **16**(5): 1577–1586.

[135] Leidinger P, Keller A, Borries A, Reichrath J, Rass K, Jager SU, Lenhof HP, Meese E. High-throughput miRNA profiling of human melanoma blood samples. BMC Cancer. 2010; **10**: 262.

[136] Fleming NH, Zhong J, da Silva IP, Vega-Saenz de Miera E, Brady B, Han SW, Hanniford D, Wang J, Shapiro RL, Hernando E, Osman I. Serum-based miRNAs in the prediction and detection of recurrence in melanoma patients. Cancer. 2015; **121**(1): 51–59.

[137] Friedman EB, Shang S, de Miera EVS, Fog JU, Teilum MW, Ma MW, Berman RS, Shapiro RL, Pavlick AC, Hernando E, Baker A, Shao Y, Osman I. Serum microRNAs as biomarkers for recurrence in melanoma. Journal of Translational Medicine. 2012; **10**: 155.

[138] Garbe C, Peris K, Hauschild A, Saiag P, Middleton M, Spatz A. Diagnosis and treatment of melanoma. European consensus-based interdisciplinary guideline update 2012. European Journal Cancer. 2012; **48**: 2375–2390.

[139] Harries M, Malvehy J, Lebbe C, Heron L, Amelio J, Szabo Z, Schadendorf D. Treatment patterns of advanced malignant melanoma (stage III–IV)—a review of current standards in Europe. European Journal of Cancer. 2016; **60**: 179–189.

[140] Garbe C, Peris K, Hauschild A, Saiag P, Middleton M, Bastholt L, Grob J, Malvehy J, Newton-Bishop J, Stratigos AJ, Pehamberger H, Eggermont AM. Diagnosis and treatment of melanoma. European consensus-based interdisciplinary guideline e Update 2016. European Journal of Cancer. 2016; **63**: 201–217.

[141] Su MY, Fisher DE. Immunotherapy in the precision medicine era: melanoma and beyond. PLoS Medicine. 2016; **13**: 1–6.

[142] Tang T, Eldabaje R, Yang L. Current status of biological therapies for the treatment of metastatic melanoma. Anticancer Research. 2016; **36**: 3229–3242.

[143] Lin WM, Fisher DE. Signaling and immune regulation in melanoma development and responses to therapy. Annual Review of Pathology Mechanisms of Disease. 2016; **5**: 1–28.

[144] Kirkwood JM, Tarhini AA. Biomarkers of therapeutic response in melanoma and renal cell carcinoma: potential in roads to improved immunotherapy. Journal of Clinical Oncology. 2009; **27**: 2583–2585.

[145] Drake CG, Lipson EJ, Brahmer JR. Breathing new life into immunotherapy: melanoma, lung and kidney cancer. Nature Review Clinical Oncology. 2014; **11**: 24–37.

[146] Luke J J, Ott PA. New developments in the treatment of metastatic melanoma role of dabrafenib–trametinib combination therapy. Drug Health Patient. 2014; **6**: 77–88.

[147] Amann VC, Ramelyte E, Thurneysen S, Pitocco R, Bentele-Jaberg N, Goldinger SM, Dummer R, Mangana J. Developments in targeted therapy in melanoma. European Journal of Surgical Oncology. 2016; 43(3): 581–593.

[148] Heppt MV, Dietrich C, Graf SA, Ruzicka T, Tietze JK, Berking C. The systemic management of advanced melanoma in 2016. Oncology Research Treatment. 2016; **39**: 635–642.

[149] Andtbacka RHI, Kaufman HL, Collichio F, Amatruda T, Senzer N, Chesney J, Delman KA, Spitler LE, Puzanov I, Agarwala SS, Milhem M, Cranmer L, Curti B, Lewis K, Ross M, Guthrie T, Linette GP, Daniels GA, Harrington K, Middleton MR, Miller Jr WH, Zager JS, Ye Y, Yao B, Li A, Doleman S, Vander Walde A, Gansert J, Coffin RS. Talimogene laherparepvec improves durable response rate in patients with advanced melanoma. Journal of Clinical Oncology. 2015; **33**: 2780–2788.

[150] Al-Jadidi HSK, Hossain MA. Determination of the total phenols, flavonoids and antimicrobial activity of the crude extracts from locally grown neem stems. Asian Pacific Journal of Tropical Disease. 2016; **6**(5): 376–379.

[151] Hoensch HP, Oertel R. The value of flavonoids for the human nutrition: short review and perspectives. Clinical Nutrition Experimental. 2015; **3**(2015): 8–14.

[152] Fiol M, Adermann S, Neugart S, Rohn S, Mügge C, Schreiner M, Kroh LW. Highly glycosylated and acylated flavonols isolated from kale (*Brassica oleracea* var. sabellica) – Structure-antioxidant activity relationship. Food Research International. 2012; **47**(1): 80–89.

[153] Olsen H, Aaby K, Borge GIA. Characterization, quantification, and yearly variation of the naturally occurring polyphenols in a common red variety of curly kale (*Brassica oleracea* L. convar. acephala var. sabellica cv. 'Redbor'). Journal of Agricultural and Food Chemistry. 2010; **58**(21): 11346–11354.

[154] Chanput W, Krueyos N, Ritthiruangdej P. Anti-oxidative assays as markers for anti-inflammatory activity of flavonoids. International Immunopharmacology. 2016; **40**(2016): 170–175.

[155] Guan LP, Liu BY. Antidepressant-like effects and mechanisms of flavonoids and related analogues. European Journal of Medicinal Chemistry. 2016; **121**(4): 47–57.

[156] Venturelli S, Burkard M, Biendl M, Lauer UM, Frank J, Busch C. Prenylated chalcones and flavonoids for the prevention and treatment of cancer. Original Research Article Nutrition. 2016; **32**: 1171–1178.

[157] Priyadarshani G, Amrutkar S, Nayak A, Banerjee UC, Kundu CN, Guchhait SS. Scaffold-hopping of bioactive flavonoids: Discovery of aryl-pyridopyrimidinones as potent anticancer agents that inhibit catalytic role of topoisomerase IIα. European Journal of Medicinal Chemistry. 2016; **122**: 43–54.

[158] Hatahet T, Morille M, Hommoss A, Dorandeu C, Müller RH, Bégu S. Dermal quercetin smartCrystals®: formulation development, antioxidant activity and cellular safety. European Journal of Pharmaceutics and Biopharmaceutics. 2016; **102**: 51–63.

[159] Nunes BC, Martins MM, Chang R, Morais SAL, Nascimento EA, Oliveira A, Cunha LCS, Silva CV, Teixeira TL, Ambrósio MALV, Martins CHG, Aquino FJT. Antimicrobial activity, cytotoxicity and selectivity index of *Banisteriopsis laevifolia* (A. Juss.) B. Gates leaves. Industrial Crops and Products. 2016; **92**: 277–289.

[160] Seleem D, Pardi V, Murata RM. Review of flavonoids: a diverse group of natural compounds with Anti-Candida albicans activity in vitro. Archives of Oral Biology. 2016; **27**: 1–26.

[161] Guidi L, Brunettib C, Finic A, Agatid G, Ferrinic F, Goric A, Tattini M. UV radiation promotes flavonoid biosynthesis, while negatively affecting the biosynthesis and the de-epoxidation of xanthophylls: Consequence for photoprotection? Environmental and Experimental Botany. 2016; **127**(2016): 14–25.

[162] Li F, Awale S, Tezuka Y, Kadota S. Cytotoxic constituents from Brazilian red propolis and their structure–activity relationship. Bioorganic and Medicinal Chemistry. 2008; **16** (2008): 5434–5440.

[163] Serafino A, Vallebona PS, Lazzarino G, Tavazzi B, Rasi G, Pierimarchi P, Andreola F, Moroni G, Galvano G, Galvano F, Garaci E. Differentiation of human melanoma cells induced by cyanidin-3-O-β-glucopyranoside. The FASEB Journal. 2004; 18(15): 1940–1942.

[164] Chen ND, Chen NF, Chen CW, Zhang L. A Novel Bihomoflavanonol with an Unprecedented Skeleton from *Pteridium aquilinum*. Chinese Herbal Medicines. 2013; **5**(2): 96–100.

[165] Chen X, Zhang B, Yuan X, Yang F, Liu J, Zhao Z, Liu L, Wang Y, Wang Z, Zheng Q. Isoliquiritigenin-induced differentiation in mouse melanoma B16F0 cell line. Oxidative Medicine and Cellular Longevity. 2012; **2012**: 1–11.

[166] Funari CS, Passalacqua TG, Rinaldo D, Napolitano A, Festa M, Capasso A, Piacente S, Pizza C, Young MCM, Durigan G, Silva DHS. Interconverting flavanone glucosides and other phenolic compounds in *Lippia salviaefolia* Cham. ethanol extracts. Phytochemistry. 2011; **72**(2011): 2052–2061.

[167] Nagao T, Abe F, Kinjo J, Okabe H. Antiproliferative Constituents in Plants 10. Flavones from the leaves of *Lantana montevidensis* BRIQ and consideration of structure-activity relationship. Biological and Pharmaceutical Bulletin. 2002; **25**(7): 875–879.

[168] Arung ET, Yoshikawa K, Shimizu K, Kondo R. Isoprenoid-substituted flavonoids from wood of *Artocarpus heterophyllus* on B16 melanoma cells: cytotoxicity and structural criteria. Fitoterapia. 2010; **81**(2010): 120–123.

[169] Hasnat MA, Pervin M, Lim JH, Lim BO. Apigenin attenuates melanoma cell migration by inducing anoikis through integrin and focal adhesion kinase inhibition. Molecules. 2015; **20**: 21157–21166.

[170] Spoerlein C, Mahal K, Schmidt H, Schobert R. Effects of chrysin, apigenin, genistein and their homoleptic copper(II) complexes on the growth and metastatic potential of cancer cells. Journal of Inorganic Biochemistry. 2013; **127**(2013): 107–115.

[171] Dar AA, Dangroo NA, Raina A, Qayum A, Singh S, Kumar A, Sangwan PL. Biologically active xanthones from *Codonopsis ovata*. Phytochemistry. 2016; **132**(2016): 102–108.

[172] Cao HH, Chu JH, Kwan HY, Su T, Yu H, Cheng CY, Fu XQ, Guo H, Li T, Tse AKW, Chou GX, Mo HB, Yu ZL. Inhibition of the STAT3 signaling pathway contributes to apigenin-mediated anti-metastatic effect in melanoma. Nature Scientific Reports. 2016; **6**(21731): 1–12.

[173] Choi EO, Cho EJ, Jeong JW, Park C, Hong SH, Hwang HJ, Moon SK, Son CG, Kim WJ, Choi YH. Baicalein inhibits the migration and invasion of B16F10 mouse melanoma cells through inactivation of the PI3K/Akt signaling pathway. Biomolecules and Therapeutics. 2016; **2016**: 1–9.

[174] Martınez C, Yanez A, Vicente V, Alcaraz M, Benavente-Garcıa O, Castillo J, Lorente J, Lozano JA. Effects of several polyhydroxylated flavonoids on the growth of B16F10 melanoma and Melan-a melanocyte cell lines: influence of the sequential oxidation state of the flavonoid skeleton. Melanoma Research. 2003; **13**: 3–9.

[175] Banskota AH, Nagaoka T, Sumioka LY, Tezuka Y, Awale S, Midorikawa K, Matsushige K, Kadota S. Antiproliferative activity of the Netherlands propolis and its active principles in cancer cell lines. Journal of Ethnopharmacology. 2002; **80**(2002): 67–73.

[176] Sánchez NA, Conesa CM, Ortega VV. Effects of IFN-α and diosmin on metastasic murine-lung melanoma. Revista Española de Patología. 2008; 41(2): 123–129.

[177] Alvarez N, Vicente V, Martınez C. Synergistic effect of diosmin and interferon-α on metastatic pulmonary melanoma. Cancer Biotherapy and Radiopharmaceuticals. 2008; **24**(3): 347–352.

[178] Martínez C, Vicente V, Yáñez J, Alcaraz M, Castells MT, Canteras M, Benavente-García O, Castillo J. The effect of the flavonoid diosmin, grape seed extract and red wine on the pulmonary metastatic B16F10 melanoma. Histology and Histopathology. 2005; **20**: 1121–1129.

[179] Conesa CM, Ortega VV, Gascón MJY, Baños MA, Jordana MC, Garcia OB, Castillo JN. Treatment of metastatic melanoma B16F10 by the flavonoids tangeretin, rutin, and diosmin. Journal of Agricultural and Food Chemistry. 2005; **53**: 6791–6797.

[180] Zater H, Huet J, Fontaine V, Benayache S, Stevigny C, Duez P, Benayache F. Chemical constituents, cytotoxic, antifungal and antimicrobial properties of *Centaurea diluta* Ait. subsp. algeriensis (Coss. & Dur.) Maire. Asian Pacific Journal of Tropical Medicine. 2016; **9**(6): 554–561.

[181] Tundis R, Deguin B, Loizzo MR, Bonesi M, Statti GA, Tillequin F, Menichini F. Potential antitumor agents: Flavones and their derivatives from *Linaria reflexa* Desf. Bioorganic and Medicinal Chemistry Letters. 2005; **15**(2005): 4757–4760.

[182] George VC, Kumar DRN, Suresh PK, Kumar S, Kumar RA. Comparative studies to evaluate relative in vitro potency of luteolin in inducing cell cycle arrest and apoptosis in HaCaT and A375 cells. Asian Pacific Journal of Cancer Prevention. 2013; **14**(2): 631–637.

[183] Kim JK, Kang KA, Ryu YS, Piao MJ, Han X, Oh MC, Boo SJ, Jeong SU, Jeong YJ, Chae S, Na SY, Hyun JW. Induction of endoplasmic reticulum stress via reactive oxygen species mediated by luteolin in melanoma cells. Anticancer Research. 2016; **36**: 2281–2290.

[184] Ruan JS, Liu YP, Zhang L, Yan LG, Fan FT, Shen CS, Wang AY, Zheng SZ, Wang SM, Lu Y. Luteolin reduces the invasive potential of malignant melanoma cells by targeting β3 integrin and the epithelial-mesenchymal transition. Acta Pharmacologica Sinica. 2012; **33**: 1325–1331.

[185] Krajnovic T, Kaluderovic GN, Wessjohann LA, Mijatovic SA, Ivanic DM. Versatile antitumor potential of isoxanthohumol: enhancement of paclitaxel activity in vivo. Pharmacological Research. 2016; **105**(2016): 62–73.

[186] Syed DN, Chamcheu JC, Khan MI, Sechi M, Lall RK, Adhami VM, Mukhtar H. Fisetin inhibits human melanoma cell growth through direct binding to p70S6K and mTOR: findings from 3-D melanoma skin equivalents and computational modeling. Biochemical Pharmacology. 2014; **89**(2014): 349–360.

[187] Pal HC, Diamond AC, Strickland LR, Kappes JC, Katiyar SK, Elmets CA, Athar M, Afaq F. Fisetin, a dietary flavonoid, augments the anti-invasive and anti-metastatic potential of sorafenib in melanoma. Oncotarget. 2015; **7**(2): 1227–1241.

[188] Syed DN, Afaq F, Maddodi N, Johnson JJ, Sarfaraz S, Ahmad A, Setaluri1 V, Mukhtar H. Inhibition of human melanoma cell growth by the dietary flavonoid fisetin is associated with disruption of Wnt/b-catenin signaling and decreased MITF levels. Journal of Investigative Dermatology. 2011; **131**: 1291–1299.

[189] Tundis R, Loizzo MR, Menichini F, Bonesi M, Colica C, Menichini F. In vitro cytotoxic activity of extracts and isolated constituents of *Salvia leriifolia* Benth. against a panel of human cancer cell lines. Chemistry and Biodiversity. 2011; **8**(2011): 1152–1162.

[190] Moon SS, Rahman AA, Manir M, Ahamed J. Kaempferol glycosides and cardenolide glycosides, cytotoxic constituents from the seeds of *Draba nemorosa* (Brassicaceae). Archives of Pharmaceutical Research. 2010; **33**(8): 1169–1173.

[191] Syed DN, Lall RK, Chamcheu JC, Haidar O, Mukhtar H. Involvement of ER stress and activation of apoptotic pathways in fisetin induced cytotoxicity in human melanoma. Archives of Biochemistry and Biophysics. 2014; **563**: 108–117.

[192] Zhang W, Lan Y, Huang Q, Hua Z. Galangin induces B16F10 melanoma cell apoptosis via mitochondrial pathway and sustained activation of p38 MAPK. Cytotechnology. 2013; **65**: 447–455.

[193] Zhang W, Tang B, Huang Q, Hua Z. Galangin inhibits tumor growth and metastasis of B16F10 melanoma. Journal of Cellular Biochemistry. 2013; **114**: 152–161.

[194] Lu YH, Tao L, Wang ZT, Wei DZ, Xiang HB. Mechanism and inhibitory effect of galangin and its flavonoid mixture from *Alpinia officinarum* on mushroom tyrosinase and B16 murine melanoma cells. Journal of Enzyme Inhibition and Medicinal Chemistry. 2007; **22**(4): 433–438.

[195] Wu J, Du J, Fu X, Liu B, Cao H, Li T, Su T, Xu J, Tse AKW, Yu ZL. Icaritin, a novel FASN inhibitor, exerts anti-melanoma activities through IGF-1R/STAT3 signaling. Oncotarget. 2016; **7**(32): 51251–51269.

[196] Kim YK, Kim YS, Choi SU, Ryu SY. Isolation of flavonol rhamnosides from *Loranthus tanakae* and cytotoxic effect of them on human tumor cell lines. Archives of Pharmaceutical Research. 2004; **27**(1): 44–47.

[197] Pradhan SJ, Mishra R, Sharma P, Kundu GC. Quercetin and sulforaphane in combination suppress the progression of melanoma through the down-regulation of matrix metalloproteinase-9. Experimental and Therapeutic Medicine. 2010; **1**: 915–920.

[198] Cao HH, Tse AKW, Kwan HY, Yu H, Cheng CY, Su T, Fong WF, Yu ZL. Quercetin exerts anti-melanoma activities and inhibits STAT3 Signaling. Biochemical Pharmacology. 2014; **87**(2014): 424–434.

[199] Cao HH, Cheng CY, Su T, Fu XQ, Guo H, Li T, Tse AKW, Kwan HY, Yu H, Yu ZL. Quercetin inhibits HGF/c-Met signaling and HGF stimulated melanoma cell migration and invasion. Molecular Cancer. 2015; **14**(103): 1–12.

[200] Martin S, Lamb HK, Brady C, Lefkove B, Bonner MY, Thompson P, Lovat PE, Arbiser JL, Hawkins AR, Redfern CPF. Inducing apoptosis of cancer cells using small-molecule plant compounds that bind to GRP78. British Journal of Cancer. 2013; **109**: 433–443.

[201] Li LH, Wu LJ, Jiang YY, Tashiro SI, Onodera S, Uchiumi F, Ikejima T. Silymarin enhanced cytotoxic effect of anti-Fas agonistic antibody CH11 on A375-S2 cells. Journal of Asian Natural Products Research. 2014; **9**(7): 593–602.

[202] Russo A, Cardile V, Lombardo L, Vanella L, Acquaviva R. Genistin inhibits UV light-induced plasmid DNA damage and cell growth in human melanoma cells. Journal of Nutritional Biochemistry. 2006; **17**(2006): 103–108.

[203] Song NR., Lee E, Byun S, Kim JE, Mottamal M, Park JHY, Lim SS, Bode AM, Lee HJ, Lee KW, Dong Z. Isoangustone A. A novel licorice compound, inhibits cell proliferation by targeting PI3K, MKK4, and MKK7 in human melanoma. Cancer Prevention Research. 2013; **6**(12):1293–303.

[204] Casagrande F, Darbon JM. Effects of structurally related flavonoids on cell cycle progression of human melanoma cells: regulation of cyclin-dependent kinases CDK2 and CDK1. Biochemical Pharmacology. 2001; **61**(2001): 1205–1215.

Chapter 9

An Update On Natural Compounds and Their Modern Formulations for the Management of Malignant Melanoma

Danciu Corina, Soica Codruta, Antal Diana,
Alexandra Popescu, Roxana Ghiulai,
Ioana Zinuca Pavel, Stefana Avram,
Minda Daliana and Cristina Dehelean

Additional information is available at the end of the chapter

http://dx.doi.org/10.5772/67647

Abstract

The chapter includes a brief presentation of the types of skin cancer. The most aggressive type of skin cancer, melanoma, is discussed from the point of view of incidence, molecular, and immunohistochemical mechanism along with the most important biomarkers for identification. Recent studies containing active phytocompounds with chemopreventive activity pointing toward phytochemicals used for melanoma prevention and therapy are reviewed. Modern physicochemical formulations for the enhancement of bioavailability of some active phytochemicals with chemopreventive activity for malignant melanoma are discussed.

Keywords: malignant melanoma, mechanism, biomarkers, active phytocompounds, modern formulations

1. Introduction

Skin cancer, with its many forms, is one of the most prevalent diseases today. In the last decades, there was a rising incidence in the reported cases of skin cancer and is estimated that one out of three Caucasians may develop a type of skin cancer in their lifetime [1, 2]. There are three common types of skin cancer, namely basal cell carcinoma (BCC), squamous cell carcinoma (SCC), and melanoma. Basal and squamous cell carcinomas are also known as non-melanoma skin cancer (NMSC) [1, 3].

Melanoma and non-melanoma skin cancers represent the most common malignancies worldwide [2, 3]. Wehner et al. indicated that approximately 30% of white people are likely to develop NMSC in their lifetime as a result of increased exposure to ultraviolet radiation [4]. It is considered that exposure to high doses of ultraviolet B radiation can cause basal cell carcinoma, while squamous cell carcinoma can be triggered after a chronic exposure to UV [2]. Melanoma in the first place and squamous cell carcinoma in the second place are tumor types with a high risk of metastasis, while basal cell carcinoma rarely does. Usually, these types of cancer affect people with white skin, blue eyes, and red hair [5]. Regarding gender, men are more likely to develop a type of NMSC in their lifetime than women [1].

As already mentioned above, one of the most important risk factors for developing skin cancer is considered exposure to ultraviolet radiation (UV) [6]. There are three types of UV radiation depending on the wavelength: UVA, UVB, and UVC. UV radiation especially ultraviolet B radiation is known to cause oxidative stress, inflammation, DNA damage, and apoptotic cell death in the skin [6, 7]. UV exposure also determines immunosuppression and photoaging of the skin [8]. People who use indoor tanning especially at an early age (before 25 years) are exposed to a higher risk of developing a form of skin cancer in their lifetime [4]. Among UV exposure, ozone depletion, genetics, and immune suppression are also incriminated in the rising incidence of skin cancer [9]. Another factor considered responsible for skin cancer growth is long-term exposure to arsenic, a class I human carcinogen found in industrial, agricultural, and medicinal substances [10, 11]. PUVA therapy is a treatment used for severe skin diseases which consists of psoralens (P) and exposure to ultraviolet A radiation (UVA). PUVA may induce skin cancer by photomutagenicity and photoinduced immunosuppression. It is important to evaluate the risk-benefit ratio before starting with the PUVA therapy [10, 12, 13]. Exposure to ionizing radiation, inorganic metals, and polycyclic hydrocarbons are also risk factors for skin cancer development [10].

1.1. Basal cell carcinoma

Basal cell carcinoma (BCC) is considered the most common type of skin cancer affecting people worldwide [5, 3]. It develops in the basal layer of the skin, from keratinocyte stem cells. Usually BCC appears *de novo* on hair-bearing skin, more often in adults. The most frequent BCC is considered the nodular/nodulo-ulcerative type which is commonly found on the neck and head. It looks like a red or pink papule with raised edges, telangiectasias, pearly appearance, and central small ulcers. Nodular BCC develops slowly but in time it can invade the tissue around it producing significant damage [14].

Exposure to high doses and intermittent UV radiation can trigger BCC [5]. Most cases of BCC were reported in Australia and are mainly attributed to UV radiation [3]. UVB is considered the most harmful environmental factor that can induce DNA mutations after exposure. BCC can develop through alteration of p53 and PTCH1 tumor-suppressor genes.

In general, BCC is found on the arms, head, neck, or the back and is more prevalent in people with light hair, blue or green eyes, and freckles. Other factors reported to increase the risk of BCC are genetic conditions, ionized radiation, genodermatoses, exposure to chemical carcinogens, organic and inorganic solvents, and organophosphate compounds [14, 15]. In some cases of superficial BCC, human papillomavirus (HPV) is considered to be a risk factor in cancer growth. Also, immunosuppression caused by other diseases is considered to have a role in NMSC development [14].

There are various types of treatment options for BCC. The therapeutic approach depends on the location and the size of the tumor. Also, it is important to know the morphology and histologic subtype of the tumor and whether or not it has spread to nearby tissues. The most common therapeutic option is surgical excision of the skin [14, 15]. In most of the cases, the method is applicable if the lesion is less than 2 cm in diameter and is found in the trunk or extremities. An advantage of surgical excision is that after surgery, the lesion can be histologically analyzed and the tumor subtype can be determined. Also, there are disadvantages of using this method, including the possibility of infection and the presence of scars [14]. When surgery is not possible due to tumor location or because it is locally advanced, radiation therapy is an option [15]. The method can be used when the tumor is located on the ears, nose, eyelids, and lips. Other therapeutical options include photodynamic therapy, cryosurgery [14, 16], and topical therapies with imiquimod, an immune response modifier or 5-fluorouracil, a pyrimidine analog [15]. It is important to properly treat BCC because it has a high tendency to reappear if it remains untreated. Even if treated, in 18% of the cases, BCC will reappear in a few years after treatment [14].

1.2. Squamous cell carcinoma

Squamous cell carcinoma (SCC) also arises from keratinocytes and is the second most common type of skin cancer [17, 18]. SCC can be localized in the epidermis, known as *in situ* SCC, or it can extend to the dermis or deeper in the skin, known as invasive SCC. UV exposure is the main risk factor incriminated for SCC development. Cumulative high doses of UV radiation are responsible for SCC evolution [17], also non-healing wounds or chronic lesions that were linked with previous cases of chronic immuno-inflammation are associated with SCC [5]. SCC is found at a higher prevalence at people who smoke, compared to non-smokers, probably as a result of the immunosuppressive effects caused by smoking. Viruses, such as human papillomavirus (HPV), human immunodeficiency virus (HIV), or human herpes virus (HHV), also increase the risk for SCC. Exposure to chemical agents, including arsenic and polycyclic aromatic hydrocarbons, can lead in time to SCC. People with genetic disorders, such as xeroderma pigmentosum and oculocutaneous albinism, are more likely to develop SCC [17].

This type of cancer is usually found in people older than 50 years and is located on the head and neck, being more frequent in males, than in females [17]. Usually, it does not metastasize, but when it does, the survival rate is poor, between 25 and 40% [18].

SCC treatment depends on the location of the tumor, the size, and whether or not it has metastasized. For high-risk tumors, Mohs micrographic surgery (microscopically oriented histographic surgery) is considered the best method, while for low-risk SCC, surgical excision is the most common therapeutic option. In order to have a low recurrence rate, safety margins must be also excised. They vary between 4 and 10 mm according to tumor size. Cryosurgery is another surgical method used for small tumors [17, 19]. Nonsurgical treatments are also effective therapies for SCC, namely radiation therapy, topical application of 5-fluorouracil and imiquimod, and photodynamic therapy. There are studies, which indicate that non-steroidal anti-inflammatory drugs are useful in the prevention and treatment of SCC [17]. Other drugs used rather in the prevention than in the treatment of SCC are retinoids. The results of Tran et al. showed that the topical administration of retinoids neutralizes vitamin A depletion induced by exposure to UVB radiation and thus has a beneficial role on recovery [20]. Recurrence rate is around 5 years after treatment, so it is important that the patients are closely monitorized [17].

1.3. Melanoma

Melanoma is a melanocytic neoplasia, and it is thought to be the rarest form of skin cancer and the most aggressive one [1]. It is considered that melanocytic nevi are precursors for melanoma. They are benign nevi, usually found in body areas exposed to the sun and can undergo transformation due to several risk factors and then progress into dysplastic nevi, which can further turn into melanoma [21].

In order to establish whether or not a melanocytic nevus has a malignant transformation, five characteristics can be followed, also known as the ABCDE of melanoma. The first is ***Asymmetry*** —usually a benign melanocytic nevus is symmetric; ***Border***—the margins of the nevus are irregular; ***Color***—the pigmentation is not equable on the entire surface of the nevus; ***Diameter*** —the melanocytic nevus is bigger than 6 mm, ***Evolution*** [1].

Exposure to UV radiation is considered one of the most important factors in melanoma development. Among it, genetic conditions, multiple nevi, and exposure to some chemical agents are incriminated as risk factors [22, 23]. People who have first-degree relatives with melanoma are exposed to a higher risk in developing this type of skin cancer. Immunosuppression is also thought to have a role in melanoma growth. Other risk factors include the exposure to some pesticides, such as parathion, carbaryl, maneb/mancozeb, and benomyl [23].

Commonly, melanoma appears on males older than 54 years and females older than 45 years and is mostly found on the trunk, face, and ears. In the last years, the number of melanomas found in women aged 15–24 has increased [23]. Indoor tanning is considered to have an important role in this higher incidence rate [24].

There are different forms of melanoma, the most common being melanoma of intermittently sun-exposed skin, acral (and mucosal) melanoma, lentigo maligna melanoma, and nodular melanoma. Melanoma of intermittently sun-exposed skin is generally found in Caucasian people and is related with BRAF mutations and melanocytic nevi. It affects more women than men, and is located in the lower extremities and the trunk [22]. Acral (and mucosal) melanomas can appear in areas of the body that are not frequently exposed to UV radiation such as the soles of the feet and the palms of the hands. This type is found in black people and is associated with chromosomal aberrations [5, 22]. Lentigo maligna (solar) melanoma develops after chronic exposure to UV radiation. It is found in people older than 60 years and is correlated with genomic aberrations and the lack of BRAF mutations. Nodular melanoma is a rapid growing tumor that can have pagetoid spread, commonly found in people older than 30 years [22].

Tumor thickness (mm)	Excisional margins (cm)
in situ melanoma	0.5
<1.0	1.0
1.0–4.0	2.0
>4.0	≥2.0

Melanoma has a high metastatic potential through lymphatic and vascular channels. Early diagnosis is very important because in the early stages it can be removed surgically. In order to reduce the risk of tumor recurrence, along with the tumoral tissue, part of the surrounding normal structure is also removed. The American Academy of Dermatology recommends the following excisional margins (cm) according to tumor thickness (mm) [1]:

When there is evidence of metastasis, systemic chemotherapy is used. Frequently used drugs are cisplatin, mitomycin, doxorubicin, and temozolomide. Immunotherapies are also an option for metastatic melanomas. This includes administration of interferon-alpha or interleukin 2 [1].

Patients with high-risk melanomas must be physically monitored every 3 months for the first 3 years, considered the period when metastases are more likely to appear and thereafter biannually or annually [22].

2. Melanoma: incidence, molecular, and immunohistochemical mechanism

2.1. Incidence and mortality of melanoma

From the total number of all skin cancer cases, melanoma represents less than 2%, nevertheless being the major cause of death from skin cancer. Despite this steadily increasing incidence of melanoma, the mortality caused by this pathology stabilized in the last 20 years, on the strength of advances in medical care. At present, the survival rate of 5 years exceeds 90%, being associated with the moment of diagnosis [25].

It was predicted that 73,870 patients would be diagnosed with this condition in 2015. The most affected segment was the white people of non-Hispanic origin. According to *American Cancer Society*, the incidence rates vary from 1 per 100,000 annual cases in blacks to 4 in Hispanics, and 25 in non-Hispanic whites. Although it can appear independently of age, usually the elders are more affected by melanoma, being diagnosed at an average age of 62 years [25]. By the age of 50, women are more affected than men; however, by age 65 the incidence is two times higher in men than in women, tripling by the age of 80. These disparities are pursuant to ultraviolet radiation, either solar or artificial. During 1930, the incidence of melanoma was 1 in 1500 American people, reaching 1 in 68 in 2002. Through the years 2002–2012, the incidence extended with 1.8% per year. This enhancement of new cases of melanoma is partially linked to the development of new, modern, diagnostic methods, and also to the rising of the average life expectancy [25, 26].

In the US, during the year 2015, there were estimated 73,870 new cases of melanoma from which 42,670 cases were in male and 31,200 in female. The total melanoma deaths in US, in 2015, reached 9940, whence 6640 cases in men and 3300 in women. In the State of California, the total number of new melanoma cases reaches the upper limit (8560 cases), being followed by Florida (5480 cases), while the minimum was observed in the District of Columbia (80 cases), followed by Alaska (100) [27].

In Europe, 100,000 new cases of melanoma were diagnosed during 2012, mostly in the central and eastern part. The incidence of melanoma deaths was high in these regions of Europe (36%); from a total of 22,000 deaths, 8000 cases were found in the Central and Eastern Europe. However, the most cases of melanoma in Europe were in the Nordic regions and the Netherlands [28].

A recent study has compared the incidence and mortality rate in 11 countries from Europe: Bosnia and Herzegovina, Bulgaria, Croatia, Cyprus, Czech Republic, Malta, Romania, Serbia, Slovenia, and Turkey. Regarding the distribution of incidence upon age and sex, it was observed that younger females and males had the same incidence rates, although it increased in middle-aged and older men in comparison with females from the same category. The incidence rate of melanoma was increased in most of the countries, the higher trend concerning the young people (25–49 years) being observed in Slovenia, though in men aged 50–69, the incidence was important in Slovenia, Slovakia, Bulgaria, and Serbia. After the age of 70, the rate was raised in men, independently on the level of the incidence in the country. In women, the rate of melanoma was increased in most regions of Europe, especially in Slovenia, whatever the age. For 50–69 aged females, the incidence was higher in Bulgaria and Romania, while for women older than 70 years, a greater incidence in Serbia and Slovakia was remarked. For this category of women, the incidence was also significant in Bulgaria, Croatia, and the Czech Republic. Regarding the melanoma mortality rates in the 11 countries of Europe previously mentioned, men were more affected than women in most countries. In younger groups, the mortality rate was non-significantly decreased, in both men and women. Men of middle and older age had a relevant mortality in Serbia. Also, the elders were affected in Turkey and Czech Republic. On the other hand, women aged 50–69 had elevated rates of mortality in most countries, particularly in Slovenia. The mortality increased with age, mainly in Serbia and Slovenia [29].

2.2. Molecular and immunohistochemical mechanism in melanoma

From the embryonic neural crest cells, throughout development, melanoblasts are first taken into dermis, and then these precursors migrate toward the epidermis to settle in its basal epithelial layer, on the basal lamina. Melanoblasts arise into dermis by 11 weeks. Melanin pigment is produced at around 12 weeks [30].

Differentiated melanocytes are hold tightly in the basement membrane, when they arrive in contact with keratinocytes. At higher epidermal layers, they are unable to survive, unless turned into nevi or melanomas. Keratinocytes play an important role in the maintenance of melanocytes homeostasis. The impairment of this homeostasis affects the epidermal melanin unit, giving rise to an unceasing proliferation of melanocytes. It is presumed that melanoma cells get rid of the keratinocytes control by several mechanisms: (a) down-regulation of some molecules (like E-cadherin) that play a role in their communication and adhesion to keratinocytes; (b) up-regulation of certain molecules that participate in cell signaling significant for melanoma-melanoma and melanoma-fibroblast interplays, like N-cadherin, zonula occludens protein-1, and MCAM (*melanoma cell adhesion molecule*); and (c) impaired expression of several proteins that bind the extracellular matrix with the repercussions for the retention into the basement membrane [31, 32].

Recent studies revealed the up-regulation of CCN3 protein in melanocyte-keratinocyte co-culture, influencing some important characteristics in the physiology of melanocytes. This matricellular protein is overexpressed in some malignant diseases being related to the evolution of prostate cancer, carcinoma of renal cells, and Ewing's sarcoma; moreover, its expression is linked to the differentiation of tumors in rhabdomyosarcoma and cartilage malignancies [33–35]. Depending on the type of cancer, CCN3 influence divergently the genesis of tumor. Therefore, in gliomas it manifests antiproliferative effects, as well as in chronic myeloid leukemia cells. By contrast, it stimulates the invasion of Ewing's sarcoma cells [36, 37]. Regarding the effects of CCN3 on melanocytes, it reduces their proliferation and is essential for the melanocyte network organization [38]. In addition to this, it enhances the adherence of melanocytes to the type-IV collagen from basement membrane. Studies *in vivo* show that CCN3 overexpression is associated with an extremely attenuated invasion of melanoma cells, through the inhibition of MMP (*matrix metalloproteinase*) expression [31, 39].

The progression of melanoma comprises five distinct phases. First of all, hyperplasia of melanocytes gives rise to nevi; these can be acquired or congenital. The second phase is characterized by dysplastic nevi along with cytological and architectural abnormality. The third one corresponds to radial growth phase (RGP) melanoma, distinguished by the presence of tumor cells within the epidermis, or their invasion through the superficial dermis, having a reduced ability to spread from the primary site. The last stage is the vertical growth phase (VGP), which is featured by the profound invasion of tumor cells into the dermis and hypodermic tissue, augmenting the systemic dissemination risk. Lastly, metastasis occurs, being the most advanced phase of this condition, as a result of the altered homeostasis in the skin. The impaired mechanisms of homeostatic control determine the development of melanoma, since these mechanisms control the proliferation of cells, as well as their differentiation and apoptosis [33, 41].

Throughout the development stages of melanoma, CCN3 protein expression is down-regulated. Immunohistochemical techniques performed on melanoma cells evidentiated the inversely proportional interdependence between CCN3 expression and tumor dimension. The transduction of CCN3 in progressive melanomas inhibited the activity of matrix metalloproteinases MMP 2 and 9, resulting in an intense reduction of tumor invasion. Hence, the absence of CCN3 expression in melanomas is related to an invasive phenotype [31].

Melanomas can appear from melanocytes that have the role in the production of melanin pigment, and also in its storage and distribution to keratinocytes. There are other melanomas that arise from nevi, particularly dysplastic or giant congenital nevi. Melanomas are divided into four clinic-histological types: superficial-spreading melanoma, nodular form, lentigo maligna, and acral lentiginous type. Different factors are involved in the development of melanoma, such as genetic triggers, methylation of DNA, acetylation, or milieu factors [40, 41].

Impairment in tumor-suppressor genes such as mutation, deletion, translocation, or activation of proto-oncogenes has a significant role in mutagenesis. Mutation or deletion of CDKN2A anti-oncogene and CDK4 proto-oncogene is related to the development of familial melanoma, which constitute 8–12% of total melanomas [42]. This type of melanoma is characterized by an abnormal regulation of cell cycle by cyclin-dependent enzymes. In this case, the 9p21 chromosome has a germline mutation in the locus of CDKN 2A gene, affecting two proteins p16 and p14 or Arf that have a suppressive role. The p16 protein has an inhibitory effect on cyclin D/CDK4 and CDK6, influencing therefore pRB (*retinoblastoma protein*) which, through liberation of E2F, change the G1 phase of cell cycle into S phase [43, 44]. It was discovered lately that E2F1 protein, as well, manifests a suppressor function through p53 or p73. Between 10 and 30% of familial melanoma cases are due to CDKN2A mutation. NRAS and p16 mutations are also incriminated in some isolated cases of melanoma. Mutation of CDKN2A can lead to multiple melanomas. This alteration seldom appears in actinic keratosis, skin carcinomas, and other types of cancers [45, 46].

The p14 protein, encoded by CDKN2A reading frame, affects the p53 protein through the influence on other protein, Mdm2. The p14 deprivation lowers the activity of p53 [47]. Studies taken on mice models have shown that p14 can determine apoptosis of oncogene-activated melanocytes [48, 49].

It is known that pigmentation of the skin that depends on the amount of melanin is in direct relation with the development of melanoma. It is 10 times more frequently in whites than in blacks; however, people affected by albinism are exceptionally affected. The highly polymorphic melanocortin 1-receptor gene (MC1R) situated on 16q24 chromosome controls sun sensitivity [50, 51]. It codifies the transmembrane receptor coupled with G protein. The pituitary polypeptide POMC (*pro-opiomelanocortin*) is cleaved to give rise to different peptide hormones, including MSH (*melanocyte-stimulating hormone*), that acts through this receptor, enhancing cAMP and therefore stimulating tyrosinase enzyme activity. As a fact, keratinocytes can also produce these molecules. The synthesis of dark eumelanin and yellow cysteine-abundant pheomelanin is augmented by MSH. It was observed that people with MC1R variations evolve to earlier melanoma [52]. New studies have revealed that MITF (*microphthalmia-associated transcription factor*) gene found on 3p14 chromosome has a role in the promotion of melanocyte cell cycle progression [53].

3. The most important biomarkers for the identification of malignant melanoma

In order to diagnose malignant melanoma, there are several methods and techniques that when combined can give a certain degree of surety to the diagnosis.

As previously discussed, the first step in diagnosing malignant melanoma is the visual inspection of the lesion and the assessment of the well-known **ABCDE** signs (**A**symmetry, irregular **B**orders, uneven **C**olor, large **D**iameter, **E**volution) [54]. These findings are combined with dermatoscopical inspection of the lesion in order to confirm or to infirm the naked eye observations. If these findings lead to a suspicion of malignancy, then most likely a wide-excision surgery is performed and upon the assessment, a sentinel lymph node biopsy is also performed

http://dx.doi.org/10.5772/67647

[55]. In order to establish a certain diagnosis, there are various sets of markers specific for this type of cancer, which enable the obtaining of a definite diagnosis and/or the prognosis and staging of the disease, which can be identified by several methods [56].

There are different types of biomarkers to investigate malignant melanoma such as the microscopical markers identified upon the examination of the tumor and the immunohistochemical biomarkers identified upon isolation from the tumor/tissue section. Another type of malignant melanoma markers is the serological biomarkers that are identified from the peripheral blood samples of the patients by various methods.

3.1. Microscopical biomarkers in malignant melanoma

Breslow thickness refers to the thickness of the tumor and was demonstrated to be the most important prognostic histopathological factor. This parameter is of great importance and is used to stage malignant melanoma [57].

Tumor ulceration is the loss of epidermal integrity of the melanoma and is used for staging malignant melanoma and was linked to rapid tumor growth and metastasis [58].

The mitotic rate refers to the number of mitoses per square millimeter. A high mitotic rate is correlated with high metabolic cell activity and predicts rapid tumor growth and metastasis. Also, increased mitotic rate was linked with decreased survival [59].

3.2. Immunohistochemical and serological biomarkers in malignant melanoma

Immunohistochemical biomarkers		
Biomarker type	**Significance/location**	**Specificity/involvement in prognosis**
2.1 **HMB 45** (human melanoma black 45)	Monoclonal antibody for the premelanosome protein (Pmel antigen) [60]	Very specific for melanoma, especially for primary lesions, not being able to identify other types of tumors [61, 62]
2.2 **Melan A**	Antigen recognized by T cells 1 or MART-1 (membrane protein of melanosomes and endoplasmic reticulum found in melanocytes, melanoma, and endoplasmic reticulum) [63, 64]	Higher sensitivity for primary melanomas compared to metastatic ones [65]
2.3 **S 100**	Family of proteins expressed in Schwann cells, melanocytes, glial cells, is involved in many cellular functions such as the activation of cell processes along the $Ca2+$ signal-transduction pathway [66, 67]	Low specificity, used together with other biomarkers [65]
2.4 **Tyrosinase**	Oxidative enzyme involved in melanin production in melanocytes and melanoma; detected with T311 monoclonal IgG antibody [68]	Elevated sensitivity for primary melanoma than for later stage tumors [68]
2.5 **Ki-67**	Protein biomarker for cellular proliferation [69]	Adjunctive diagnostic biomarker [70]
2.6 **Nestin**	Filament protein associated with migration and metastasis [71]	Advanced stages of the disease (T3 and T4) [71]

Immunohistochemical biomarkers		
Biomarker type	**Significance/location**	**Specificity/involvement in prognosis**
2.7 **Vimentin**	Ectodermal, neural, and pancreatic progenitor cell marker, overexpression in cancer [72]	Tumor growth, invasion, and poor prognosis [72]
2.8 **Chondroitin sulfate proteoglycan 4**	Located in melanocytes, promotes cell adhesion, growth, migration, motility [65]	Invasion and metastasis [65]
2.9 **EFGR** (epidermal growth factor receptor)	BRAF transmembrane tyrosine kinase [73]	Progression and metastasis [74]
2.10 **P53** (cellular tumor antigen p53)	Tumor suppressor "guardian of the genome" (promotes cell cycle arrest, apoptosis, senescence, and DNA repair) [75, 76]	Inactivated or functionally impaired in melanoma [75]
Serological biomarkers		
3.1 **LDH** (lactate dehydrogenase)	Enzyme that converts lactate into pyruvate in anaerobic conditions [77]	High levels are correlated with metastasis, decreased survival rate, negative outcome after treatment [77]
3.2 **CRP** (C-reactive protein)	Nonspecific marker of inflammation, infection, cancer [65]	Predictor for disease progression in high levels [65]
3.3 **MIA** (melanoma-inhibiting activity)	Protein associated with *in vitro* increased invasiveness, extravasation, and metastasis [77]	Elevated levels, marker for advanced stage (III and IV) and poorer prognosis [77]
3.4 **VEGF** (vascular endothelial growth factor)	Protein that stimulates vasculogenesis and angiogenesis [78]	Elevated levels linked to poor progression-free survival [78]
3.5 **BRAF**	Raf kinases family involved in RAF-MEK-ERK signal transduction pathway (cell growth, proliferation, and differentiation) [79]	BRAF mutation, BRAF-V600E, associated with increased tumor thickness, ulceration, and reduced survival [80]
3.6 **miRNA** (MicroRNAs)	RNA molecules involved in proliferation, differentiation, stress responses, apoptosis [77, 78]	Disease progression and risk of recurrence [77, 78]
3.7 **GM3**	Ganglioside (glycosphingolipid) involved in cell proliferation, differentiation, apoptosis, embryogenesis, and oncogenesis [81]	Low levels (early stage) linked to invasive proliferation; higher levels (late stage) linked to cell migration and invasion [81]
3.8 **OPN** (osteopontin)	Glycol-phosphoprotein implicated in reduction of apoptosis, promotion of tumor growth, tumor-promoting stromal cell in the bone marrow [82]	Rapid melanoma growth, angiogenesis, and aggressive metastasis [83]
3.9 **IL-8** (interleukin-8)	Chemokine produced by malignant cells [82]	Associated with tumor burden, stage of the disease, survival, and response to therapy [82]
3.10 **YKL-40**	Heparin secreted during the late stages of cell differentiation [84]	Overexpression associated with poor survival [84]
3.11 **CTC** (circulating tumor cells)	Cells from melanoma metastatic tumors [77]	Linked to inferior survival; predictive marker for selecting the systemic therapy [77]
3.12 **Melanoma-initiating cells**	Cancer stem cells [85]	Can lead the specific targeted systemic therapy [85]

4. Recent studies concerning active phytocompounds targeting malignant melanoma

Although synthesized to serve the plant in modulating its interaction with the environment, many natural compounds act as drugs when used by humans by binding to various enzymes and receptors. In the area of anticancer medications, it has been shown that about 75% of the medications are naturally derived or inspired [86]. Phytocompounds hold an important potential in the chemoprevention and treatment of melanoma, including metastasis [87, 88]. The main advantage of natural products relies in their multi-target activity, with one compound being able to interact with multiple proteins and receptors. Anti-melanoma activities have been pointed out for both phytocompounds from nutraceuticals (polyphenols, polysaccharides, and carotenoids), as well as for highly active secondary metabolite classes like the alkaloids or the terpenes. Additionally, there are a number of crude extracts or enriched fractions with anti-melanoma actions, for which the active compound(s) could not be singled out yet. A promising field in the actual usage of plant-derived compounds is their synergistic activity when administered in combination with synthetic anticancer medications [89].

4.1. Polyphenols

The potential of polyphenolic compounds (**Figure 1**) as anti-melanoma agents was recognized as early as 1995, when Menon and coworkers found that orally administered curcumin, catechin, and rutin significantly prolonged the life span of animals with experimental melanoma [90]. The anticancer potential of these food constituents is supported by epidemiological studies [91]. Their general mechanisms of action may be summarized as follows: antioxidative, photoprotectant, induction of apoptosis, and inhibition of angiogenesis. Antioxidative capacities are seminal for the protective activity against UV-induced oxidative stress [92]. The ability to act as UV filters is related to the physiologic function of certain flavonoids present in epicuticular waxes protecting the plant epidermis against UV radiation [93]. Apoptosis is mainly promoted by polyphenols via regulation of Bcl-2 family proteins and caspase-3 activation, while the anti-migratory effects are mainly obtained by down-regulation of MMPs expression.

Intensely researched polyphenols in the context on melanoma include flavonoids (quercetin, apigenin, silymarin, genistein, catechins, anthocyanins, biflavonoids), curcumin, and resveratrol [94]. Quercetin (**1**), an abundant dietary flavonol, acts via all above-cited mechanisms. It decreases the viability and promotes the apoptosis of ultraviolet UVB-irradiated B16F10 melanoma cells by several mechanisms: it increases the levels of reactive oxygen species, depolarizes mitochondrial membrane potential, induces the imbalance of calcium homeostasis, attenuates MEK-ERK signaling, and changes the ratio of Bcl-2, Bax, and Bim expression in favor of cell death elicitation [95]. It offers photoprotection against melanogenesis through a regulatory effect on the Nrf2-ARE pathway [96]. Furthermore, quercetin inhibits melanoma cell migration in a setup of experimentally activated receptor tyrosine kinase c-Met, known to be involved in the acquisition of metastatic phenotypes [97].

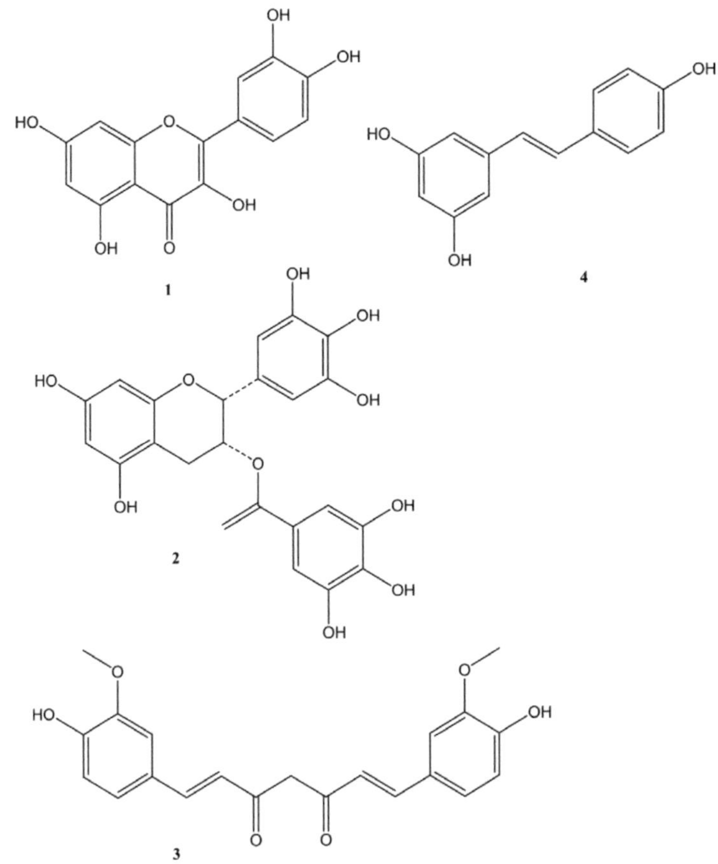

Figure 1. Chemical structure of representative polyphenols targeting malignant melanoma. 1: quercetin, 2: (–)-epigallocatechin-3-gallate, 3: curcumin; 4: resveratrol.

Apigenin, a flavone from the point of view of chemical structure, offers an effective photoprotection against UVA- and UVB-induced skin carcinogenesis [98], fights metastasis by preventing the activation of MMP-2, MMP-9, VEGF, and Twist1 genes through down-regulation of STAT2 signaling [99], promotes apoptosis via caspase-3 and cleaved poly(ADP-ribose) polymerase [100]. In addition, apigenin blocks the COX-2 pathway and increases terminal differentiation in the epidermis [101].

Silymarin, a complex of flavonolignans from the achenes of milk thistle, is a natural product known especially for its hepatoprotective, anti-oxidative and anti-inflammatory effects [102]. When applied locally, silymarin was able to inhibit carcinogenesis induced by UV-radiation and to decrease tumor multiplicity and growth. It produces cell cycle arrest in melanoma cells via inhibition of kinase activities of (MEK)-1/2 and RSK-2 [103], induces apoptosis and counteracts metastasis via down-regulation of MMPs expression [104]. Silymarin is a prominent inhibitor of Wnt/β-catenin translocation in melanoma cells, beside few other phytocompounds like the flavonoid fisetin, the triterpene lupeol, and the alkaloid tryptanthrin; aberrant Wnt signaling occurs in one-third of melanomas [105].

Catechins are flavanols devoid of the 3-oxo group specific to other flavonoids; they may especially be found in woody plants like wine and the tea plant. Catechins as well as their esters with gallic acid, in particular epigallocatechin-3-gallate (EGCG, **2**), are the subject of intense research in cancer prevention and treatment. In the field of anti-melanoma activities, the chemopreventive effect of ECGC is mainly achieved by a photoprotective effect exerted through interleukin 12 induction followed by DNA repair, inhibition of angiogenesis, and the stimulation of cytolytic T cells [106]. The proapoptotic effects are exerted by EGCG through down-regulation of inhibitory proteins such as Bcl-2, D1, and cdk2, as well as the up-regulation of the proapoptosis protein Bax. Important tumor-suppressor proteins (p16, p21, and p2) are induced by EGCG [107, 108]. More recently, the discussed polyphenol was shown to bind to the cell surface receptor 67LR, overexpressed in melanoma [109]. As an agonist of 67LR, EGCG is able to suppress melanoma tumor growth by activating a specific signaling pathway (cAMP/PKA/PP2A) via regulation of miRNA-let-7b expression in melanoma cells [110]. Moreover, EGCG displays an excellent anti-metastatic profile, reducing the number of lung metastases in mice [111]. Molecular targets in this regard are COX-2, PGE2 receptors, the impairment of epithelial-to-mesenchymal transition [112], reduction of angiogenesis promoters and down-regulation of MMP2 activity and ERK1/2 pathway [113].

Curcumin (**3**), an orange-colored constituent of turmeric rhizomes (*Curcuma* sp.), is an extensively investigated compound with anti-inflammatory and anticancer activities. In human melanoma cell lines (A375 and C8161), it reduces cell viability, has an antiproliferative effect arresting mitosis at the transition of G2/M phase, suppresses cell invasion, and induces autophagy [114]. The anti-metastatic effect was demonstrated *in vivo* using C57BL/6 mice; the down-regulation of metalloproteinases and collagenases activities, modulation of integrin receptors [115] and interference with the STAT3 pathway support this observation [116].

Resveratrol (**4**), a stilbene found mainly in grapes and *Polygonum cuspidatum*, inhibits melanoma proliferation *in vitro*, arresting cell divisions at the G1/S transition and induces apoptosis targeting Bcl-2-associated X protein, B-cell lymphoma 2, and caspases -9 and -3 [117]. Through the suppression of β-catenin and STAT3-pathway, resveratrol reduces the levels of survivin, a protein which is essential for the survival of melanoma cells. Furthermore, the compound has anti-migratory activities mediated by the deactivation of the proto-oncogenic Akt [118]. The low bioavailability of resveratrol triggered the obtainment of several analogs, as well as the preference for the use of the natural pterostilbene having a longer half-life [87].

4.2. Polysaccharides

The potential of polysaccharide fractions obtained from terrestrial and marine organisms in cancer treatment receives an increasing attention. These compounds are potent immunomodulators, leading to the release of cytokines which may play important roles in the defense against cancer [119]. Their main mechanism of action includes activation of natural killer cells, induction of inflammatory caspases, and down-regulation of MMPs expression, but as a general feature their mechanism of action is much less known than in the case of plant polyphenols. An important advantage of polysaccharides is their very low toxicity.

The sulfated and partially acetylated fucoidans from brown algae *Coccophora langsdorfii* and *Fucus evanescens*, consisting of (1→3)- and (1→4)-linked α-l-fucopyranose residues, produced a significant inhibition of colony formation of SK-MEL-5 and SK-MEL-28 melanoma cells [120].

Beta-glucans are constituents of cell walls in certain fungi, algae, and vascular plants such as oat or barley. Oral administration of yeast-derived beta-glucan to mice inoculated with B16 murine melanoma cells significantly reduced tumor weight, pulmonary metastasis, and survival rate. These effects are mediated by the activation of NK cells. An important finding was that beta-glucan supplementation was devoid of hematopoietic toxicity, unlike chemotherapeutic drugs such as 5-fluorouracil [121]. Low-molecular-weight beta-glucan prepared from oat decreased the cell viability of cancer cell lines Me45 and A431, while normal keratinocytes were not affected. The cytotoxic effect was mediated by induction of caspase-12 expression. This natural product had the advantage of a good solubility in water and a low viscosity, in comparison with other glucans [122]. Polysaccharides from higher plants, like raspberry fruits, have as well been shown to inhibit melanoma growth, and to have a synergistic activity with docetaxel *in vivo*, reducing at the same time liver and kidney injuries inflicted by the latter [123]. Pectins from corn demonstrated their ability to inhibit cancer cell growth and metastasis by modulating specific markers such as galectin-3, VEGF, MMP-2 and MMP-9, and NF-κB [124].

4.3. Volatile oils

Volatile oils are complex mixtures of monoterpenes, sesquiterpes, aromatic compounds, and their derivatives, which are produced by plants in order to protect themselves against pathogens, herbivores, or, on the contrary, to act as signals for pollinators and disseminators [125]. In the search for innovative strategies in melanoma treatment, these natural products have as well been investigated. The main mechanisms of action known so far are represented by induction of apoptosis (via increasing the expression of p53 and caspase-3) and reduction of angiogenesis with down-regulation of MMPs.

The volatile oil of the tea tree plant (*Melaleuca alternifolia*) and its main component terpinen-4-ol (5) were evaluated in an experimental setting of human melanoma M14 WT cells and M14 adriamycin-resistant cells. Concentration as low as 0.005–0.03% proved to induce apoptosis, and conversely the resistant cell variant was more sensitive [126]. More recently, Greay and coworkers [127] applied a topical formulation containing 10% tea tree oil and found a significant delay in the growth of established subcutaneous B16-F10 melanoma, while systemic toxicity was absent. The volatile oil of *Tridax procumbens*, a common annual

Asteraceae in most tropical regions, displayed anti-metastatic effects by the inhibition of lung nodule formation by B16F-10 cells in C57BL/6 mice. Furthermore, it induced apoptosis increasing the expression of p53 and caspase-3 and reduced angiogenesis [128]. *Curcuma zedoaria* volatile oil suppressed as well melanoma growth and lung metastasis, with the down-regulation of MMPs [129].

4.4. Alkaloids

Alkaloids are nitrogen-containing plant metabolites with usually very intense pharmacologic effects at even low dosages. Consequently, their safety profile is very different from the one of compounds discussed above. The main compounds from this class, which are able to target melanoma, include berberine, harmine, paclitaxel, and glycoalkaloids from Solanaceae. While the number of reports on the anti-melanoma potential of alkaloids is rather scarce in comparison with that of polyphenols, the mechanisms of action are well studied. The anti-migratory properties of alkaloids in malignant melanoma have been the subject of a comprehensive review [87]. Alkaloids may induce apoptosis via the inhibition of the Ras-signaling cascade at various downstream points, blocking both PI3K/AKT and MAP/ERK pathways. Metastasis is mainly counteracted by blocking the COX pathway and angiogenesis. NF-κB inhibition is as well a target of anti-melanoma alkaloids.

Berberine, an isoquinoline alkaloid (**6**), occurs in several medicinal plants of the Berberidaceae, Ranunculaceae, and Papaveraceae families [130]. While best known for antimicrobial, anti-inflammatory, anti-hyperglycemic, and anti-hyperlipidemic effects [131], berberine is one of the most active alkaloids in melanoma. It has been shown to inhibit kinases like PI3K, ERK, and GSK3β [132]. Moreover, in combination with doxorubicin, it intensely reduces proliferation and increases apoptosis, effect demonstrated both *in vitro* and *in vivo* [133]. Berberine inhibits the migration of melanoma cells via the reduction of COX-2/PGE2 receptors expression [134] and has anti-angiogenetic properties [135]. Harmine is an indole alkaloid contained by only a few plant species, including *Peganum harmala* and *Banisteriopsis caapi*. While its ability to bind monoamino-oxidase A and to elicit psychoactive effects is known since several decades, the potential anticancer properties of this compound have only been explored in recent years. In melanoma, it displays important anti-migratory effects through the inhibition of NF-κB and other transcription factors (CREB, ATF-2) [136]; it reduces lung metastasis in C57BL/6 mice and down-regulates the expression of pro-metastatic genes (MMP-9, ERK, and VEGF) [137].

Paclitaxel is a pseudoalkaloid, first isolated from the bark of the Pacific yew (*Taxus brevifolia*), approved for the clinical treatment of several solid tumors with poor prognosis including melanoma [138]. It stabilizes microtubules, disrupting the dynamic equilibrium between free and polymerized tubulin; as a consequence, cell division is arrested in the G2/M transition of mitosis [139]. Additionally, paclitaxel has antiangiogenic effects, which are potentiated by COX-2 inhibitors [140]. Disadvantages of this compound include its extreme hydrophobicity, which could be overcome in modern nanoformulations, as well as drug resistance to paclitaxel due to the induction of the efflux protein P-gp and unusual expression of class III isotype of β-tubulin [139].

Glycoalkaloids from Solanaceae, including α-solanine and solamargine, displayed anti-melanoma effects in recent reports. Interestingly, solamargine inhibited selectively the growth of WM239 and WM115 melanoma cells, in comparison to benign WM35 cells. Cellular necrosis occurred upon permeabilization of the lysosomal membrane, which triggered, in turn, the extrinsic pathway of mitochondrial destruction. The intrinsic apoptosis pathway was as well disrupted by this compound [141]. α-Solanine displays anti-proliferative effects, induces apoptosis, and suppresses melanoma cell invasion, mainly via the reduction of MMP-2 and MMP-9 activities. The potential of this compound in the treatment of metastatic melanoma is further substantiated by the inhibition of JNK and PI3K kinases as well as the reduction of NF-κB activity [142]. Two chemical structures of representative natural compounds targeting melanoma, other than polyphenols, are presented in **Figure 2**.

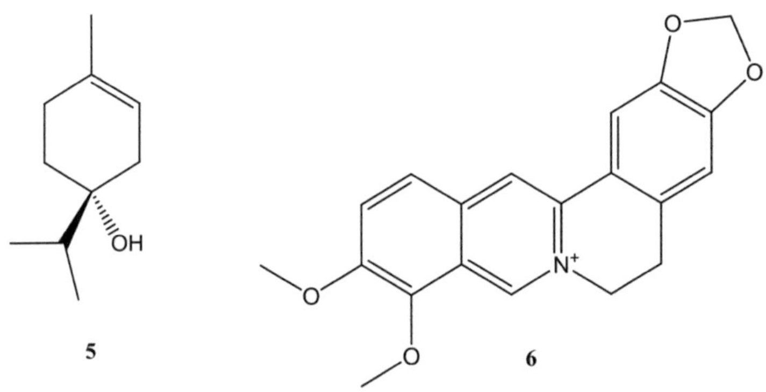

Figure 2. Chemical structures of representative natural compounds targeting melanoma, other than polyphenols. 5: Terpinen-4-ol, the major monoterpene in tea tree volatile oil, 6: Berberine, an intensely researched alkaloid.

5. Modern physicochemical formulations for the enhancement of bioavailability of selected active phytochemicals with chemopreventive activity for malignant melanoma

Formulation development can be regarded as a determining aspect in the delivery of antineoplastic natural compounds due to their physicochemical properties, in particular water solubility, which limit their bioavailability [143]. A variety of formulation strategies have been reported highlighting the main challenges that arise in the development of optimized drug delivery in the anticancer field [144], including skin cancer. The most studied natural anticancer compounds in terms of bioavailability improvement are different types of polyphenols (curcumin, silymarin, and resveratrol) and alkaloids (paclitaxel). In **Tables 1–4**, we aim to summarize the main reported attempts to increase the bioavailability of the above-mentioned compounds through various modulations of their physicochemical parameters as well as modern pharmaceutical formulations.

Curcumin formulations	Components	Method of application	Indications/remarks	Ref.
Curcumin + piperine	-curcumin -piperine	Oral administration to male Wistar rats (epilepsy model) (2 g/kg curcumin, +20 mg/kg piperine)	20-fold higher curcumin bioavailability compared to curcumin alone (piperine decrease hepatic and intestinal glucuronidation)	[145]
Curcuminoids (curcumin, demethoxycurcumin, bis-demethoxycurcumin) + Sesamin Ferulic acid Naringenin Xanthohumol (simultaneous administration) Curcuminoids micellar solubilized + Sesamin Ferulic acid Naringenin Xanthohumol; Curcuminoids micellar solubilized	2:2:1:1:1 (*w/w*): -Curcumin powder: (82% curcumin +16% demethoxycurcumin +2% bis-demethoxycurcumin) -sesamin -ferulic acid -naringenin -xanthohumol -95.1% Tween-80 -1.4% curcumin -1.4% sesamin -0.7% naringenin -0.7% ferulic acid -0.7% xanthohumol -7% curcuminoid powder (=6% curcumin) -93% Tween-80	Oral capsule administered to healthy humans (98 mg curcuminoids, single dose)	8-fold increase in bioavailability; 73-fold increase in bioavailability; 88-fold increase in bioavailability	[146]
Liquid micelles of curcumin Micronized powder of curcumin Native curcumin powder	- 7% curcumin powder (equivalent to 6% curcumin) -93% Tween-80 -25 % curcumin powder -58.3% triacetin -16.7% panodan -82% curcumin -16% dimethoxy-curcumin - 2% bis-dimethoxy-curcumin	Oral administration to healthy humans (500 mg curcuminoids, single dose)	277-, 114-, 185-fold increase in bioavailability in women/men/all subjects compared to native curcumin powder; 14-, 5-, 9-fold increase in bioavailability in women/men/all subjects compared to native curcumin powder; Women absorbed curcumin much more efficiently than men	[147]
Curcumin nanosuspension	-10% curcumin - 2% polyvinyl alcohol -88% water	Oral capsules administered to male Wistar rats, 100 mg/kg	Increased oral absorption and bioavailability -> significant increased concentration in selective organs; -direct uptake from the gastrointestinal tract; -increased permeability induced by surfactants;	[148]

Curcumin formulations	Components	Method of application	Indications/remarks	Ref.
			-increased resistance to degradation and elimination.	
Sustained-release formulation of curcumin	*MicroActive® Curcumin* (patented formulation): -25% micronized curcuminoids -polyglycerol esters of fatty acids -medium-chain triglycerides -hydroxypropyl-methylcellulose -sodium alginate -microcrystalline cellulose	Oral capsules administered to healthy humans, 500 mg curcumin (single dose)	9.7-fold increase in bioavailability (test period: 12 h)	[149]
Curcumin + phosphatidylcholine	*Meriva®*, (patented complex of curcumin with soy phosphatidylcholine): -20% curcuminoid mixture - 75% curcumin - 15% demethoxycurcumin - 10% bisdemethoxycurcumin -40% soy phosphatidylcholine -40% microcrystalline cellulose	Oral administration to male Wistar albino rats, 340 mg/kg	Reduced curcumin concentration in the gastrointestinal mucosa; Significant increased plasma/liver levels (compared to an unformulated curcumin); *Indications:* Chemoprophylaxis intervention studies targeting sites other than the gastrointestinal tract	[150]
Curcumin + PVP (polyvinylpyrrolidone) + cellulosic derivatives +antioxidant agents	*CurcuWIN*, -minimum 20% curcuminoids - PVP (polyvinylpyrrolidone) - cellulosic derivatives - antioxidant agents	Randomized, double-blind, crossover human study in healthy volunteers (hard gel capsules, 376 mg curcuminoids)	-45.9-fold increase in curcumin oral absorption compared to unformulated standard curcumin, 5.8-fold increase over a phytosome formulation, 34.9-fold increase over (curcumin + volatile oils from turmeric rhizome) formulation	[151]
Lipid based nanoparticles: phospholipid vesicles/lipid-nanospheres	*Phospholipid vesicles:* -DMPC/SA/PEG-DSPE/curcumin (molar ratio 10/1/0.06/1.9): DMPC = 1,2-Dimyristoyl-sn-glycero-3-phosphocholine; SA = l-glutamic acid, N-(3-carboxy-1-oxopropyl)-, 1,5-dihexadecyl ester);	IV administration to male Wistar rats (2 mg/kg)	Selectively delivered to macrophages in spleen and bone marrow; Potential intravenous delivery system for antioxidant and anti-inflammatory therapies	[152]

Curcumin formulations	Components	Method of application	Indications/remarks	Ref.
	PEG-DSPE = (1,2-distearoyl-sn-glycero-3-phosphoethanolamine-N-[monomethoxy poly(ethylene glycol) (5000)] -*t*-butyl alcohol/benzene, (1/1,*v*/*v*) -physiological saline 70 mg/mL; *Lipid-nanospheres:* -curcumin + soybean oil (10 mg/mL) -DMPC/SA/PEG-DSPE (10/1/0.06, molar ratio) + soybean oil (280 mg/mL) -2.5% glycerin solution			
Liposomal curcumin	-10:1 (*w*/*w*)-total lipids:curcumin; *Lipids*: -1,2-dimyristoyl-sn-glycero-3-phosphocholine/1,2-dimyristoyl-*sn*-glycero-3-[phospho-*rac*-(1-glycerol)] (sodium salt) or a pegylated version of 1,2-dimyristoyl-*sn*-glycero-3-phosphocholine/cholesterol/1,2-dimyristoyl-*sn*-glycero-3-phosphoethanolamine-N-[methoxy-(polyethylene glycol)-2000]	IV administration to female athymic *nu*/*nu* mice (human colorectal tumor xenografts in nude mice models) (liposomal curcumin 40 mg/kg, oxaliplatin 5 mg/kg); *in vitro* studies (LoVo and Colo205 cells)	Equivalent or greater growth-inhibitory and apoptotic effects with oxaliplatin both *in vitro* and *in vivo* in colorectal cancer	[153]
Self nanoemulsion of curcumin and silymarin	-15 mg curcumin -25 mg silymarin - 1 g oil phase (glycerin monooleate; Tween 20:PEG 400, 1:8:1 ratio) - deionized water:oil phase, 5:1 (self-nanoemulsifying method)	Stability study	Higher stability of silymarin and curcumin in comparison with a conventional emulsion Efficient drug delivery system	[154]

Table 1. Curcumin formulations.

Silymarin formulations	Components	Method of application	Indications/remarks	Ref.
Self-microemulsifying drug delivery system (SMEDDS)	-10% ethyl linoleate -30% Cremophor EL -60% ethyl alcohol (% *w/w*)	Oral administration to male mongrel dogs (50 mg/kg, single dose)	3 months stability; Faster release; 2.2-fold enhanced oral absorption, increased bioavailability; *Indication:* Oral administration of silymarin	[155]
Semisolid dispersion binary system using Gelucire 44/14 as carrier	Silymarin:Gelucire 1:1 and 1:3 (*w/w*)	Oral administration to New Zealand albino rabbits (280 mg/kg)	Linear increase of silymarin solubility and dissolution degree depending on the career concentration -> significant superior pharmacokinetic profile	[156]
Solid dispersion of silymarin with a hydrophilic polymer (HPMC E15 LV)	-silymarin powder -78.7 % silymarin -20.3 % silybin -isosilybin) -HPMC E 15LV (1:1, 1:3, and 1:5 (*w/w*)) (kneading, spray drying and co-precipitation method of preparation)	Influence of preparation methodology of solid dispersions of silymarin	Co-precipitation method revealed the best soluble and stable amorphous solid dispersion; The best results: 1:1 for the kneading method and 1:3 for other methods; Increased silymarin dissolution: co-precipitation (2.5-fold) > spray drying (1.9-fold) > kneading (1.5-fold); Mean dissolution time: 8.3 min for co-precipitation, 14.2 min for spray drying and 17.4 min for kneading	[157]
Silymarin loaded chitosan nanoparticles	-40 mg chitosan -10 mg silymarin - 2% acetic acid solution - 1mL ethanol -10 mg sodium tripolyphosphate -1M NaOH 1M/0.1M HCl (for pH adjustment) -5% D-mannitol solution (ionic gelation method of preparation)	Oral administration to Swiss Albino mice (CCl_4 hepatotoxicity model), 50 mg/kg	Sustained release Improved pharmacological activity	[158]
Solid dispersion and silica nanoparticles of silymarin with slow-release matrix material and release enhancer	- silymarin solid dispersion: -silymarin:povidone K30:soy bean lecithin: acrylic resin IV: 1–3:0.3–0.8:0.2–0.5 (*w:w*) -silymarin solid dispersion:	Oral administration in Beagle dogs	Continuous controlled release for 72 h; Half-life 2.3 times longer	[159]

http://dx.doi.org/10.5772/67647

Silymarin formulations	Components	Method of application	Indications/remarks	Ref.
	silymarin-loaded silica nanoparticles:slow-release matrix material:release enhancer: 0.5–1.25:0.1–0.3:0.1–0.3 (*w/w*)			
Silymarin glyceryl monooleate/ Poloxamer 407 liquid crystalline matrices	-20 g glyceryl monooleate -2.4 g poloxamer 407 -silymarin 2%, 4%, 8% (melting/ congealing method of preparation)	Oral capsules administered to Beagle dogs (14.4 mg/kg silybin)	*In vitro* limited release of silymarin; 3.46-fold enhancement in oral bioavailability in comparison with Legalon® (as a result of the liquid crystalline phase formed in the digestive tract)	[160]
Silymarin-loaded liquid proliposome	- 1.0 g silymarin -10.0 g soy lecithin - 5.0 g cholesterol - 0.5 g sodium oleate -100.0 mL propylene glycol simple dissolving process)	Oral administration to Kunming mice (hepatitis experimental models ; 75, 150, or 300 mg/kg)	Improved bioavailability and hepatoprotection; Efficient oral drug-delivery system for silymarin	[161]
Liposomal lecithin-based carrier system of phytosomal silymarin	-lecithin:cholesterol 6:1 (maximum entrapment-55%) (film hydration method of preparation)	*In vitro* study on Chang liver cells; Oral administration to Wistar rats	3.5-fold enhanced oral bioavailability; Higher hepatoprotective and anti-inflammatory effects in comparison with a silymarin suspension	[162]
Bile salt (sodium deoxycholate) containing liposomes of silymarin	-ethanol:dichloromethane (12/13, *v/v*) -liposomes 20 mg/mL different methods of preparation: thin-film dispersion, reversed-phase evaporation, supercritical fluid technology)	Oral administration to male Wistar rats (20 mg/kg)	Supercritical fluid technology -> adequate for liposomes preparation (the best stability of liposomes, the highest entrapment efficiency and drug loading, the smallest particle dimension); Enhanced *in vitro* drug release; Increased oral bioavailability	[163]

Table 2. Silymarin formulations.

Paclitaxel formulations	Components	Method of application	Indications/Remarks	Ref.
Paclitaxel (microemulsion/Taxol®)+ silymarin	-Taxol® -paclitaxel microemulsion -silymarin *(insufficient data)*	Oral administration to rats: -Taxol® +10–20 mg/kg silymarin; -paclitaxel microemulsion +20 mg/kg silymarin	Silymarin association increased the oral bioavailability of paclitaxel; The highest absolute bioavailability (19%) -> for silymarin + paclitaxel microemulsion; Faster absorption for paclitaxel microemulsion compared to Taxol®	[164]
Paclitaxel (nanoemulsion) + curcumin	-paclitaxel nanoemulsion -curcumin *(insufficient data)*	Oral administration to SKOV3 tumor-bearing *nu/nu* mice (50 mg/kg curcumin +20 mg/kg paclitaxel)	5.2-fold increased oral relative bioavailability and anti-tumor activity of paclitaxel (3.2-fold enhanced accumulation in the tumor tissue)	[165]
Paclitaxel (Genetaxyl®) + cyclosporin A	Genetaxyl® (paclitaxel 6 mg/mL) + cyclosporin A; Genetaxyl®: -20% (*v/v*) Cremophor EL Genaxol®: -50% (*v/v*) Cremophor EL	Oral administration to cancer patients (60/120/180 $mg/m^{2)}$ +oral cyclosporin A, 10 mg/kg IV: 175 mg/m^2, 3 h infusion	Less than proportional increase in systemic exposure with increasing doses; Limited paclitaxel bioavailability by micellar entrapment; Cremophor EL ↓ concentration: -↓ median time to peak concentration; -↑ absorption of paclitaxel; -↑ metabolism of paclitaxel	[166]
Paclitaxel + Cremophor EL	Taxol®: Paclitaxel in Cremophor EL – dehydrated ethanol (1:1, *v/v*)	Intraperitoneal administration to cancer patients	↓ Plasma concentration and bioavailability; Prolonged peritoneal activity	[167]
Crystalline nanosuspension	-paclitaxel (20 mg/mL): -0.1% (*w/w*) Cremophor EL in phosphate saline	IV administration to tumor bearing xenograft female SCID-beige mice (20 mg/kg)	Weaker antiproliferative effects than the Cremophor standard formulations	[168]
Self micro emulsifying oily formulations (SMEOFs) +cyclosporine A	*Paclitaxel 1.5% (% w/v):* -paclitaxel 1.5 % -vitamin E 5.00%	-Oral administration to wild-type and P-glycoprotein knockout mice [169]; -oral administration to humans [170]	Satisfying oral bioavailability -> the systemic exposure and oral bioavailability of paclitaxel was comparable to Taxol® (40%);	[169], [170]

Paclitaxel formulations	Components	Method of application	Indications/Remarks	Ref.
	-TPGS 29.95% (d-alpha-tocopheryl polyethylene glycol 1000 succinate) -tyloxapol 33.05% -ethanol 30.5% *Paclitaxel 3%* *(% w/v):* -paclitaxel 3.0% -vitamin E 5.0% -TPGS 29.45% -tyloxapol 32.55% -ethanol 30%		Higher dose of paclitaxel->less effective uptake (saturation of the first-pass metabolism); SMEOF = suitable vehicle for oral administration of paclitaxel associated with cyclosporine A	
Supersaturable self-emulsifying drug delivery system of paclitaxel (S-SEDDS) containing HPMC (precipitation inhibitor); +cyclosporine A	*-lack of data*	Oral administration to male Sprague-Dawley rats (10 mg/kg paclitaxel; 5 mg/kg cyclosporine A)	5-fold higher oral bioavailability, 10-fold higher maximum concentration for S-SEDDS formulation compared to Taxol®; Association of cyclosporin A=> further increase in oral bioavailability; Slow crystallization of paclitaxel (*in vitro* dilution)	[171]
Solid-nanoemulsion preconcentrate (surfactant-co-surfactant system based on Tween 20 and PEG)	*Nanoemulsion preconcentrate:* -50 mg paclitaxel - 1 mL of different combinations of oil, surfactant, and cosurfactant; Optimized formulation: oil:surfactant:cosurfactant (μL) - 175:350:175; *Nanocarrier:* -Oil: -propylene glycol monocaprylate/ glycerol monooleate, 4:1 (*w/w*), -Surfactant: -polyoxyethylene 20 sorbitan monooleate/ polyoxyl 15 hydroxystearate, 1:1 (*w/w*),	Oral administration to Wistar albino rats (10 mg/kg)	Increased oral bioavailability; High cumulative *in vitro* drug release; Significant antiproliferative effect on breast cancer cell line MCF7	[172]

Paclitaxel formulations	Components	Method of application	Indications/Remarks	Ref.
	-Cosurfactant: -diethylene glycol monoethyl ether/ polyethylene glycol 300, 1:1(*w/w*)			
Niosomal formulation: Niosomes with nonionic surfactants	*Organic phase:* -Span 40 (M) – 0.0475 -cholesterol (M) – 0.0475 -DCP (dicetyl phosphate) (M) – 0.005 -paclitaxel (mM) – 0.234 -chloroform (Ml) – 10; *Water phase:* -ultrapure water (mL) q.s. 10 (niosomes prepared through film hydration method)	*In vitro* studies	Diffusion controlled release; Low toxicologic profile; Gastrointestinal stability Suitable formulation for oral drug delivery	[173]
Paclitaxel-loaded pegylated ethosomes	-paclitaxel -cholesterol -PEG3350 -phosphatidylcholine (1:6.5:9:28, *w/w*) -deionized water and ethanol 99.4% (67.5:32.5, *v/v*) (pegylated ethosomes prepared by reverse phase evaporation technique)	*In vitro* studies	Longer half life, slower release rate; 4.5-fold increase in cytotoxicity on human melanoma SK-MEL-3 cell line, in comparison with the free drug; Possible alternative to the conventional therapy	[174]
Paclitaxel-loaded lipid nanocapsules	(mg/g): - 1.9 paclitaxel - 51.9 Solutol®HS15 -842.6 water - 90.7 Captex® 8000 - 8.1 Lipoid® S100-3 - 4.8 NaCl powder	Oral administration to male Sprague-Dawley rats (10 mg/kg)	3-fold higher oral bioavailability (same results for Taxol®-verapamil (=P-glycoprotein inhibitor) association); Potential formulation to augment the oral bioavailability of the drug, avoiding verapamil association	[175]
Solid lipid nanoparticles surface-modified with hydroxypropyl-β-cyclodextrin (HPCD)	- 100 mg stearic acid - 5 mg paclitaxel -0.25 mL ethanol - 75 mg lecithin - 75 mg poloxamer 188	Oral administration to male Sprague-Dawley male rats (25 mg/kg)	Oral administration: -fast release of paclitaxel (nearly complete release); -high cellular uptake by	[176]

Paclitaxel formulations	Components	Method of application	Indications/Remarks	Ref.
	- 3 mL distilled water -HPCD (modified hot sonication method of preparation)		Caco-2 cells; -high concentrations in the lymph nodes (increased bioavailability); Role of HPCD in reducing the nanoparticle size and enhancing the solubility and dissolution of the drug; HPCD may inhibit P-glycoprotein; Alternative formulation for oral administration of the drug	
Solid lipid nanoparticles (=specific colloidal carriers)	-paclitaxel: stearic acid+DPPG.NA – 1:10, 1:15, 1:20 (micro-emulsification technique)	Female Swiss Albino mice (7.5 mg/kg)	Increased anticancer effect; Increased specificity on breast cancer cells (for 1:20 formulation); Release profile delayed with the enhancement of lipid concentration; Entrapment efficiency, particle size and zeta potential value raised as lipid concentration was augmented	[177]
Solid lipid nanoparticles modified with 2-hydroxypropyl-β-cyclodextrin	- 5 mg paclitaxel - 100 mg stearic acid -0.25 mL ethanol - 75 mg lecithin - 75 mg poloxamer 188 - 400 mg HPCD (hot-melted sonication technique)	Intratumoral administration in female BALB/c nude mice for evaluation of antitumor activity (10 mg/kg) IV administration to male Sprague Dawley rats for pharmacokinetic study (5 mg/kg)	*IV delivery:* -diminished burst release; -low nephrotoxicity; -prolonged antiproliferative activity, increased absorption; *Intratumoral administration:* -high antitumor efficiency (sustained release, high cellular uptake); -reduced toxicity to normal organs; Potential therapeutic formulation for breast cancer with reduced nephrotoxicity	[178]
Biocompatible and biodegradable polymeric nanoparticles	*Organic phase:* -1 mg paclitaxel	*In vitro* studies	Initial burst release followed by 7-days sustained release;	[179]

Paclitaxel formulations	Components	Method of application	Indications/Remarks	Ref.
	- PLGA – 2%, 3%, 4% (*w/v*) (Poly(lactic-co-glycolic acid)) -10 mL acetone; *Aqueous phase:* -PVA (polyvinyl alcohol) 1%, 3%, 5% (*w/v*) (emulsification-solvent diffusion method)		Higher antiproliferative activity on Caco-2-cell-line when compared to blank nanoparticles but similar to paclitaxel solution	
Stabilized Pluronic micelles	*-lack of data* (solvent/evaporation technique)	Oral/IV administration in rats/mice	Prolonged gastrointestinal release; High oral absorption; Optimized pharmacokinetic profile after IV administration; *Indication*: delivery vehicles (carriers) for oral or intravenous paclitaxel administration	[180]

Table 3. Paclitaxel formulations.

http://dx.doi.org/10.5772/67647

Resveratrol formulations	Components	Method of application	Indications/remarks	Ref.
Liposomal formulation	-DPPC (dipalmitoyl-phosphatidylcholine) -PEG_{2000}-DSPE –poly(ethyleneglycol)-distearoylphosphatidyl ethanolamine) -cholesterol dissolved in ethanol, 1.85:0.15:1 (molar ratio) -resveratrol (maximum incorporation): ~5 mg/μmol of total lipid (equivalent to 10 mg/μmol total lipids added).	IV administration to nude Balb/c female mice (murine tumor model); 5 mg/kg	Inhibition of tumor growth by 70%; Improved chemical stability (prevention of inactivating cis-trans isomerization)	[181]
β-cyclodextrin-based nanosponges (BNS) formulation	-1:5 and 1:10 (*w/w*) resveratrol:BNS; -1:2 and 1:4 (molar ratio) cyclodextrin:cross- linker (carbonyldiimidazole)/BNS	*In vitro* studies	Increased release and stability (in comparison with plain drug); Improved cytotoxicity on HCPC-I cell; Good penetration in pigskin; Better accumulation in rabbit mucosa. *Indication*: buccal and topical administration	[182]
Monodisperse cyano-functionalized porous polymeric microspheres	- 4 g cyano-functionalized porous particles -0.2 *wt*% Tween 20 aqueous solution (86g) -0.2 g resveratrol - 10 g ethanol; *Cyano-functionalized porous particles:* *a. Seed dispersion:* -0.50 g polystyrene - 40 g 0.25 *wt*% sodium lauryl sulfate in water/EtOH (5/1, *w/w*) solution (=SE solution); *b. CD (Chlorododecane) swelling:* -0.5 g 1-CD - 10 g SE solution; *c. The second monomer swelling:* -7 g/5 g/2 g styrene -1 g/3 g/6 g divinylbenzene - 2 g acrylonitrile -10 g toluene/heptane (porogen): 0/100, 30/70,	*In vitro* studies	Antioxidant activity preserved for 5 weeks	[183]

Resveratrol formulations	Components	Method of application	Indications/remarks	Ref.
	60/40, 100/0 *wt%* -0.1 g benzoyl peroxide - 40 g SE solution; *d. Stabilization:* -50 g polyvinyl alcohol 5% solution (seeded polymerization technique)			
Encapsulation within yeast cell	*Lack of data*	*In vitro* studies	Increased DPPH-radical scavenging activity; Good stability, enhanced bioavailability (increased solubility, sustained release)	[184]
Zinc pectinate beads	Zinc acetate = cross-linking agent; -cross-linking solution pH 1.5 -zinc acetate concentration 5% (% *w/v*) -crosslinking time 0.5 h -drying at room temperature -pectin concentration 5% (% *w/v*) -pectin to resveratrol ratio of 3:1 (ionotropic gelation method)	*In vitro* studies	Better delayed release for zinc-pectinate beads than calcium-pectinate beads; Encapsulation of a great amount of resveratrol in zinc-pectinate beads	[185]
Zinc-pectin-chitosan composite microparticles	-pectin:resveratrol, 3:1 -1% chitosan	*In vivo* studies on rats	Specific drug release in the colon	[186]
Resveratrol+quercetin+curcumin	-quercetin -resveratrol -curcumin (applied alone/in combination, at 50 μM)	*In vitro* studies	Increased oral absorption of resveratrol and curcumin, without interfering with the absorption of quercetin	[187]

Table 4. Resveratrol formulations.

Author details

Danciu Corina[1]*, Soica Codruta[2], Antal Diana[3], Alexandra Popescu[4], Roxana Ghiulai[2], Ioana Zinuca Pavel[1], Stefana Avram[1], Minda Daliana[1] and Cristina Dehelean[5]

*Address all correspondence to: corina.danciu@umft.ro

1 Department of Pharmacognosy, Faculty of Pharmacy, University of Medicine and Pharmacy "Victor Babes", Timisoara, Romania

2 Department of Pharmaceutical Chemistry, Faculty of Pharmacy, University of Medicine and Pharmacy "Victor Babes", Timisoara, Romania

3 Department of Pharmaceutical Botany, Faculty of Pharmacy, University of Medicine and Pharmacy "Victor Babes", Timisoara, Romania

4 Department of Physical Chemistry, Faculty of Pharmacy, University of Medicine and Pharmacy "Victor Babes", Timisoara, Romania

5 Department of Toxicology, Faculty of Pharmacy, University of Medicine and Pharmacy "Victor Babes", Timisoara, Romania

References

[1] Almeida CA, Barry SA. Cancer basic science and clinical aspects, 1st ed. West Sussex, UK: Wiley-Blackwell; 2010, pp. 262–293.

[2] Leiter U, Eigentler T, Garbe C. Epidemiology of skin cancer. Adv Exp Med Biol. 2014; **810**:120–140.

[3] Lomas A, Leonardi-Bee J, Bath-Hextall F. A systematic review of worldwide incidence of nonmelanoma skin cancer. Br J Dermatol. 2012;**166**:1069–1080.

[4] Wehner MR, Shive ML, Chren MM, Han J, Qureshi AA, Linos E. Indoor tanning and non-melanoma skin cancer: systematic review and meta-analysis. BMJ. 2012;**345**:e5909. doi:10.1136/bmj.e5909.

[5] Feller L, Khammissa RA, Kramer B, Altini M, Lemmer J. Basal cell carcinoma, squamous cell carcinoma and melanoma of the head and face. Head Face Med. 2016;**12**(1):11. doi:10.1186/s13005-016-0106-0.

[6] Reichrath J, Rass K. Ultraviolet damage, DNA repair and vitamin D in nonmelanoma skin cancer and in malignant melanoma: an update. Adv Exp Med Biol. 2014;**810**:208–233.

[7] Ichihashi M, Ueda M, Budiyanto A, Bito T, Oka M, Fukunaga M, Tsuru K, Horikawa T. UV-induced skin damage. Toxicology. 2003;**189**(1–2):21–39.

[8] Zhan JY, Wang XF, Liu YH, Zhang ZB, Wang L, Chen JN, Huang S, Zeng HF, Lai XP. Andrographolide sodium bisulfate prevents UV-induced skin photoaging through inhibiting oxidative stress and inflammation. Mediators Inflamm. 2016;**2016**:3271451. doi:10.1155/2016/3271451.

[9] Leiter U, Garbe C. Epidemiology of melanoma and non-melanoma skin cancer: the role of sunlight. Adv Exp Med Biol. 2008;**624**:89–103. doi:10.1007/978-0-387-77574-6_8.

[10] Gonzales M, Erdei E, Berwick M. Epidemiology of skin cancer. In: Nouri K, editor. Skin cancer. New York, USA: McGraw-Hill; 2008, pp. 32–38. doi:10.1036/0071472568.

[11] Muenyi CS, Ljungman M, States JC. Arsenic disruption of DNA damage responses-potential role in carcinogenesis and chemotherapy. Biomolecules. 2015;**5**(4):2184–2193. doi:10.3390/biom5042184.

[12] Maiorino A, De Simone C, Perino F, Caldarola G, Peris K. Melanoma and non-melanoma skin cancer in psoriatic patients treated with high-dose phototherapy. J Dermatolog Treat. 2016;**27**(5):443-7. doi: 10.3109/09546634.2015.1133882. [Epub 2016 Jan 28].

[13] Archier E, Devaux S, Castela E, Gallini A, Aubin F, Le Maître M, Aractingi S, Bachelez H, Cribier B, Joly P, Jullien D, Misery L, Paul C, Ortonne JP, Richard MA. Carcinogenic risks of psoralen UV-A therapy and narrowband UV-B therapy in chronic plaque psoriasis: a systematic literature review. J Eur Acad Dermatol Venereol. 2012;**26**(Suppl 3):22–31. doi:10.1111/j.1468-3083.2012.04520.x.

[14] Nouri K, Ballard CJ, Patel AR, Anadolu-Brasie R. Basal cell carcinoma. In: Nouri K, editor. Skin cancer. New York, USA: McGraw-Hill; 2008, pp. 61–85. doi:10.1036/0071472568.

[15] Alter M, Hillen U, Leiter U, Sachse M, Gutzmer R. Current diagnosis and treatment of basal cell carcinoma. J Dtsch Dermatol Ges. 2015;**13**(9):863–75. doi:10.1111/ddg.12798.

[16] Griffin LL, Ali FR, Lear JT. Non-melanoma skin cancer. Clin Med (Lond). 2016;**16**(1):62–65. doi:10.7861/clinmedicine.16-1-62.

[17] Anadolu-Brasie R, Patel AR, Patel SS, Singh A, Nouri K. Squamous cell carcinoma of the skin. In: Nouri K, editor. Skin cancer. New York, USA: McGraw-Hill; 2008, pp. 86–114. doi:10.1036/0071472568.

[18] van der Pols JC. Epidemiology of basal cell and squamous cell carcinoma of the skin. In: Dummer R, Pittelkow MR, Iwatsuki K, Green A, Elwan NM, editors. Skin cancer-a worldwide perspective. Verlag-Berlin-Heidelberg, Germany: Springer; 2011, pp. 3–12. doi:10.1007/978-3-642-05072-5.

[19] Bahner JD, Bordeaux JS. Non-melanoma skin cancers: photodynamic therapy, cryotherapy, 5-fluorouracil, imiquimod, diclofenac, or what? Facts and controversies. Clin Dermatol. 2013;**31**(6):792–798. doi:10.1016/j.clindermatol.2013.08.020.

[20] Tran C, Sorg O, Carraux P, Didierjean L, Saurat JH. Topical delivery of retinoids counteracts the UVB-induced epidermal vitamin A depletion in hairless mouse. Photochem Photobiol. 2001;**73**(4):425–431.

[21] Bosserhoff A, Strizzi L. Introduction. In: Bosserhoff A, editor. Melanoma development-molecular biology, genetics and clinical application. Wien and New York: Springer; 2011, pp. 1–7. doi:10.1007/978-3-7091-0371-5.

[22] Barnhill RL, Mihm MC, Elgart G. Malignant melanoma. In: Nouri K, editor. Skin cancer. New York, USA: McGraw-Hill; 2008, pp. 140–167. doi:10.1036/0071472568.

[23] Berwick M. Melanoma epidemiology. In: Bosserhoff A, editor. Melanoma development-molecular biology, genetics and clinical application. Wien and New York: Springer; 2011, pp. 35–57. doi:10.1007/978-3-7091-0371-5.

[24] Lazovich D, Isaksson Vogel R, Weinstock MA, Nelson HH, Ahmed RL, Berwick M. Association between indoor tanning and melanoma in younger men and women. JAMA Dermatol. 2016. doi:10.1001/jamadermatol.2015.2938. [Epub ahead of print].

[25] Wolf Horrell Erin M., Wilson Kalin, D'Orazio John A. Melanoma: epidemiology, risk factors, and the role of adaptive pigmentation. In: Murph M, editor. Melanoma: current clinical management and future therapeutics. Rijeka, Croatia: InTech; 2015, pp. 1–19, ISBN 978-953-51-2036-0, doi:10.5772/58994.

[26] Rigel, D.S. The effect of sunscreen on melanoma risk. Dermatol Clin. 2002;**20**(4):601–606.

[27] Cancer facts & figures. Atlanta: American Cancer Society Inc.; 2015. https://www.cancer.org

[28] Ferlay J, Soerjomataram I, Dikshit R, Eser S, Mathers C, Rebelo M, et al. Cancer incidence and mortality worldwide: sources, methods and major patterns in GLOBOCAN 2012. Int J Cancer 2015;**136**(5):E359–E386. doi:10.1002/ijc.29210.

[29] Barbaric J, Sekerija M, Agius D, Coza D, Dimitrova N, Demetroiu A, Diba CS, Eser S, Gavric Z, Zakelj MP, Zivkovic S, Zvolsky M, Bray F, Coebergh JW, Znoar A. Disparities in melanoma incidence and mortality in South-Eastern Europe: increasing incidence and divergent mortality patterns. Is progress around the corner? EJC. 2016;**55**:47–55. doi:10.1016/j.ejca.2015.11.019.

[30] Parichy DM, Reedy MV, Erickson CA. Regulation of melanoblast migration and differentiation. In: Nordland JJ, Boissy RE, Hearing VJ, King RA, Ortonne JP, editors. The pigmentary system: physiology and pathophysiology, 2nd ed. Oxford University Press; 2006, pp. 108–139. doi:10.1002/9780470987100.ch5.

[31] Kalabis MF, Martinez G, Telson SM, Liu ZJ, Balint K, Juhasz I, Elder DE, Perbal B, Herlyn M. Downregulation of CCN3 expression as a potential mechanism for melanoma progression. Oncogene. 2008;**27**:2552–2560. doi:10.1038/sj.onc.1210896.

[32] Haass NK, Smalley KS, Li L, Herlyn M. Adhesion, migration and communication in melanocytes and melanoma. Pigment Cell Res. 2005;**18**:150–159. doi:10.1111/j.1600-0749.2005.00235.x.

[33] Maillard M, Cadot B, Ball RY, Sethia K, Edwards DR, Perbal B, Tatoud R. Differential expression of the ccn3 (nov) protooncogene in human prostate cell lines and tissues. Mol Pathol. 2001;**54**:275–280. doi:10.1136/mp.54.4.275.

[34] Glukhova L, Angevin E, Lavialle C, Cadot B, Terrier-Lacombe MJ, Perbal B, Bernheim A, Goguel AF. Patterns of specific genomic alterations associated with poor prognosis in highgrade renal cell carcinomas. Cancer Genet Cytogenet. 2001;**130**:105–110. doi:10.1016/S0165-4608(01)00477-0.

[35] Manara MC, Perbal B, Benini S, Strammiello R, Cerisano V, Perdichizzi S, Serra M, Astolfi A, Bertoni F, Alami J, Yeger H, Picci P, Scotlandi K. The expression of CCN3 (nov) gene in musculoskeletal tumors. Am J Pathol. 2002;**160**:849–859. doi:10.1016/S0002-9440(10)64908-5.

[36] Gupta N, Wang H, McLeod TL, Naus CC, Kyurkchiev S, Advani S, Yu J, Perbal B, Weichselbaum RR. Inhibition of glioma cell growth and tumorigenic potential by CCN3 (NOV). Mol Pathol. 2001;**54**:293–299. doi:10.1136/mp.54.5.293.

[37] McCallum L, Price S, Planque N, Perbal B, Pierce A, Whetton AD, Irvine AE. A novel mechanism for BCR-ABL action: stimulated secretion of CCN3 is involved in growth and differentiation regulation. Blood. 2006;**108:**1716–1723. doi:10.1182/blood-2006-04-016113.

[38] Fukunaga-Kalabis M, Martinez G, Liu ZJ, Kalabis J, Mrass P, Weninger W, Firth SM, Planque M, Perbal B, Herlyn M. CCN3 controls 3D spatial localization of melanocytes in the human skin through DDR1. J Cell Biol. 2006;**175**:563–569. doi:10.1083/jcb.200602132.

[39] Haass NK, Smalley KS, Herlyn M. The role of altered cell–cell communication in melanoma progression. J Mol Histol. 2004;**35**:309–318. doi:10.1023/B:HIJO.0000032362.35354.bb.

[40] Weber B, Stresemann C, Brueckner B, Lyko F. Methylation of human microRNA genes in normal and neoplastic cells. Cell Cycle. 2007;**6**:1001–1005.

[41] Esteller M. Epigenetics in cancer. Eng J Med. 2008;**358**:1148–1159. doi:10.1056/NEJMra072067.

[42] Polsky D, Cordon Carlo C. Oncogenes in melanoma. Oncogene. 2003;**22**:3087–3091. doi:10.1038/sj.onc.1206449.

[43] Zigmund M, Nikuseva-Martic T, Cacic M, Pecina-Slaus N. New insights on genetics of malignant melanoma. Lijec Vjesn. 2005;**127**:89–93.

[44] Hashemi J, Platz A, Ueno T, Stierner V, Ringborn V, Hansson J. CDKN2A germ-line mutations in individuals with multiple cutaneous melanomas. Cancer Res. 2000;**60**:6864–6867.

[45] Wang J, Shen WH, Jin YJ, Brand-Rauf PW, Yin Y. A molecular link between E2F-1 and the MAPK cascade. J Biol Chem. 2007;**282**:18521–18531.

[46] Eskandapour M, Hashemi J, Kanter L, Ringborg U, Platz A, Hansson J. Frequency of UV-inducible NRAS mutations in melanomas of patients with germline CDKN2A mutations. J Natl Cancer Inst. 2005;**95**:790–798.

[47] Boukamp P. UV-induced skin cancer: similarities – variations. JDDG. 2005;**3**:493–503. doi:10.1111/j.1610-0387.2005.05037.x.

[48] Chin L. The genetics of malignant melanoma: lessons from mouse and man. Nature Rev. 2003;**3**:559–570.

[49] HA L, Ichikawa T, Anver M, Dickins R, Lowe S, Sharpless NE, Krimpenfort P, DePinho RA, Bennett DC, Sviderskaya EV, Merlino G. ARF functions as a melanoma tumor suppressor by inducing p53-independent senescence. PNAS. 2002;**104**:10968–10973. doi:10.1073/pnas.0611638104.

[50] Rees JL. The genetics of sun sensitivity in humans. Am J Hum Genet. 2004;**75**:739–751. doi:10.1086/425285.

[51] Duffy DL, Box NF, Chen W, Palmer JS, Montgomery GW, James MR, Hairward NK, Martin NG, Sturm RA. Interactive effects of MC1R and OCA2 on melanoma risk phenotypes. Hum Mol Genet. 2004;**13**:447–461. doi:10.1093/hmg/ddh043.

[52] Van der Velden PA, Sandkuijl LA, Bergman W, Pavel S, Van mourik L, Frants RR, Gruis NA. Melanocortin-1 receptor variant R151C modifies melanoma risk in Dutch families with melanoma. Am J Hum Genet. 2001;**69**:774–779.

[53] Gao L, Zhao H, Cornelius LA. The molecular mechanisms of melanoma tumorigeneis: an update. G Ital Dermatol Venereol. 2007;**142**:71–82.

[54] Abbasi NR, Shaw HM, Rigel DS, et al. Early diagnosis of cutaneous melanoma: revisiting the ABCD criteria. JAMA. 2004;**292**(22):2771–2776. doi:10.1001/jama.292.22.2771.

[55] Morton DL, Thompson JF, Cochran AJ, Mozzillo N, Elashoff R, et al. Sentinel-node biopsy or nodal observation in melanoma. N Engl J Med. 2006;**355**:1307–1317. doi:10.1056/NEJMoa060992.

[56] Balch CM, Gershenwald JE, Soong SJ, Thompson JF, Atkins MB, et al. Final version of 2009 AJCC melanoma staging and classification. J Clin Oncol. 2009;**27**:6199–6206. doi:10.1200/JCO.2009.23.4799.

[57] Breslow A. Thickness, cross-sectional areas and depth of invasion in the prognosis of cutaneous melanoma. Ann Surg. 1970;**172**:902–908.

[58] Grande Sarpa H, Reinke K, Shaikh L, Leong SP, Miller JR, et al. Prognostic significance of extent of ulceration in primary cutaneous melanoma. Am J Surg Pathol. 2006;**30**:1396–1400.

[59] Francken AB, Shaw HM, Thompson JF. The prognostic importance of tumor mitotic rate confirmed in 1,317 patients with primary cutaneous melanoma and long follow-up. Ann. Surg. Oncol. 2004;**11**:426–433.

[60] Gown AM, Vogel AM, Hoak D, Gough F, McNutt MA. Monoclonal antibodies specific for melanocytic tumors distinguish subpopulations of melanocytes. Am J Pathol. 1986;**123**(2):195–203.

[61] Fernando SS, Johnson S, Bate J. Immunohistochemical analysis of cutaneous malignant melanoma: comparison of S-100 protein, HMB-45 monoclonal antibody and NKI/C3 monoclonal antibody. Pathology. 1994;**26**(1):16–19.

[62] Ordonez NG, Ji XL, Hickey RC. Comparison of HMB-45 monoclonal antibody and S-100 protein in the immunohistochemical diagnosis of melanoma. Am J Clin Pathol. 1988;**90**:385–390.

[63] Chen YT, Stockert E, Jungbluth A, et al. Serological analysis of Melan-A(MART-1), a melanocyte-specific protein homogeneously expressed in human melanomas. Proc Natl Acad Sci U S A. 1996;**93**(12):5915–5919.

[64] Kawakami Y, Eliyahu S, Delgado CH, et al. Cloning of the gene coding for a shared human melanoma antigen recognized by autologous T cells infiltrating into tumor. Proc Natl Acad Sci U S A. 1994;**91**:3515–3519.

[65] Weinstein D, Leininger J, Hamby C, Safai B. Diagnostic and prognostic biomarkers in melanoma. J Clin Aesthet Dermatol. 2014;**7**(6):13–24.

[66] Bonfrer JM, Korse CM, Nieweg OE, Rankin EM. The luminescence immunoassay S-100: a sensitive test to measure circulating S-100B: its prognostic value in malignant melanoma. Br J Cancer. 1998;**77**(12):2210–2214.

[67] Nakajima T, Watanabe S, Sato Y, et al. Immunohistochemical demonstration of S100 protein in malignant melanoma and pigmented nevus, and its diagnostic application. Cancer. 1982;**50**:912–918.

[68] Hofbauer GF, Kamarashev J, Geertsen R, et al. Tyrosinase immunoreactivity in formalin-fixed, paraffin-embedded primary and metastatic melanoma: frequency and distribution. J Cutan Pathol. 1998;**25**:204–249.

[69] Gerdes J, Lemke H, Baisch H, et al. Cell cycle analysis of a cell proliferation-associated human nuclear antigen defined by the monoclonal antibody Ki-67. J Immunol. 1984;**133**:1710–1715.

[70] Gimotty PA, Van Belle P, Elder DE, Murry T, et al. Biologic and prognostic significance of dermal Ki67 expression, mitoses, and tumorigenicity in thin invasive cutaneous melanoma. JCO. 2005;**23**(31):8048–8056. doi:10.1200/JCO.2005.02.0735.

[71] Akiyama M, Matsuda Y, Ishiwata T, Naito Z, Kawana S. Nestin is highly expressed in advanced-stage melanomas and neurotized nevi. Oncol Rep. 2013;**29**(4):1595–1599.

[72] Lai S, Piras F, Mura E, Spiga S, et al. Nestin and vimentin intermediate filaments expression in cutaneous melanoma. Ital J Anat Embryol. 2011;**116**(2):96. doi:10.13128/IJAE-10066.

[73] Gross A, Niemetz-Rahn A, Nonnenmacher A, Tucholski J, et al. Expression and activity of EGFR in human cutaneous melanoma cell lines and influence of vemurafenib on the EGFR pathway. Target Oncol. 2015;**10**(1):77-84. doi:10.1007/s11523-014-0318-9.

[74] Boone B, Jacobs K, Ferdinande L, Taildeman J, Lambert J, Peeters M, Bracke M, Pauwels P. Brochez L. EGFR in melanoma: clinical significance and potential therapeutic target. J Cutan Pathol. 2011;**38**:492–502. doi:10.1111/j.1600-0560.2011.01673.x.

[75] Surget S, Khoury MP, Bourdon JC. Uncovering the role of p53 splice variants in human malignancy: a clinical perspective. OncoTargets Therapy. 2013;**7**:57–68. doi:10.2147/OTT.S53876.

[76] Houben R, Hesbacher S, Schmid CP, et al. High-level expression of wild-type p53 in melanoma cells is frequently associated with inactivity in p53 reporter gene assays. PLoS One. 2011;**6**(7):e22096. doi:10.1371/journal.pone.0022096.

[77] Palmer SR, Erickson LA, Ichetovkin I, Knauer DJ, Markovic SN. Circulating serologic and molecular biomarkers in malignant melanoma. Mayo Clinic Proc. 2011;**86**(10):981–990. doi:10.4065/mcp.2011.0287.

[78] Verykiou S, Ellis RA, Lovat PE. Established and emerging biomarkers in cutaneous malignant melanoma. Healthcare. 2014;**2**(1):60–73. doi:10.3390/healthcare2010060.

[79] Wan PTC, Garnett MJ, Roe SM, Lee S, et al. Mechanism of activation of the RAF-ERK signaling pathway by oncogenic mutations of B-RAF. Cell. 2004;**116**(6):855–867. doi:10.1016/S0092-8674(04)00215-6.

[80] Hugdahl E, Kalvenes MB, Puntervoll HE, Ladstein RG, Akslen LA. BRAF-V600E expression in primary nodular melanoma is associated with aggressive tumor features and reduced survival. Br J Cancer. 2016. doi:10.1038/bjc.2016.44.

[81] Wang P, Guan P, Xu S, Wang Z, et al. Emerging GM3 regulated biomarkers in malignant melanoma, recent advances in the biology, therapy and management of melanoma. In: Dr. Lester Davids, Editor, Melanoma — Epidemiology, Genetics and Risk Factors. Rijeka, Croatia: InTech; 2013. doi:10.5772/54941.

[82] Karagiannis P, Fittall M, Karagiannis SN. Evaluating biomarkers in melanoma. Front Oncol. 2014;**4**:383. doi:10.3389/fonc.2014.00383.

[83] Kumar S, Sharma P, Kumar D, Chakraborty G, Gorain M, Kundu GC. Functional characterization of stromal osteopontin in melanoma progression and metastasis. PLoS One. 2013;8(7):e69116. doi:10.1371/journal.pone.0069116.

[84] Gogas H, Eggermont AMM, Hauschild A, et al. Biomarkers in melanoma. Ann Oncol. 2009;**20**(Suppl 6):vi8–vi13. doi:10.1093/annonc/mdp251.

[85] Boiko AD, Razorenova OV, van de Rijn M, et al. Human melanoma initiating cells express neural crest nerve growth factor receptor CD271. Nature. 2010;**466**(7302):133–137. doi:10.1038/nature09161.

[86] Cragg GM., Newman DJ. Natural products: a continuing source of novel drug leads. Biochim Biophys Acta. 2013;**1830**(6):3670–3695.

[87] AlQathama A, Prieto JM. Natural products with therapeutic potential in melanoma metastasis. Nat Prod Rep. 2015, **32**(8):1170–1182.

[88] Pal HC, Hunt KM, Diamond A, Elmets CA, Afaq F. Phytochemicals for the management of melanoma. Mini Rev Med Chem. 2016;**16**:1–27. doi:10.2174/ 1389557516666160211120157.

[89] Chinembiri TN, du Plessis LH, Gerber M, Hamman JH, du Plessis J. Review of natural compounds for potential skin cancer treatment. Molecules. 2014;**19**:11679–11721.

[90] Menon LG, Kuttan R, Kuttan G. Inhibition of lung metastasis in mice induced by B16F10 melanoma cells by polyphenolic compounds. Cancer Lett. 1995;**95**(1–2):221–225.

[91] Steinmetz KA, Potter JD. Vegetables, fruit and cancer. II. Mechanisms. Cancer Causes Control. 1991;**2**(6):427–442.

[92] Solovchenko A., Merzlyak M. Optical properties and contribution of cuticle to UV protection in plants: experiments with apple fruit. Photochem Photobiol Sci. 2003;**2**:861–866.

[93] Liu-Smith F., Meyskens F. Molecular mechanisms of flavonoids in melanin synthesis and the potential for the prevention and treatment of melanoma. Mol Nutr Food Res. 2016. doi:10.1002/mnfr.201500822.

[94] Dzialo M, Mierziak J, Korzun U, Preisner M, Szopa J, Kulma A. The potential of plant phenolics in prevention and therapy of skin disorders. Int J Mol Sci. 2016;**17**(2). doi:10.3390/ijms17020160.

[95] Rafiq RA, Quadri A, Nazir LA, Peerzada K, Ganai BA, Tasduq SA. A potent inhibitor of phosphoinositide 3-kinase (PI3K) and mitogen activated protein (MAP) kinase signalling, quercetin (3, 3′, 4′, 5, 7-pentahydroxyflavone) promotes cell death in ultraviolet (UV)-B-irradiated B16F10Melanoma cells. PLoS One. 2015;**10**(7):e0131253.

[96] Chaiprasongsuk A., Onkoksoong T, Pluemsamran T, Limsaengurai S, Panich U. Photoprotection by dietary phenolics against melanogenesis induced by UVA through Nrf2-dependentantioxidantresponses. Redox Biol. 2016;**8**:79–90.

[97] Cao HH, Cheng CY, Su T, Fu XQ, Guo H, Li T, Tse AK, Kwan HY, Yu H, Yu ZL. Quercetin inhibits HGF/c-Met signaling and HGF-stimulated melanoma cell migration and invasion. Mol Cancer. 2015;**14**:103.

[98] Saewan N., Jimtaisong A. Photoprotection of natural flavonoids. J Appl Pharm Sci. 2013;**3**(9):129–141.

[99] Cao HH, Chu JH, Kwan HY, Su T, Yu H, Cheng CY, Fu XQ, Guo H, Li T, Tse AK, Chou GX, Mo HB, Yu ZL. Inhibition of the STAT3 signaling pathway contributes to apigenin-mediated anti-metastatic effect in melanoma. Sci Rep. 2016;**6**:21731. doi:10.1038/srep21731.

[100] Hasnat MA, Pervin M, Lim JH, Lim BO. Apigenin attenuates melanoma cell migration by inducing anoikis through integrin and focal adhesion kinase inhibition. Molecules. 2015;**20**(12):21157–21166. doi:10.3390/molecules201219752.

[101] Kiraly AJ, Soliman E, Jenkins A, Van Dross RT. Apigenin inhibits COX-2, PGE2, and EP1 and also initiates terminal differentiation in the epidermis of tumor bearing mice. Prostaglandins Leukot Essent Fatty Acids. 2016;**104**:44–53. doi:10.1016/j.plefa.2015.11.006.

[102] Ghosh A., Ghosh T, Jain S. Silymarin – a review on the pharmacodynamics and bioavailability enhancement approaches. J Pharm Sci Technol. 2010;**2**(10):348–355.

[103] Lee MH, Huang Z, Kim DJ, Kim SH, Kim MO, Lee SY, Xie H, Park SJ, Kim JY, Kundu JK, Bode A, Surh YJ, Dong Z. Direct targeting of MEK1/2 and RSK2 by silybin induces cell-cycle arrest and inhibits melanoma cell growth. Cancer Prev Res (Phila). 2013;**6**(5):455–465. doi:10.1158/1940-6207.

[104] Vaid M, Singh T, Prasad R, Katiyar SK. Silymarin inhibits melanoma cell growth both in vitro and in vivo by targeting cell cycle regulators, angiogenic biomarkers and induction of apoptosis. Mol Carcinog. 2015;**54**(11):1328–1339.

[105] Gajos-Michniewicz A, Czyz M. Modulation of WNT/β-catenin pathway in melanoma by biologically active components derived from plants. Fitoterapia. 2016;**109**:283–292.

[106] Katiyar S, Elmets CA, Katiyar SK. Green tea and skin cancer: photoimmunology, angiogenesis and DNA repair. J Nutr Biochem. 2007;**18**(5):287–296.

[107] Nihal M, Ahmad N, Mukhtar H, Wood GS. Anti-proliferative and proapoptotic effects of (-)-epigallocatechin-3-gallate on human melanoma: possible implications for the chemoprevention of melanoma. Int J Cancer. 2005;**114**:513–521.

[108] Chung SY, Hong W, Guang Xun L, Zhihong Y, Fei G, Huanyu J. Review: cancer prevention by tea: evidence from laboratory studies. Pharm Res. 2011;**64:**113–122.

[109] Umeda D, Yano S, Yamada K, Tachibana H. Green tea polyphenol epigallocatechin-3-gallate signaling pathway through 67-kDa laminin receptor. J Biol Chem 2008;**283**:3050–3058.

[110] Yamada S, Tsukamoto S, Huang Y, Makio A, Kumazoe M, Yamashita S, Tachibana H. Epigallocatechin-3-O-gallate up-regulates microRNA-let-7b expression by activating 67-kDa laminin receptor signaling in melanoma cells. Sci Rep. 2016;**6**:19225.

[111] Takahashi A, Watanabe T, Mondal A, Suzuki K, Kurusu-Kanno M, Li Z, Yamazaki T, Fujiki H, Suganuma M. Mechanism-based inhibition of cancer metastasis with (-)-epigallocatechin gallate. Biochem Biophys Res Commun. 2014;**443**(1):1–6. doi:10.1016/j.bbrc.2013.10.094.

[112] Singh T, Katiyar SK. Green tea catechins reduce invasive potential of human melanoma cells by targeting COX-2, PGE2 receptors and epithelial-to-mesenchymal transition. PLoS One. 2011;**6**(10):e25224. doi:10.1371/journal.pone.0025224.

[113] Chang CW, Hsieh YH, Yang WE, Yang SF, Chen Y, Hu DN. Epigallocatechingallate inhibits migration of human uveal melanoma cells via downregulation of matrix metalloproteinase-2 activity and ERK1/2 pathway. Biomed Res Int. 2014;**2014**:141582. doi:10.1155/2014/141582. [Epub 12 Aug 2014].

[114] Zhao G, Han X, Zheng S, Li Z, Sha Y, Ni J, Sun Z, Qiao S, Song Z. Curcumin induces autophagy, inhibits proliferation and invasion by downregulating AKT/mTOR signaling pathway in human melanoma cells. Oncol Rep. 2016;**35**(2):1065–1074.

[115] Ray S, Chattopadhyay N, Mitra A, Siddiqi M, Chatterjee A. Curcumin exhibits antimetastatic properties by modulating integrin receptors, collagenase activity, and expression of Nm23 and E-cadherin. J Environ Pathol Toxicol Oncol. 2003;**22**(1):49–58.

[116] Zhang YP, Li YQ, Lv YT, Wang JM. Effect of curcumin on the proliferation, apoptosis, migration, and invasion of human melanoma A375 cells. Genet Mol Res. 2015;**14** (1):1056–67.

[117] Wu Z, Liu B, E C, Liu J, Zhang Q, Liu J, Chen N, Chen R, Zhu R. Resveratrol inhibits the proliferation of human melanoma cells by inducing G1/S cell cycle arrest and apoptosis. Mol Med Rep. 2015;**11**(1):400–404. doi:10.3892/mmr.2014.2716.

[118] Bhattacharya S, Darjatmoko SR, Polans AS. Resveratrol modulates the malignant properties of cutaneous melanoma through changes in the activation and attenuation of the antiapoptotic protooncogenic protein Akt/PKB. Melanoma Res. 2011;**21**(3):180–187.

[119] Chan GC, Chan WK, Sze DM. The effects of beta-glucan on human immune and cancer cells. J Hematol Oncol. 2009;**2**:25. doi:10.1186/1756-8722-2-25.

[120] Imbs TI, Ermakova SP, Malyarenko Vishchuk OS, Isakov VV, Zvyagintseva TN. Structural elucidation of polysaccharide fractions from the brown alga Coccophora langsdorfii and in vitro investigation of their anticancer activity. Carbohydr Polym. 2016;**135**:162–168.

[121] Vetvicka V, Vetvickova J. Glucan supplementation has strong anti-melanoma effects: role of NK cells. Anticancer Res. 2015;**35**(10):5287–5292.

[122] Choromanska A, Kulbacka J, Rembialkowska N, Pilat J, Oledzki R, Harasym J, Saczko J. Anticancer properties of low molecular weight oat beta-glucan – an in vitro study. Int J Biol Macromol. 2015;**80**:23-28.

[123] Yang YJ, Xu HM, Suo YR. Raspberry pulp polysaccharides inhibit tumor growth via immunopotentiation and enhance docetaxel chemotherapy against malignant melanoma in vivo. Food Funct. 2015;**6**(9):3022–3034.

[124] Jayaram S, Kapoor S, Dharmesh SM. Pectic polysaccharide from corn (Zea mays L.) effectively inhibited multi-step mediated cancer cell growth and metastasis. Chem Biol Interact. 2015;**235**:63–75.

[125] Raguso RA, Pichersky E. A day in the life of a linalool molecule: chemical communication in a plant-pollinator system. Part 1: linalool biosynthesis in flowering plants. Plant Spec Biol. 1999;**14**:95–120.

[126] Calcabrini A, Stringaro A, Toccacieli L, Meschini S, Marra M, Colone M, Salvatore G, Mondello F, Arancia G, Molinari A. Terpinen-4-ol, the main component of *Melaleuca alternifolia* (tea tree) oil inhibits the in vitro growth of human melanoma cells. J Invest Dermatol. 2004;**122**(2):349–360.

[127] Greay SJ, Ireland DJ, Kissick HT, Heenan PJ, Carson CF, Riley TV, Beilharz MW. Inhibition of established subcutaneous murine tumor growth with topical *Melaleuca alternifolia* (tea tree) oil. Cancer Chemother Pharmacol. 2010;**66**(6):1095–1102.

[128] Manjamalai A, Kumar MJ, Grace VM. Essential oil of Tridax procumbens L. induces apoptosis and suppresses angiogenesis and lung metastasis of the B16F-10 cell line in C57BL/6 mice. Asian Pac J Cancer Prev. 2012;**13**(11):5887–5895.

[129] Chen W, Lu Y, Gao M, Wu J, Wang A, Shi R. Anti-angiogenesis effect of essential oil from *Curcuma zedoaria* in vitro and in vivo. J Ethnopharmacol. 2011;**133**(1):220–226.

[130] Mantena SK, Sharma SD, Katiyar SK. Berberine inhibits growth, induces G1 arrest and apoptosis in human epidermoid carcinoma A431 cells by regulating Cdki-Cdk-cyclin cascade, disruption of mitochondrial membrane potential and cleavage of caspase 3 and PARP. Carcinogenesis. 2006;**27**(10):2018–2027. [Epub 18 Apr 2006].

[131] Barbagallo CM, Cefalu AB, Noto D, Averna MR. Role of nutraceuticals in hypolipidemic therapy. Front Cardiovasc Med. 2015;**2**:22.

[132] Song YC, Lee Y, Kim HM, Hyun MY, Lim YY, Song KY, Kim BJ. Berberine regulates melanin synthesis by activating PI3K/AKT, ERK and GSK3β in B16F10 melanoma cells. Int J Mol Med. 2015;**35**(4):1011–1016.

[133] Mittal A, Tabasum S, Singh RP. Berberine in combination with doxorubicin suppresses growth of murine melanoma B16F10 cells in culture and xenograft Phytomedicine. 2014;**21**(3):340–347.

[134] Singh T, Vaid M, Katiyar N, Sharma S, Katiyar SK. Berberine, an isoquinoline alkaloid, inhibits melanoma cancer cell migration by reducing the expressions of cyclooxygenase-2, prostaglandin E2 and prostaglandin E2 receptors. Carcinogenesis. 2011;**32**(1):86–92.

[135] Hamsa TP, Kuttan G. Antiangiogenic activity of berberine is mediated through the downregulation of hypoxia-inducible factor-1, VEGF, and proinflammatory mediators. Drug Chem Toxicol. 2012;**35**(1):57–70.

[136] Hamsa TP, Kuttan G. Harmine inhibits tumor specific neo-vessel formation by regulating VEGF, MMP, TIMP and pro-inflammatory mediators both in vivo and in vitro. Eur J Pharmacol. 2010;**649**(1–3):64–73.

[137] Hamsa TP, Kuttan G. Studies on anti-metastatic and anti-invasive effects of harmine using highly metastatic murine B16F-10 melanoma cells. J Environ Pathol Toxicol Oncol. 2011;**30**(2):123–137.

[138] Kundranda MN, Niu J. Albumin-bound paclitaxel in solid tumors: clinical development and future directions. Drug Des Devel Ther. 2015;**9**:3767–3777.

[139] Yue Q-X, Liu X, Guo D-A. Microtubule-binding natural products for cancer therapy. Planta Med. 2010;**76**:1037–1043.

[140] Merchan JR, Jayaram DR, Supko JG, He X, Bubley GJ, Sukhatme VP. Increased endothelial uptake of paclitaxel as a potential mechanism for its antiangiogenic effects: potentiation by Cox-2 inhibition. Int J Cancer. 2005;**113**(3):490–498.

[141] Al Sinani SS, Eltayeb EA, Coomber BL, Adham SA. Solamargine triggers cellular necrosis selectively in different types of human melanoma cancer cells through extrinsic lysosomal mitochondrial death pathway. Cancer Cell Int. 2016;**16**:11.

[142] Lu MK, Shih YW, Chang Chien TT, Fang LH, Huang HC, Chen PS. α-Solanine inhibits human melanoma cell migration and invasion by reducing matrix metalloproteinase-2/9 activities. Biol Pharm Bull. 2010;**33**(10):1685–1691.

[143] Abirami A, Mohamed Halith S, Pillai KK, Anbalagan C. Herbal nanoparticle for anticancer potential- a review. World J Pharm Pharm Sci. 2014;**3**:2123–2132.

[144] Srinivas NR. Formulation development for cancer compounds – biopharmaceutical issues and perspectives. Asian J Pharm. 2009;90–93. doi:10.4103/0973-8398.55044.

[145] Sharma V, Nehru B, Munshi A, Jyothy A. Antioxidant potential of curcumin against oxidative insult induced by pentylenetetrazol in epileptic rats. Methods Find Exper Clin Pharm. 2010;**2**(4):227. doi:10.1358/mf.2010.32.4.1452090.

[146] Kocher A, Schiborr C, Behnam D, Frank J. The oral bioavailability of curcuminoids in healthy humans is markedly enhanced by micellar solubilisation but not further improved by simultaneous ingestion of sesamin, ferulic acid, naringenin and xanthohumol. J Funct Foods. 2015;**14**:183–191.

[147] Schiborr C, Kocher A, Behnam D, Jandasek J, Toelstede S, Frank J. The oral bioavailability of curcumin from micronized powder and liquid micelles is significantly increased in healthy humans and differs between sexes. Mol Nutr Food Res. 2014;**58**:516–527. doi:10.1002/mnfr.201300724.

[148] Ravichandran R, Pharmacokinetic study of nanoparticulate curcumin: oral formulation for enhanced bioavailability. J Biomater Nanobiotechnol. 2013;**4**:291–299. doi:10.4236/jbnb.2013.43037.

[149] Madhavi D, Kagan D. Bioavailability of a sustained release formulation of curcumin. Integr Med (Encinitas). 2014;**13**:24–30.

[150] Marczylo TH, Verschoyle RD, Cooke DN, Morazzoni P, Steward WP, Gescher AJ. Comparison of systemic availability of curcumin with that of curcumin formulated with phosphatidylcholine. Cancer Chemother Pharmacol. 2007;**60**:171–177.

[151] Jäger R, Lowery RP, Calvanese AV, Joy JM, Purpura M, Wilson JM. Comparative absorption of curcumin formulations. Nutr J. 2014;**13**:11. doi:10.1186/1475-2891-13-11.

[152] Sou K, Inenaga S, Takeoka S, Tsuchida E. Loading of curcumin into macrophages using lipid-based nanoparticles. Int J Pharm. 2008;**352**:287–293.

[153] Li L, Ahmed B, Mehta K, Kurzrock R. Liposomal curcumin with and without oxaliplatin: effects on cell growth, apoptosis, and angiogenesis in colorectal cancer. Mol Cancer Ther. 2007;**6**:1276–1282.

[154] Rachmadi UW, Permatasari D, Rahma A, Rachmawati H. Self-nanoemulsion containing combination of curcumin and silymarin: formulation and characterization. Res Dev Nanotechnol Indones. 2015;**2**:37–48.

[155] Li X, Yuan Q, Huang Y, Zhou Y, Liu Y. Development of silymarin self-microemulsifying drug delivery system with enhanced oral bioavailability. AAPS PharmSciTech. 2010;**11**:672–678. doi:10.1208/s12249-010-9432-x.

[156] Hussein A, El-Menshawe S, Afouna M. Enhancement of the in-vitro dissolution and in-vivo oral bioavailability of silymarin from liquid-filled hard gelatin capsules of semi-solid dispersion using Gelucire 44/14 as a carrier. Pharmazie. 2012;**67**:209–214.

[157] Sonali D, Tejal S, Vaishali T, Tejal G. Silymarin-solid dispersions: characterization and influence of preparation methods on dissolution. Acta Pharm. 2010;**60**:427–443. doi:10.2478/v10007-010-0038-3.

[158] Gupta S, Kumar Singh S, Girotra P. Targeting silymarin for improved hepatoprotective activity through chitosan nanoparticles. Int J Pharm Investig 2014;**4**:156–163. doi:10.4103/2230-973X.143113.

[159] Xu X, Yu J, Tong S, Zhu Y, Cao X. Formulation of silymarin with high efficacy and prolonged action and the preparation method thereof. US Patent 20110201680 A1, 2011.

[160] Lian R, Lu Y, Qi J, Tan Y, Niu M, Guan P, Hu F, Wu W. Silymarin glyceryl monooleate/poloxamer 407 liquid crystalline matrices: physical characterization and enhanced oral bioavailability. AAPS PharmSciTech. 2011;**12**:1234–40. doi:10.1208/s12249-011-9666-2.

[161] Wang M, Xie T, Chang Z, Wang L, Xie X, Kou Y, Xu H, Gao X. A new type of liquid silymarin proliposome containing bile salts: its preparation and improved hepato-protective effects. PLoS One. 2015;**10**:e0143625. doi:10.1371/journal.pone.0143625. eCollection 2015.

[162] Kumar N, Rai A, Reddy ND, Raj PV, Jain P, Deshpande P, Mathew G, Kutty NG, Udupa N, Rao CM. Silymarin liposomes improves oral bioavailability of silybin besides targeting hepatocytes, and immune cells. Pharmacol Rep. 2014;**66**:788–798. doi:10.1016/j.pharep.2014.04.007.

[163] Yang G, Zhao Y, Zhang Y, Dang B, Liu Y, Feng N. Enhanced oral bioavailability of silymarin using liposomes containing a bile salt: preparation by supercritical fluid technology and evaluation in vitro and in vivo. 2015;**2015**:6633–6644.

[164] Park JH, Park JH, Hur HJ, Woo JS, Lee HJ. Effects of silymarin and formulation on the oral bioavailability of paclitaxel in rats. Eur J Pharm Sci. 2012;**45**:296–301. doi:10.1016/j.ejps.2011.11.021.

[165] Ganta S, Devalapally H, Amiji M. Curcumin enhances oral bioavailability and anti-tumor therapeutic efficacy of paclitaxel upon administration in nanoemulsion formulation. J Pharm Sci. 2010;**99**:4630–4641. doi:10.1002/jps.22157.

[166] Chu Z, Chen JS, Liau CT, Wang HM, Lin YC, Yang MH, Chen PM, Gardner ER, Figg WD, Sparreboom A. Oral bioavailability of a novel paclitaxel formulation (Genetaxyl) administered with cyclosporin A in cancer patients. Anticancer Drugs. 2008;**19**:275–281.

[167] Gelderblom H, Verweij J, van Zomeren DM, Buijs D, Ouwens L, Nooter K, Stoter G, Sparreboom A. Influence of Cremophor El on the bioavailability of intraperitoneal paclitaxel. Clin Cancer Res 2002;**8**:1237–1241.

[168] Chiang P-C, Gould S, Nannini M, Qin A, Deng Y, Arrazate A, Kam KR, Ran Y, Wong H. Nanosuspension delivery of paclitaxel to xenograft mice can alter drug disposition and anti-tumor activity. Nanoscale Res Lett. 2014;**9**(1):156.

[169] Oostendorp RL, Buckle T, Lambert G, Garrigue JS, Beijnen JH, Schellens JH, van Tellingen O. Paclitaxel in self-micro emulsifying formulations: oral bioavailability study in mice. Invest New Drugs. 2010;**29**:768–776.

[170] Veltkamp SA, Thijssen B, Garrigue JS, Lambert G, Lallemand F, Binlich F, Huitema ADR, Nuijen B, Nol A, Beijnen JH, Schellens JHM. A novel self-microemulsifying formulation of paclitaxel for oral administration to patients with advanced cancer. Br J Cancer. 2006;**95**:729–734.

[171] Gao P, Rush BD, Pfund WP, Huang T, Bauer JM, Morozowich W, Kuo MS, Hageman MJ. Development of a supersaturable SEDDS (S-SEDDS) formulation of paclitaxel with improved oral bioavailability. J Pharm Sci. 2003;**92**:2386–2398.

[172] Ahmad J, Mir SR, Kohli K, Chuttani K, Mishra AK, Panda AK, Amin S. Solid-nanoemulsion preconcentrate for oral delivery of paclitaxel: formulation design, biodistribution, and γ scintigraphy imaging. Biomed Res Int. 2014;**2014**:984756. doi:10.1155/2014/984756.

[173] Bayindir ZS, Yuksel N. Characterization of niosomes prepared with various nonionic surfactants for paclitaxel oral delivery. J Pharm Sci. 2010;**99**:2049–2060. doi:10.1002/jps.21944.

[174] Eskolaky EB, Ardjmand M, Akbarzadeh A. Evaluation of anti-cancer properties of pegylated ethosomal paclitaxel on human melanoma cell line SKMEL- 3. Trop J Pharm Res. 2015;**14**:1421–1425.

[175] Peltier S, Oger JM, Lagarce F, Couet W, Benoît JP. Enhanced oral paclitaxel bioavailability after administration of paclitaxel-loaded lipid nanocapsules. Pharm Res. 2006;**23**:1243–1250.

[176] Baek JS, So JW, Shin SC, Cho CW. Solid lipid nanoparticles of paclitaxel strengthened by hydroxypropyl-β-cyclodextrin as an oral delivery system. Int J Mol Med. 2012;**30**:953–959. doi:10.3892/ijmm.2012.1086.

[177] Patil SM, Joshi HP. Colloidal drug delivery system for tumor specificity of paclitaxel in mice. Der Pharm Lett. 2012;**4**:961–967.

[178] Baek JS, Kim J-H, Park J-S, Cho CW. Modification of paclitaxel-loaded solid lipid nanoparticles with 2-hydroxypropyl-β-cyclodextrin enhances absorption and reduces nephrotoxicity associated with intravenous injection. Int J Nanomed. 2015;**10**:5397–5405.

[179] Aygül G, Yerlikaya F, Caban S, Vural I, Çapan Y. Formulation and *in vitro* evaluation of paclitaxel loaded nanoparticles, Hacettepe Univ J Faculty Pharm. 2013;**33**:25–40.

[180] Yoncheva K, Calleja P, Agüeros M, Petrov P, Miladinova I, Tsvetanov C, Irache JM. Stabilized micelles as delivery vehicles for paclitaxel. Int J Pharm. 2012;**436**:258–264. doi:10.1016/j.ijpharm.2012.06.030.

[181] Coimbra M, Isacchi, B, van Bloois L, Torano JS, Ket A, Wu XJ, Broere F, Metselaar JM, Rijcken CJF, Storm G, Bilia R, Schiffelers RM. Improving solubility and chemical stability of natural compounds for medicinal use by incorporation into liposomes. Int J Pharm. 2011;**416**(2):433–442.

[182] Ansari KA, Vavia PR, Trotta F, Cavalli R. Cyclodextrin-based nanosponges for delivery of resveratrol: *in vitro* characterisation, stability, cytotoxicity and permeation study. AAPS PharmSciTech. 2011;**12**(1):279–286.

[183] Nam JB, Ryu JH, Kim JW, Chang IS, Suh KD. Stabilization of resveratrol immobilized in monodisperse cyano-functionalized porous polymeric microspheres. Polymer. 2005;**46** (21):8956–8963.

[184] Shi G, Rao L, Yu H, Xiang H, Yang H, Ji R. Stabilization and encapsulation of photosensitive resveratrol within yeast cell. Int J Pharm. 2008;**349**(1–2):83–93.

[185] Das S, Ng KY, Ho PC. Formulation and optimization of zinc-pectinate beads for the controlled delivery of resveratrol. AAPS PharmSciTech. 2010;**11**(2):729–742.

[186] Das S, Chaudhury A, Ng KY. Preparation and evaluation of zinc-pectinchitosan composite particles for drug delivery to the colon: role of chitosan in modifying in vitro and *in vivo* drug release. Int J Pharm. 2011;**406**(1–2):11–20.

[187] Lund KC, Pantuso T. Combination effects of quercetin, resveratrol and curcumin on in vitro intestinal absorption. J Restorat Med. 2014;**3**:112–120.

Section 5

Computational and Bitochenology Advancement of Phytotherapy in Cancer

Chapter 10

Computational Studies and Biosynthesis of Natural Products with Promising Anticancer Properties

Aurélien F.A. Moumbock, Conrad V. Simoben,
Ludger Wessjohann, Wolfgang Sippl,
Stefan Günther and Fidele Ntie-Kang

Additional information is available at the end of the chapter

http://dx.doi.org/10.5772/67650

Abstract

We present an overview of computational approaches for the prediction of metabolic pathways by which plants biosynthesise compounds, with a focus on selected very promising anticancer secondary metabolites from floral sources. We also provide an overview of databases for the retrieval of useful genomic data, discussing the strengths and limitations of selected prediction software and the main computational tools (and methods), which could be employed for the investigation of the uncharted routes towards the biosynthesis of some of the identified anticancer metabolites from plant sources, eventually using specific examples to address some knowledge gaps when using these approaches.

Keywords: anticancer, biosynthesis, computational prediction, natural products, plant metabolism

1. Introduction

An immense number of secondary metabolites (SMs) exist in nature, originating from plants, bacteria, fungi and marine life forms, serving as drugs for the treatment of many life-threatening diseases, including cancer [1–4]. Taxol, vinblastine, vincristine, podophyllotoxin and camptothecin, for example, are typically well-known drugs used in cancer treatment, which are of plant origin. The search for drugs against cancer has often resorted to plants and marine life for lead compounds. To illustrate this, Newmann and Cragg published a recent study in which it was shown that ~49% of drugs used in cancer treatment were either natural products

(NPs) or their derivatives [5]. We would henceforth refer to SMs and NPs interchangeably, since NPs are the products of secondary (or specialised) metabolism, as opposed to primary metabolism, which results in molecules playing a key role in physiological processes of the organism and are thus necessary for the plant's survival. It should be mentioned that SMs are important for the plant's defence against attacks by other organisms. Several efforts have also been made towards the collection of data on naturally occurring plant metabolites showing anticancer properties. As an example, Mangal and co-workers published the naturally occurring plant-based anti-cancer compound activity-target database (NPACT), containing about 1,500 NPs [6]. In addition to the experimentally verified *in vitro* and *in vivo* data for these NPs, the authors also include biological activities (in the form of IC_{50}s, ED_{50}s, EC_{50}s, GI_{50}s, etc.), along with physical, elemental and topological properties of the NPs, the tested cancer types, cell lines, protein targets, commercial suppliers and drug likeness of the NPACT compounds. A similar effort was published the following year, for NPs from African flora, resulting in a dataset of about 400 compounds, named AfroCancer [7]. A further study showed that the NPACT and AfroCancer datasets showed little intersection, thus providing us a combined dataset of about 2,000 NPs [8]. The anticancer properties of some of the most promising AfroCancer compounds have been described in detail in recent reviews [9–12]. Further curation of data from Northern African species has recently resulted in the Northern African Natural Products Database (NANPDB), a web accessible and completely downloadable vast database of NPs, with a significant proportion of anticancer metabolites [13]. The NANPDB effort was founded on the observation that the Northern Africa region is particularly highly endowed with diverse vegetation types, serving as a huge reservoir of bioactive natural products [14–16].

For decades, NPs were identified exclusively by using chemical identification based on bioactivity-guided screening approaches. Recently, it has been postulated that genomics and bioinformatics would transform the approach of natural products discovery, even though genome mining has had only little influence on the advancement of natural product discovery until now [17]. Several algorithms have been developed for the mining of the (meta)genomic data, which continue to be generated. Computational methods and tools for the identification of biosynthetic gene clusters (BGCs, which are physically clustered groups of a few genes in a particular genome that together encode a biosynthetic pathway for the production of a specialised metabolite) in genome sequences and the prediction of chemical structures of their products have been developed [18]. BGCs for SM biosynthetic pathways are important in bacteria and filamentous fungi, with examples being recently discovered in plants [19, 20], although some metabolic processes in plants, for example, the thalianol pathway for triterpene synthesis in *Arabidopsis thaliana* has been suggested to be controlled by operon-like (clusters of unrelated) gene clusters [21]. This, coupled with the rapid progress in sequencing technologies has led to the development of new screening methods, which focus on whole genome sequences of the organisms producing the NPs. Genome mining approaches for NP discovery basically focus on:

- identifying the genes of the organism involved in the biosynthesis of the NPs,
- identifying the metabolic pathways by which the NPs are biosynthesised and
- predicting the products of the identified pathways (**Figure 1A**).

http://dx.doi.org/10.5772/67650

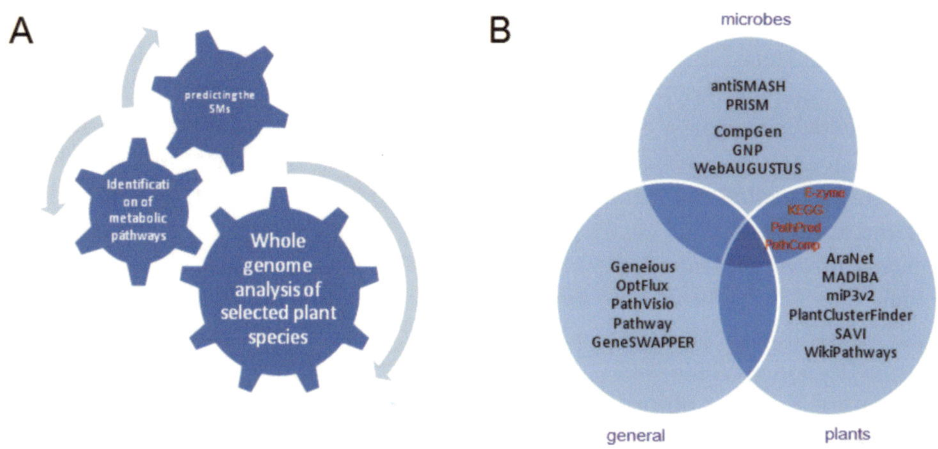

Figure 1. (A) Summary of genome mining approaches for the discovery of SMs and (B) classification of tools by applicability domain.

The four main strategies that are mostly employed to identify such pathways are based on processes involved in the production of plant secondary metabolites, for example, physical clustering, co-expression, evolutionary co-occurrence and epigenomic co-regulation of the genes [22–25]. Such approaches have been successfully applied for the investigation of fungal and microbial metabolites [26–28]. Since the discovery of the first gene cluster for secondary metabolism in *Zea mays*, the corn species [29], BGCs for plant secondary metabolism have become an emerging theme in plant biology [30]. It is even believed that synthetic biology technologies will eventually lead to the effective functional reconstitution of candidate pathways using a variety of genetic systems [25]. A knowledge of BGCs and their manipulation is therefore important in understanding how to activate a number of 'silent' gene clusters observed from the investigation of whole-genome sequencing of organisms. This would make available a wealth of new chemical entities (NCEs), which could be evaluated as drug leads and biologically active compounds [20].

This chapter aims at discussing the metabolic pathways by which plants biosynthesise compounds with anticancer activities, with a focus on selected very promising anticancer SMs from the African flora. We also aim to provide an overview of computational tools, which have been used to predict metabolic pathways and eventually address knowledge gaps when using the former. Additionally, we will present some databases for the retrieval of useful genomic data, discuss the strengths and limitations of selected computational (prediction) tools, which could be employed for the investigation of the uncharted routes towards the biosynthesis of some of the identified anticancer metabolites from plant sources, with specific examples. It is believed that properly addressing knowledge gaps that exist would lay the foundation for proper future investigations.

2. Natural products and plant genomic data

Genome data mining indicates that the vast majority of plant-based NPs have not yet been discovered [24, 25]. In addition, SMs are normally produced only at later growth stages of plant metabolism and are frequently found only at low concentrations within complex mixtures in plant extracts, due to several factors. Some of these factors include physiological variations, geographic variations, environmental conditions and genetic factors [25, 31, 32]. The aforementioned factors are the main drawbacks in the isolation and purification of NPs in meaningful quantities for either research or commercial aims. Nowadays, BGCs can be investigated using computational methodologies and used to predict the NPs present in microbial, fungal and floral matter [18, 20, 33, 34]. It is current knowledge that more than 70 genome sequences for several plant species have been made available, along with a wealth of transcriptome data [25]. However, the interpretation of such data, for example, the translation of predicted sequences into enzymes, pathways and SMs remains challenging. Advances in bioinformatics and synthetic biology have permitted the cheap and efficient overproduction of secondary metabolites of medicinal interest in heterologous (non-native) host organisms by reengineering of BGCs [35]. This is carried out through reengineering of BGCs as well as the activation of silent BGCs to yield unreported natural products of the target chemical space [17, 36], for example, an engineered *Escherichia coli* strain was used as the heterologous host organism for the production of taxadiene (a vital precursor of paclitaxel, an anticancer agent isolated from the bark of *Taxus brevifolia*), a precursor of the anticancer agent taxol [37]. In this way, quite a number of interesting SMs of plant origin (e.g. resveratrol, vanillin, conolidin, etc.) have been objects of pathway engineering in bacteria, yeast and other plants [38]. Thus, chemical libraries of diverse and novel hybrid natural products analogues can now be generated through combinatorial biosynthesis by manipulation of biosynthetic enzymes [39], for example, several analogues of the antibiotic erythromycin were obtained *via* combinatorial biosynthesis [40]. Such bioengineered libraries of 'unnatural' natural products show promises in drug discovery campaigns against multidrug-resistant cancer cells.

3. Some database resources for retrieving secondary metabolism prediction information

A summary of databases for retrieving information on BGCs is provided in **Table 1**. A majority of them focus on microbial BGCs, for example, ClusterMine360, ClustScan, DoBISCUIT, IMG-ABC and the Recombinant ClustScan Database. Details on the utility of the aforementioned databases have been provided in excellent recent reviews [26–28, 53]. Further efforts towards the construction of plant-based BGC and genomic databases include those of the Medicinal Plants Genomics and Metabolomics Resource consortium [47]. This effort has been focused on 14 medicinal plants and includes a BLAST search module, a genome browser, a genome putative search function tool and transcriptome search tools. While the entire database is available for download, similar efforts from the Plant Metabolic Network (PMN) have the advantage of having included several plant metabolic pathway databases, mostly among food crops [49, 50]. The PMN, for example, currently houses one multi-species reference database called PlantCyc and 22 species/taxon-specific databases, providing access to manually curated and/or computationally predicted information about enzymes, pathways, and more for individual species.

Database	Description	Web accessibility	Advantages	Disadvantages	Reference
ClusterMine360	A database of microbial polyketide and non-ribosomal peptide gene clusters.	http://www.clustermine360.ca/	Users can make contributions. Automation leads to high data consistency and quality data.	Focuses only on microbial PKS/NRPS biosynthesis	[41, 42]
ClustScan Database	A database for *in silico* detection of promising new compounds.	http://csdb.bioserv.pbf.hr/csdb/ClustScanWeb.html	Allows easy extraction of DNA and protein sequences of polypeptides, modules, and domains.	Currently includes data for only 57 SMs (PKS), 51 SMs (NRPS) and 62 SMs (PKS-NRPS hybrid) biosynthesis.	[43, 44]
DoBISCUIT	A database of secondary metabolite biosynthetic gene clusters.	http://www.bio.nite.go.jp/pks/	Provides standardised gene/module/domain descriptions related to the gene clusters. Available for download	Contains mostly data relating to bacterial species, mostly of the genus *Streptomyces*.	[45]
GenomeNet	A network of databases and computational services for genome research and related research areas in biomedical sciences.	http://www.genome.jp/	Provides several web accessible tools, e.g. KEGG, E-zyme, etc. See **Table 2**.		
IMG-ABC	A knowledge base for biosynthetic gene clusters for the discovery of novel SMs.	https://img.jgi.doe.gov/cgi-bin/abc-public/main.cgi	Integrates structural and functional genomics with annotated BGCs and associated SMs.	Not available for download. Limited to data on microbes	[46]
Medicinal Plants Genomics Resource	A database for medicinal plants genome sequence data.	http://medicinalplantgenomics.msu.edu/	Available for download	Only genomic data for 14 species are currently available.	[47]
Medicinal Plants Metabolomics Resource	A database for medicinal plants metabolomics data.	http://metnetweb.gdcb.iastate.edu/mpmr_public/	Available for download	Currently limited to metabolite data for 2 medicinal plant species.	[48]

Database	Description	Web accessibility	Advantages	Disadvantages	Reference
Minimum Information about a Biosynthetic Gene cluster (MIBiG)	A community standard for annotations and metadata on biosynthetic gene clusters and their molecular products.	http://mibig.secondarymetabolites.org/index.html	Facilitates the standardised deposition and retrieval of biosynthetic gene cluster data. Useful for the development of comprehensive comparative analysis tools. Available for download		[18]
Plant Metabolic Network (PMN)	Several plant metabolic pathway databases.	http://www.plantcyc.org/	Includes species/taxon-specific data for more than 22 plant species.		[49, 50]
Plant Reactome/"Cyc" Pathways	A pathway database for several crops and model plant species.	http://gramene.org/pathways	Currently includes gene homology-based pathway projections to 62 plant species.		[51]
Recombinant ClustScan Database	A database of gene cluster recombinants and their corresponding chemical structures.	http://csdb.bioserv.pbf.hr/csdb/RCSDB.html	Provides a virtual compound library, which could be a useful resource for computer-aided drug design of pharmaceutically relevant chemical entities.	Currently contains only 47 cluster combinations	[44, 52]
SMBP	Secondary metabolites bioinformatics portal.	http://www.secondarymetabolites.org/	Includes hand-curated links to all major tools and databases commonly used in the field		[53]

Table 1. Summary of currently available database resources for retrieving genomic data for biosynthesis prediction.

It provides a broad network of plant metabolic pathway databases that contain curated information from the literature and computational analyses about the genes, enzymes, compounds, reactions and pathways involved in primary and secondary metabolism in the included plant species. The PlantCyc database also provides access to manually curated or reviewed information about shared and unique metabolic pathways present in over 350 plant species. On the other hand, Plant Reactome is a pathway database for several crops and model plant species, making use of a framework of a eukaryotic cell model. Currently, it uses rice as a reference species and gene homology-based pathway projections have been made to 62 plant species [51].

4. Some computational tools for the analysis of genomic data and specialised metabolism prediction

Some computational tools for biochemical pathway prediction have been summarised in excellent reviews [54]. We have provided a more detailed summary of the main tools that could be useful in analysing plant and microbial genomic data for metabolism prediction in **Table 2**. Some of the tools are designed for the detection and analysis of specialised metabolism in microbes (e.g. antiSMASH, CompGen, GNP, PRISM and WebAUGUSTUS). Others are specially designed for plant metabolism prediction or may only include data for some specific organisms (e.g. AraNet, MADIBA, miP3v2, PlantClusterFinder, SAVI and WikiPathways for plants), while others are more general tools, useful for both microbial and plant metabolism prediction and BGC analysis (e.g. E-zyme, KEGG, PathPred and PathComp) and others are more useful for developers (e.g. Geneious, OptFlux, PathVisio and Pathway GeneSWAPPER), **Figure 1B**. We could also classify the tools according to their respective tasks; prediction and analysis of BGCs (e.g. antiSMASH, MADIBA, Pathway GeneSWAPPER, WebAUGUSTUS), searching, visualisation and prediction of biosynthetic pathways and reaction paths (e.g. BioCyc, CycSim, FMM, GNP, KEGG, MetaCyc, PathComp, PathPred, PathSearch, PathVisio, Pathway GeneSWAPPER, PlantClusterFinder, SAVI, WikiPathways for plants), prediction of SMs (PRISM), metabolic engineering (OptFlux), other functions (miP3v2). Among the tools for specialised metabolism in plants, AraNet is a probabilistic functional gene network (with currently a total of 27,029 protein-encoding genes) of *A. thaliana*. It is based on a modified Bayesian integration of data from multiple organisms, each data type being weighted based on how well it links genes that are known to function together in *A. thaliana*. Each interaction is associated with a log-likelihood score (LLS), which is a measure of the probability of an interaction representing a true functional linkage between two genes [56]. On the other hand, MADIBA facilitates the interpretation of *Plasmodium* and plant (data currently available for *Oryza sativa* and *A. thaliana*) gene clusters [64]. This tool eases the task by automating the post-processing stage during the assignment of biological meaning to gene expression clusters. MADIBA is designed as a relational database and has stored data from gene to pathway for the aforementioned species. Tools within the GUI allow the rapid analyses of each cluster with the view of identifying the Gene Ontology terms, as well as visualising the metabolic pathways where the genes are implicated, their genomic localisations, putative common

Tool	Utility	Web accessibility	Advantage	Disadvantage	Reference
antiSMASH*	A web server and tool for the automatic genomic identification and analysis of biosynthetic gene clusters.	http://antismash.secondarymetabolites.org.	Detects putative gene clusters of unknown types. Identifies similarities of identified clusters to any of 1172 clusters with known end products, etc.	Designed for analysis of BGCs in microbes.	[55]
AraNet	Gene function identification and genetic dissection of plant traits.	http://www.functionalnet.org/aranet/	Had greater precision than literature-based protein interactions (21%) for 55% of tested genes. Is highly predictive for diverse biological pathways.	Applicability is limited to one species - *A. thaliana.*	[56]
BioCyc/CycSim/MetaCyc	Online tools for genome-scale metabolic modelling.	https://biocyc.org/http://www.genoscope.cns.fr/cycsim https://metacyc.org/	Support the design and simulation of knockout experiments, e.g. deletions mutants on specified media, etc.		[57, 58]
CompGen	Carry out *in silico* homologous recombination between gene clusters.	http://csdb.bioserv.pbf.hr/csdb/RCSDB.html		Focuses on gene clusters encoding PKSs in *Streptomyces* sp. and related bacterial genera.	[52]
E-zyme	Assignment of EC numbers.	http://www.genome.jp/tools/e-zyme/	Classifies enzymatic reactions and links the enzyme genes or proteins to reactions in metabolic pathways.		[59]
From Metabolite to metabolite (FMM)	A web server to find biosynthetic routes between two metabolites within the KEGG database.	http://FMM.mbc.nctu.edu.tw/	Both local and global graphical views of the metabolic pathways are designed.		[60]
Geneious	Organisation and analysis of sequence data.	http://www.geneious.com/basic	Includes a public application programming interface (API) available for developers. Freely available for download.		[61]
Genomes-to-Natural Products platform (GNP)	Prediction, combinatorial design and identification of PKs and NRPs from biosynthetic assembly lines.	http://magarveylab.ca/gnp/	Uses LC–MS/MS data of crude extracts to make predictions in a high-throughput manner.	Focuses on bacterial NPs.	[62]

Tool	Utility	Web accessibility	Advantage	Disadvantage	Reference
Gene Regulatory network inference ACcuracy Enhancement (GRACE)	An algorithm to enhance the accuracy of transcriptional gene regulatory networks.	https://dpb.carnegiescience.edu/labs/rhee-lab/software	Focuses on plant species. Available for download.	Only algorithm is available. Lacks a graphical user interface	
KEGG Mapper	A tool to search a biosynthetic pathway.	http://www.kegg.jp/kegg/tool/map_pathway1.html?rn	KEGG is applicable to all organisms and enables interpretation of high-level functions from genomic and molecular data.		[63]
MicroArray Data Interface for Biological Annotation (MADIBA)	A webserver toolkit for biological interpretation of *Plasmodium* and plant gene clusters.	http://www.bi.up.ac.za/MADIBA	It allows rapid gene cluster analyses and the identification of the relevant Gene Ontology terms, visualisation of metabolic pathways, genomic localisations, etc.	Only 2 plant species are currently considered [rice (*Oryza sativa*), and *A. thaliana*].	[64]
miP3v2	Predicts microproteins in a sequenced genome.	https://github.com/npklein/miP3	Sheds light on the prevalence, biological roles, and evolution of microProteins.	Only the algorithm is available. Lacks a graphical user interface	[65]
OptFlux	A software platform for *in silico* metabolic engineering.	http://www.optflux.org/	Open source platform. Integrates visualisation tools. Allows users to load a genome-scale model of a given organism. Wild type and mutants can be simulated. Available for download.		[66]
PathComp	Possible reaction path computation.	http://www.genome.jp/tools/pathcomp/			
PathPred	Prediction of biodegradation and/or biosynthetic pathways.	http://www.genome.jp/tools/pathpred/	Specifically designed for biosynthesis of SMs (in plants) and xenobiotics biodegradation of environmental compounds (by bacteria).		[67]
PathSearch	Search for similar reaction pathways.	http://www.genome.jp/tools/pathsearch/			

Tool	Utility	Web accessibility	Advantage	Disadvantage	Reference
PathVisio	A biological pathway analysis software that allows users to draw, edit and analyse biological pathways.	http://www.pathvisio.org/	Plugins are included, which provide advanced analysis methods, visualisation options or additional import/export functionality. Available for download.		[68, 69]
Pathway GeneSWAPPER	Maps homologous genes from one species onto the PathVisio pathway diagram of another species.	http://jaiswallab.cgrb.oregonstate.edu/software/PGS	Improves the functionalities of PathVisio and WikiPathways for plants.		[70]
PlantClusterFinder	Predicts metabolic gene clusters from plant genomes.	https://dpb.carnegiescience.edu/labs/rhee-lab/software	Focuses on plant species. Available for download.	Only the algorithm is available. Lacks a graphical user interface	
Prediction informatics for secondary metabolomes (PRISM)	Genomes to natural products prediction informatics for secondary metabolomes.	http://magarveylab.ca/prism/	Open-source, user-friendly web available application.	Focuses on microbial SMs.	[71]
RetroPath	A webserver for retrosynthetic pathway design.	http://www.jfaulon.com/bioretrosynth/	Integrates pathway prediction and ranking, prediction of compatibility with host genes, toxicity prediction and metabolic modeling.		[72, 73]
Semi-Automated Validation Infrastructure (SAVI)	Predicts metabolic pathways using pathway metadata (e.g. taxonomic distribution, key reactions, etc.).	https://dpb.carnegiescience.edu/labs/rhee-lab/software	Decides which pathways to keep, remove or validate manually. Available for download.	Only the algorithm is available. Lacks a graphical user interface.	
WebAUGUSTUS	Gene prediction tool.	http://bioinf.uni-greifswald.de/webaugustus	One of the most accurate tools for eukaryotic gene prediction.	Focuses on eukaryotes.	[74]
WikiPathways for plants	A community pathway curation portal.	http://plants.wikipathways.org	Freely available.	Currently limited to rice and *Arabidopsis* sp.	[70, 75, 76]

*Currently provided detection rules for 44 classes and subclasses of SMs.

Table 2. Summary of current computational tools which could be useful for the plant genomic data analysis.

transcriptional regulatory elements in the upstream sequences, and an analysis specific to the organism being studied.

PlantClusterFinder, SAVI and WikiPathways for plants are all purpose tools designed to assist in the prediction of metabolic gene cluster from plant genomes, although WikiPathways for plants has currently included mostly data for rice and *Arabidopsis* sp. SAVI has the added advantage of offering the user the possibility of including pathway metadata (e.g. taxonomic distribution, key reactions, etc.) and offering the possibility to decide which pathway(s) to keep and which to remove or validate manually.

5. Some computational methods for efficient production and the *de novo* engineering of natural products

Two main areas for computational tools can be distinguished: on the one hand the rational modification of genomes for the production of molecules by host organisms, and on the other hand the modification or the *de novo* design of gene clusters for the biosynthesis of novel NPs. For both genetic engineering approaches, the already known genomes of bacteria, fungi and more and more plants provide the basic datasets. A very important computational approach for a rational modification of NP-producing host organisms is the genome-scale metabolic modelling [77, 78].

Automatic assignments of functional annotations of all genes in a genome are ideally proven by manual curation and enriched by current knowledge about the metabolic network of subjected organisms. The curated genomes are then applied to a complete automatic reconstruction of the metabolic pathways of the cell. These metabolic models are normally encoded in the Systems Biology Markup Language (SBML) and are compatible with various software tools, for example, Cytoscape [79], which can be applied for static network analyses. For instance, missing enzymes (gaps) within the network become apparent by substrates that are not taken up or have not been produced by the cell, as well as products that are not consumed by other reactions and are not secreted from cell. The RAST annotation pipeline provides a full automatic server for predicting all gene functions and discovering new pathways in microbial genomes of bacteria [80]. Such models can then be used to predict the turnover rate of each reaction in a Flux Balance Analysis (FBA) [81]. Several tools have been built, which apply FBA to identify enzymes that should be either introduced or knocked-out in the organism to increase production rate in the host organisms. A widely used FBA package is the MATLAB-based COBRA Toolbox [82]. With CycSim [58], BioMet [83] and FAME [84] powerful web-based FBA applications were published that do not require any software installation.

Within the last 10 years, FBA was applied to support numerous genetic engineering approaches, for example, for the determination of minimal media in *Helicobacter pylori* [85], for growth rate predictions in *Bacillus subtilis* [86] or for the development of metabolic engineering strategies in *Pseudomonas putida* [87]. Based on FBA, it was possible to increase vanillin production in baker's yeast by twofold and enhance sesquiterpene production in the same species [88, 89].

The rational modification of a given genome to design novel molecules needs a detailed understanding of the producing gene clusters. Well-studied gene clusters such as polyketide synthases consist of specific domain types that can be identified by trained hidden Markov models that are stored in related databases, for example, PFAM [90]. Gene cluster analysis tools such as antiSMASH [55, 91] or PRISM [71] analyse a given gene cluster to predict the specific domains and to describe the architecture of a gene cluster. However, the prediction of the structure of the resulting natural products is a difficult task because substrate recognition of active sites and the correct ordering of enzymatic reactions has to be predicted. If subjected enzymes are catalysing multiple substrates, the availability of each substrate has to be predicted. Most frequently, the automatic analysis of a cluster is based on the deduction of information from gene clusters similar to the queried one. If well-annotated similar gene clusters do not exist, the prediction of the structure of the biosynthesised NP is challenging. With more and more knowledge about the structure of natural products and the encoding sequences, the relation between the composition of the active sites and substrate binding will be better understood. Existing algorithms are often based on machine-learning approaches and predict the correct substrates for a selected set of enzyme families [92]. For the prediction of NPs synthesised by non-ribosomal peptide synthetases, such a sequence-based prediction method is integrated in the related webserver NRPSpredictor2 [93]. Rational substitution of residues to generate novel molecules still requires a detailed manual analysis of the encoding gene cluster, and new software tools that propose mutations leading to novel molecules might accelerate this approach considerably in future.

6. Selected natural products with promising anticancer properties from African sources

Recent reviews on the anticancer potential of African flora have discussed the anticancer, cytotoxic, antiproferative and antitumour activities of about 500 NPs [9–12]. In this section, we focus on the most promising (recent) results for anticancer SMs from African flora (**Table 3**, **Figure 2**), published after the last reviews. The isolation of two new lignans; 3α-O-(β-*D*-glucopyranosyl) desoxypodophyllotoxin (**1**) and 4-O-(β-*D*-glucopyranosyl) dehydropodophyllotoxin (**2**), alongside other known lignans (**3** and **4**), have been reported from the species, *Cleistanthus boivinianus* (Phyllanthaceae), collected in Madagascar (coordinates 13°06′37″S 049°09′39″E) [94]. These compounds showed potent to moderate antiproliferative activities against the A2780 ovarian cancer cell line, with compound **1** showing potent antiproliferative activity against the HCT-116 human colon carcinoma cell line (IC_{50} = 0.03 μM). The known compounds with promising activities from this species included the lignans; (±)-β-apopicropodophyllin (**3**, PubChem CID: 6452099), (−)-desoxypodophyllotoxin (**4**, PubChem CID: 345501). The same authors also isolated a new butanolide, macrocarpolide A (**5**, PubChem CID: 122372160) and two new secobutanolides; macrocarpolides B (**6**, PubChem CID: 122372161) and C (**7**, PubChem CID: 122372162), together with other known compounds from the ethanol extract of the roots of the Madagascan

Cpd. No.*	Molecule class	Source species (Family)	Cancer cell line	IC_{50} (μM)	Biosynthetic pathway	References
1	lignan	*Cleistanthus boivinianus* (Phyllanthaceae)	HCT-116 human colon carcinoma cell line	0.03	shikimic acid pathway, via phenylalanine	[94]
			A2780 ovarian cancer cell line	0.02		
2	″	″	″	2.10	″	″
3	″	″	″	0.06	″	
4	″	″	″	0.23	″	
5	butanolide	*Ocotea macrocarpa* (Lauraceae)	″	2.57		[95]
6	secobutanolide	″	″	1.98		″
7	″	″	″	1.67		″
8	butanolide	″	″	2.43		″
9	″	″	″	1.65		″
10	polyoxygenated cyclohexene derivative	*Cleistochlamys kirkii* (Annonaceae)	MDA-MB-231 triple-negative human breast cancer cell line	0.03	Shikimic acid pathway	[96]
11	″	″	″	0.29	″	″
12	″	″	″	0.29	″	″
13	″	″	″	0.12	″	″
14	″	″	″	0.45	″	″
15	″	″	″	2.10	″	″
16	″	″	″	0.09	″	″
17	″	″	″	2.70	″	″
18	″	″	″	0.24	″	″

*Compound number.

Table 3. Summary of recently published selected promising anticancer SMs from African flora.

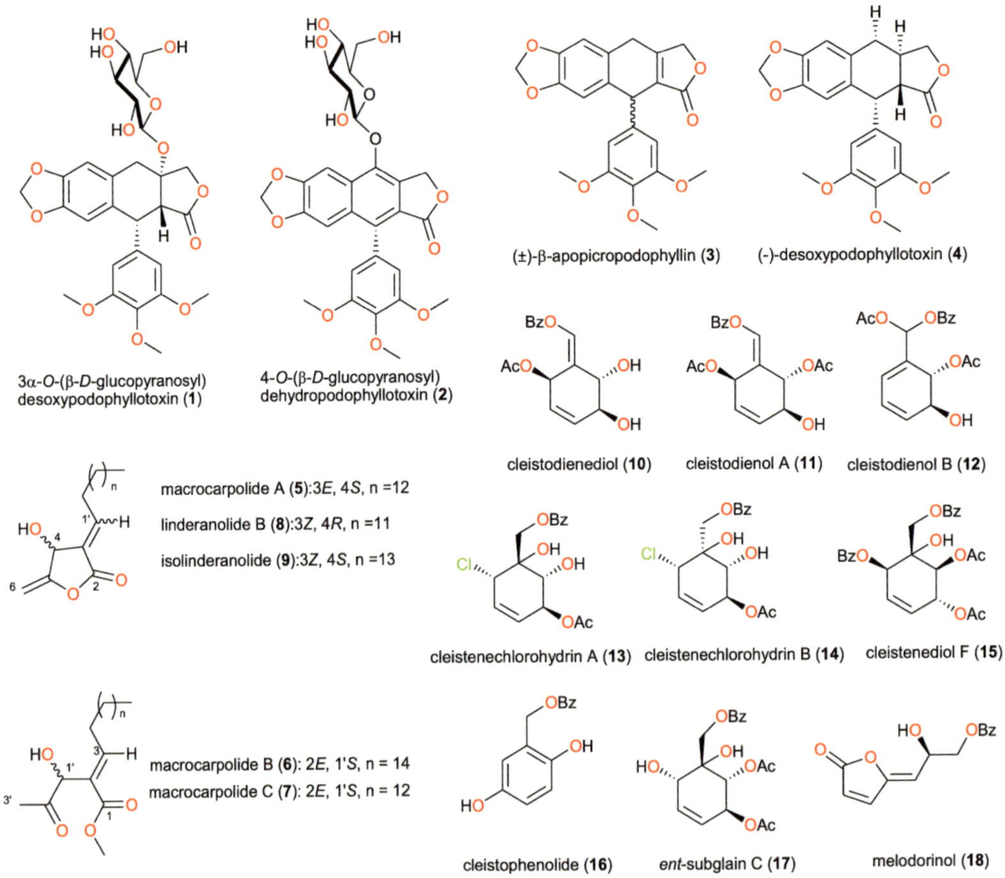

Figure 2. Chemical structures of selected anticancer SMs from African flora.

species *Ocotea macrocarpa* (Lauraceae), which showed antiproliferative activities against the A2780 ovarian cell line [95]. The known isolates included the butanolides; linderanolide B (**8**, PubChem CID: 53308122) and isolinderanolide (**9**, PubChem CID: 44576054). The anticancer activities showed IC_{50} values of 2.57 (**5**), 1.98 (**6**), 1.67 (**7**), 2.43 (**8**) and 1.65 μM (**9**) against A2780 ovarian cancer cell lines. Additionally, the leaves of *Cleistochlamys kirkii* (Annonaceae) from Tanzania have been recently shown to be a rich source of polyoxygenated cyclohexene derivatives with antiplasmodial activities, along with very potent activities against MDA-MB-231 triple-negative human breast cancer cell line [96]. The isolates; cleistodienediol (**10**), cleistodienol A (**11**), cleistodienol B (**12**), cleistenechlorohydrin A (**13**), cleistenechlorohydrin B (**14**), cleistenediol F (**15**), cleistophenolide (**16**), *ent*-subglain C (**17**) and melodorinol (**18**, PubChem CID: 6438687) showed some activities as low as IC_{50} = 0.09 μM against the aforementioned cancer cell lines. To the best of our knowledge, mode of action studies have not yet been conducted for the SMs **1** to **18** and *in vivo* activity data is currently unavailable.

7. Case studies

In this section, we shall discuss specific examples of the investigation of biosynthesis of anticancer plant-based SMs by (computational) analysis of genomic data.

7.1. Biogenesis of several anticancer metabolites by *Ocimum tenuiflorum* (Lamiaceae)

Species from the genus *Ocimum* are well known for their high medicinal values and are therefore used to cure a variety of ailments in Ayurveda, an Indian system of medicine [97, 98]. About 30 SMs have been reported from the genus *Ocimum*, with a variety of biological properties [99]. Only 14 of these SMs belong to the five basic groups of compounds having a complete biosynthetic pathway information in the PMN database [49, 50], thereby leaving us with ~15 medicinally relevant metabolites from *Ocimum* sp. with unknown pathways. This has prompted further investigation on SMs with uncharted biosynthetic pathways. Several bioactive SMs, including the anticancer compounds; apigenin (**19**, PubChem CID: 5280443), rosmarinic acid (**20**, PubChem CID: 5281792), taxol (**21**, PubChem CID: 36314), ursolic acid (**22**, PubChem CID: 64945), oleanolic acid (**23**, PubChem CID: 10494) and the plant steroid sitosterol (**24**, PubChem CID: 222284) have been identified from the herb Krishna Tulsi (*O. tenuiflorum*, Lamiaceae), with the mature leaves retaining the medicinally relevant metabolites [100]. Upadhyay et al. carried out a draft genome analysis of the species and generated paired-end and mate-pair sequence libraries for the whole sequenced genome, together with transcriptomic analysis (RNA-Seq) of two subtypes of *O. tenuiflorum* (Krishna and Rama Tulsi) and reporting the relative expression of genes in the both varieties. The authors further investigated the pathways, which lead to the biosynthesis of the identified SMs, with respect to similar pathways in *A. thaliana* and other model plants (e.g. *Oryza sativa japonica*). Six important genes (including *Q8RWT0* and *F1T282*) were expressed and identified from analysis of genome data. These were validated by q-RT-PCR on the different studied tissues (e.g. roots, mature leaves, etc.) of five closely related species (e.g. *O. gratissimum*, *O. sacharicum*, *O. kilmund*, *Solanum lycopersicum* and *Vitis vinifera*), which showed a high extent of urosolic acid-producing genes in young leaves. The other identified anticancer metabolites included eugenol and ursolic acid. As an example, the authors employed sequence search algorithms to search for the three enzymes of the three-step synthetic pathway of ursolic acid from squalene in the Tulsi genome. Each of these enzymes in Tulsi (squalene epoxidase, α-amyrin synthase and α-amyrin 2,8 monoxygenase) were queried from the PlantCyc database, starting from their protein sequences. The search for analogous enzymes in the model plants *O. sativa japonica* and *A. thaliana*, showed sequence identity covering from 50 to 80% of the query length. The whole genome and sequence analysis of *O. tenuiflorum* suggested that small amino acid changes at the functional sites of genes involved in metabolite synthesis pathways could confer special medicinal (particularly anticancer) properties to this herb.

7.2. Biosynthesis of the anticancer alkaloid noscapine by *Papaver somniferum* (Papaveraceae)

Noscapine (**25**, PubChem CID: 275196) is an antitumour phthalideisoquinoline alkaloid from opium poppy (*Papaver somniferum*, Papaveraceae). Compound **25** is known to bind stoichiometrically to tubulin, alters its conformation, affects microtubule assembly (promotes microtubule polymerisation), hence arresting metaphase and inducing apoptosis in many cell types [101]. It has been demonstrated that the compound has potent antitumour activity against solid murine lymphoid tumours (even when the drug was administered orally). This drug has also shown potency against human breast, ovarian and bladder tumours implanted in nude mice and in dividing human cells [102, 103]. Although the compound is water-soluble and absorbed after oral administration, its chemotherapeutic potential in human cancer could not be fully exploited for drug discovery projects because, like most SMs, this has been limited by the typically small amounts produced in the slow-growing plant species [104]. The quest to improve production levels of the NP is essential for drug discovery. However, such would require a proper understanding biological processes underlying the biosynthesis of this SM, known from isotope-labelling experiments to be derived from scoulerine since the 1960s [105]. Winzer et al. have carried out a transcriptomic analysis, with the aim of elucidating the biosynthetic pathway of this important metabolite for the improvement of its commercial production in both poppy and other systems [106]. The analysis of a high noscapine-producing poppy variety, HN1, showed the exclusive expression of 10 genes encoding five distinct enzyme classes, whereas five functionally characterised genes (*BBE, TNMT, SalR, SalAT* and *T6ODM*) were present in all three of the studied poppy varieties, respectively, rich in morphine, thebaine and noscapine (HM1, HN1 and HT1). The authors analysed the expressed sequence tag (EST) abundance and discovered some previously uncharacterised genes expressed in HN1, which were completely absent from the other (HM1 and HT1) EST libraries. This led to the identification of the corresponding enzymes as three *O*-methyltransferases (*PSMT1, PSMT2, PSMT3*), four cytochrome P450s (*CYP82X1, CYP82X2, CYP82Y1* and *CYP719A21*), an acetyltransferase (*PSAT1*), a carboxylesterase (*PSCXE1*) and a short-chain dehydrogenase/reductase (*PSSDR1*). Further analysis of an F2 mapping population, using HN1 and HM1 as parents, indicated that these genes are tightly linked in HN1. Moreover, bacterial artificial chromosome sequencing confirmed the existence of a complex BGC for plant alkaloids. Based on the knowledge derived from the investigation, the authors could make suggestions for the improved production of noscapine and related bioactive molecules by the molecular breeding of commercial poppy varieties or engineering of new production systems, for example, by virus-induced gene silencing, which resulted in the accumulation of pathway intermediates, thus allowing gene function to be linked to noscapine synthesis [104, 106].

7.3. Biosynthesis of vinblastine and vincristine by *Catharanthus roseus* (Apocynaceae)

Vinblastine (**26**, PubChem CID: 13342) and vincristine (**27**, PubChem CID: 5978) are chemotherapy drugs used to treat a number of cancer types. These are among the >120 known terpenoid indole alkaloids from the medicinal plant *C. roseus*, also known as the Madagascar periwinkle [107]. Since these two very important anticancer compounds have only been produced in very low amounts in *C. roseus*, as opposed to the fairly high levels of several monomeric alkaloids (e.g. ajmalicine and serpentine) [108], attempts to improve the yields of compounds **26** and **27** have led to the genome-wide transcript profiling of elicited *C. roseus* cell cultures, by cDNA-amplified fragment-length polymorphism combined with metabolic profiling [107]. This resulted in the identification of several gene-to-gene and gene-to-metabolite networks obtained by an attempt to establish correlations between the expression profiles of 417 gene tags and the accumulation profiles of 178 metabolite peaks. The results proved that different branches of terpenoid indole alkaloid biosynthesis and various other metabolic pathways are affected by differences in hormonal regulation. Thus, the investigations of Rischer et al. provided the foundations for a proper understanding of secondary metabolism in *C. roseus*, thereby enhancing the applicability of metabolic engineering of Madagascar periwinkle. This study provided the possibility of exploring a select number of genes (e.g. *STR*, *10HGO*, *T16H* and *DAT*) involved in biosynthesis of terpenoid indole alkaloids [107].

8. The way forward

The case studies show that the detailed computational analysis of the transcriptomic and metabolomic data of a plant species could reveal its metabolic capacity and hence help identify candidate genes involved in the biosynthesis of the important SMs it contains. Thus, modifying the plant genes could represent a premise for improving metabolite yield. It should be mentioned that other compounds from some of the aforementioned compound classes (**Table 3**), from both floral and microbial sources, have shown promising anticancer activities [109–113], e.g. isolinderanolide B (**28**, PubChem CID: 53308122) (**Figure 3**), a butanolide from the stems of *Cinnamomum subavenium* (Lauraceae) had shown antiproliferative activity in T24 human bladder cancer cells by blocking cell cycle progression and inducing apoptosis [112]. In addition, subamolide B (**29**, PubChem CID: 16104907), another butanolide from this same species, is known to induce cytotoxicity in human cutaneous squamous cell carcinoma through mitochondrial and CHOP-dependent cell death pathways [113]. Meanwhile, obtusilactone B (**30**, PubChem CID: 101286261), from *Machilus thunbergii* (Lauraceae), is known to target barrier-to-autointegration factor to treat cancer [111].

From the African flora, apart from the Lauraceae, Phyllanthaceae and Annonaceae, known to be rich in anticancer metabolites, the genus *Tacca* of the yam family (Dioscoreaceae) is known for the abundant presence of taccalonolides, which are microtubule stabilisers with clinical potential for cancer treatment [114]. Additionally, the genus *Tamarix* (e.g. *T. aphylla*

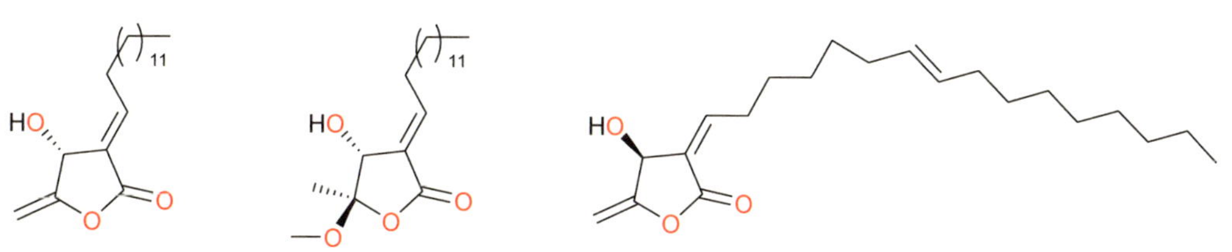

isolinderanolide B (**28**) subamolide B (**29**) obtusilactone B (**30**)

Figure 3. Chemical structures of selected anticancer butanolides from Lauraceae.

and *T. nilotica* from Northern Africa), together with the genus *Reaumuria* (Tamaricaceae) are known for the abundant presence of tannins (gallo-ellagitannin, gallotannins) with remarkable cytotoxic effects. The high salt content of the leaves of *Tamarix* species, rendering them useful locally as a fire barrier, and their adaptability to drought and high salinity are of equal interest. It therefore becomes urgent to investigate the genomics of some of the aforementioned plant species, particularly those from the *Cinnamomum* sp., *Ocotea* sp. and *Machilus* sp. (Lauraceae), *Tacca* sp. (Dioscoreaceae), *Cleistanthus* sp. (Phyllanthaceae), *Cleistochlamys* sp. (Annonaceae), *Tamarix* sp. (Tamaricaceae) and so on, and hence further investigate the genes or BGCs responsible for secondary metabolism with the view of understanding and better exploring the biosynthetic pathways of the anticancer SMs.

9. Conclusions

It has been our intention in this chapter to provide a detailed overview of the important computational tools and resources for the analysis of plant genomic data and for the prediction of biosynthetic pathways in plants. We have taken a few case studies of anticancer SMs to illustrate this. Even though it is unclear how widespread plant genes are clusters, genes that encode the biosynthesis of several small plant SMs are well known, including the vital genes for the production of some highly potent anticancer drugs. With the use of the tools and databases described, along with the drop in the cost of whole genome sequencing in plant species, the future for the discovery of new plant-based anticancer metabolites would involve the identification of one or more genes or BGCs encoding the enzymes in the biosynthetic pathway for the target compound(s), followed by the co-expression analysis, also exploiting the knowledge of the chemical structure of the target compound, for the identification of other enzymes that might be involved in this pathway. As an example, the exploration of the pathway for podophyllotoxin biosynthesis by the use transcriptome mining in *Podophyllum hexandrum* led to the identification biosynthetic genes, 29 of which were combinatorially expressed in the tobacco plant (*Nicotiana benthamiana*), leading to the identification of six pathway enzymes, among which is oxoglutarate-dependent dioxygenase responsible for closing the core cyclohexane ring of the aryltetralin scaffold [115]. An alternative approach could be, if the metabolic pathway and nature of SMs are unknown, then the identified co-expressed genes encoding the enzymes for secondary metabolism could be subjected to untargeted metabolomics for the elucidation of unknown pathways and chemical structures. As an example, a single pathogen-induced P450 enzyme, CYP82C2, with a combination of untargeted metabolomics and co-expression analysis was used to uncover the complete biosynthetic pathway, which leads to the metabolite 4-hydroxyindole-3-carbonyl nitrile, previously unknown to *Arabidopsis* sp. This rare and hitherto unprecedented plant metabolite, with a cyanogenic functionality revealed a hidden capacity of *Arabidopsis* sp. for cyanogenic glucoside biosynthesis. This was confirmed by expressing 4-OH-ICN engineering biosynthetic enzymes in *Saccharomyces cerevisiae* and *Nicotiana benthamiana*, to reconstitute the complete pathway *in vitro* and *in vivo*, thus validating the functions of the enzymes involved in the pathway [116].

Acknowledegments

FNK acknowledges a Georg Forster fellowship from the Alexander von Humboldt Foundation, Germany. CVS is currently a doctoral candidate financed by the German Academic Exchange Services (DAAD), Germany.

Competing interests

The authors declare that they have no competing interests.

Abbreviations

AfroCancer	African Anticancer Natural Products Database
BGC	Biosynthetic gene clusters
EC_{50}	Half maximal effective concentration, that is, the concentration of a drug, antibody or toxicant, which induces a response halfway between the baseline and maximum after a specified exposure time
ED_{50}	The median effective dose, a dose that produces the desired effect in 50% of a population
FBA	Flux Balance Analysis
GI_{50}	The growth inhibition of 50%, drug concentration resulting in a 50% reduction in the net protein increase.
IC_{50}	The drug concentration causing 50% inhibition of the desired activity
IMG-ABC	The Integrated Microbial Genomes Atlas of Biosynthetic gene Clusters
NANPDB	Northern African Natural Products Database
NP	Natural product
NPACT	Naturally Occurring Plant-based Anti-cancer Compound Activity-Target Database
NRP	Nonribosomal peptide
NRPS	Nonribosomal peptide synthase
PK	Polyketide
PKS	Polyketides synthase
PMN	Plant Metabolic Network
PRISM	PRediction Informatics for Secondary Metabolomes
SM	Secondary metabolite

Author details

Aurélien F.A. Moumbock[1], Conrad V. Simoben[2], Ludger Wessjohann[3], Wolfgang Sippl[2], Stefan Günther[4], and Fidele Ntie-Kang[1,2]*

*Address all correspondence to: ntiekfidele@gmail.com

1 Department of Chemistry, University of Buea, Buea, Cameroon

2 Department of Pharmaceutical Chemistry, Martin-Luther University of Halle-Wittenberg, Halle, Germany

3 Leibniz Institute of Plant Biochemistry, Halle, Germany

4 Pharmaceutical Bioinformatics, Albert-Ludwig-University Freiburg, Freiburg, Germany

References

[1] Cragg GM, Newman DJ. Plants as a source of anti-cancer and anti-HIV agents. Ann Appl Biol. 2003;143:127-133. doi:10.1111/j.1744-7348.2003.tb00278.x

[2] Cragg GM, Grothaus PG, Newman DJ. Impact of natural products on developing new anti-cancer agents. Chem Rev. 2009;109:3012-3043. doi:10.1021/cr900019j

[3] Lamari FN, Cordopatis P. Exploring the potential of natural products in cancer treatment. In: Missailidis S, editor. *Anticancer therapeutics*. West Sussex: Wiley-Blackwell; 2008, pp. 3-16.

[4] Pan L, Chai HB, Kinghorn AD. Discovery of new anticancer agents from higher plants. Front Biosci (Schol Ed). 2013;4:142-156.

[5] Newman DJ, Cragg GM. Natural products as sources of new drugs from 1981 to 2014. J Nat Prod. 2016;79:629-661. doi:10.1021/acs.jnatprod.5b01055

[6] Mangal M, Sagar P, Singh H, Raghava GPS, Agarwal SM. NPACT: naturally occurring plant-based anti-cancer compound activity-target database. Nucleic Acids Res. 2013;41:D1124-D1129. doi:10.1093/nar/gks1047

[7] Ntie-Kang F, Nwodo JN, Ibezim A, Simoben CV, Karaman B, et al. Molecular modeling of potential anticancer agents from African medicinal plants. J Chem Inf Model. 2014;54:2433-2450. doi:10.1021/ci5003697

[8] Ntie-Kang F, Simoben CV, Karaman B, Ngwa VF, Judson PN, et al. Pharmacophore modeling and *in silico* toxicity assessment of potential anticancer agents from African medicinal plants. Drug Des Dev Ther. 2016;10:2137-2154. doi:10.2147/DDDT.S108118

[9] Beutler JA, Cragg GM, Iwu M, Newman DJ, Okunji C. Anticancer potential of African plants: the experience of the United States National Cancer Institute and National

Institutes of Health. In: Gurib-Fakim A, editor. Novel plant bioresources: applications in food, medicine and cosmetics, 1st ed. Oxford: John Wiley & Sons Ltd; 2014, pp. 133-149. doi:10.1002/9781118460566.ch10

[10] Nwodo JN, Ibezim A, Simoben CV, Ntie-Kang F. Exploring cancer therapeutics with natural products from African medicinal plants, part II: alkaloids, terpenoids and flavonoids. Anticancer Agents Med Chem. 2016;16:108-127. doi:10.2174/187152061566615 0520143827

[11] Simoben CV, Ibezim A, Ntie-Kang F, Nwodo JN, Lifongo LL. Exploring cancer therapeutics with natural products from African medicinal plants, part I: xanthones, quinones, steroids, coumarins, phenolics and other classes of compounds. Anticancer Agents Med Chem. 2015;15:1092-1111. doi:10.2174/1871520615666150113110241

[12] Simoben CV, Ntie-Kang F. African medicinal plants: an untapped reservoir of potential anticancer agents. In: Prasad S, Tyagi AK, editors. Cancer preventive and therapeutic compounds: gift from mother nature. Beijing: Bentham Science Publishers; 2016. p. 78-95.

[13] Ntie-Kang F, Telukunta KK, Döring K, Simoben CV, Moumbock, et al. The Northern African Natural Products Database (NANPDB), 2016. www.african-compounds.org/nanpdb

[14] Ntie-Kang F, Yong JN. The chemistry and biological activities of natural products from Northern African plant families: from Aloaceae to Cupressaceae. RSC Adv. 2014;4:61975-61991. doi:10.1039/C4RA11467A

[15] Yong JN, Ntie-Kang F. The chemistry and biological activities of natural products from Northern African plant families: from Ebenaceae to Solanaceae. RSC Adv. 2015;5:26580-26595. doi:10.1039/C4RA15377D

[16] Ntie-Kang F, Njume LE, Malange YI, Günther S, Sippl W, et al. The chemistry and biological activities of natural products from Northern African plant families: from Taccaceae to Zygophyllaceae. Nat Prod Bioprospect. 2016;6:63-96. doi:10.1007/s13659-016-0091-9

[17] Medema MH, Fischbach M. Computational approaches to natural product discovery. Nat Chem Biol. 2015;11:639-648. doi:10.1038/nchembio.1884

[18] Medema MH, Kottmann R, Yilmaz P, Cummings M, Biggins JB, et al. Minimum information about a biosynthetic gene cluster. Nat Chem Biol. 2015;11:625-631. doi:10.1038/nchembio.1890

[19] Nützmann HW, Osbourn A. Gene clustering in plant specialized metabolism. Curr Opin Biotechnol. 2014;26:91-99. doi:10.1016/j.copbio.2013.10.009

[20] Osbourn A. Secondary metabolic gene clusters: evolutionary toolkits for chemical innovation. Trends Genet. 2010;26:449-457. doi:10.1016/j.tig.2010.07.001

[21] Osbourn AE, Field B. Operons. Cell Mol Life Sci. 2009;66:3755-3775. doi:10.1007/s00018-009-0114-3

[22] Rhee SY, Mutwil M. Towards revealing the functions of all genes in plants. Trends Plant Sci. 2014;19:212-221. doi:10.1016/j.tplants.2013.10.006

[23] Xu M, Rhee SY. Becoming data-savvy in a big-data world. Trends Plant Sci. 2014;19:619-622. doi:10.1016/j.tplants.2014.08.003

[24] Chae L, Lee I, Shin J, Rhee SY. Towards understanding how molecular networks evolve in plants. Curr Opin Plant Biol. 2012;15:177-184. doi:10.1016/j.pbi.2012.01.006

[25] Medema MH, Osbourn A. Computational genomic identification and functional reconstitution of plant natural product biosynthetic pathways. Nat Prod Rep. 2016;33:951-962. doi:10.1039/c6np00035e

[26] Weber T. *In silico* tools for the analysis of antibiotic biosynthetic pathways. Int J Med Microbiol. 2014;304:230-235. doi:10.1016/j.ijmm.2014.02.001

[27] Li YF, Tsai KJ, Harvey CJ, Li JJ, Ary BE, et al. Comprehensive curation and analysis of fungal biosynthetic gene clusters of published natural products. Fungal Genet Biol. 201689:18-28. doi:10.1016/j.fgb.2016.01.012

[28] van der Lee TA, Medema MH. Computational strategies for genome-based natural product discovery and engineering in fungi. Fungal Genet Biol. 2016;89:29-36. doi:10.1016/j.fgb.2016.01.006

[29] Frey M, Chomet P, Glawischnig E, Stettner C, Grun S, et al. Analysis of a chemical plant defense mechanism in grasses. Science. 1997;277:696-699. doi:10.1126/science.277.5326.696

[30] Osbourn A. Gene clusters for secondary metabolic pathways: an emerging theme in plant biology. Plant Physiol. 2010;154:531-535. doi:10.1104/pp.110.161315

[31] Figueiredo AC, Barroso JG, Pedro LG, Scheffer JJC. Factors affecting secondary metabolite production in plants: volatile components and essential oils. Flavour Fragr J. 2008;23:213-226. doi:10.1002/ffj.1875

[32] Leal MC, Hilario A, Munro MHG, Blunt JW, Calado R. Natural products discovery needs improved taxonomic and geographic information. Nat Prod Rep. 2016;33:747-750. doi:10.1039/c5np00130g

[33] Luo Y, Enghiad B, Zhao H. New tools for reconstruction and heterologous expression of natural product biosynthetic gene clusters. Nat Prod Rep. 2016;33:174-182. doi:10.1039/c5np00085h

[34] Carbonell P, Currin A, Jervis AJ, Rattray NJW, Swainston N, et al. Bioinformatics for the synthetic biology of natural products: integrating across the Design-Build-Test cycle. Nat Prod Rep. 2016;33:925-932. doi:10.1039/c6np00018e

[35] Song MC, Kim EJ, Kim E, Rathwell K, Nama SJ, et al. Microbial biosynthesis of medicinally important plant secondary metabolites. Nat Prod Rep. 2014;31:1497-1509. doi:10.1039/c4np00057a

[36] Zhao H, Medema MH. Standardization for natural product synthetic biology. Nat Prod Rep. 2016;33:920-924. doi:10.1039/c6np00030d

[37] Ajikumar PK, Xiao WH, Tyo KE, Wang Y, Simeon F, et al. Isoprenoid pathway optimization for Taxol precursor overproduction in *Escherichia coli*. Science. 2010;330:70-74. doi:10.1126/science.1191652

[38] De Luca V, Salim V, Atsumi SM, Yu F. Mining the biodiversity of plants: a revolution in the making. Science. 2012;336:1658-1661. doi:10.1126/science.1217410

[39] Kim E, Moore BS, Yoon YJ. Reinvigorating natural product combinatorial biosynthesis with synthetic biology. Nat Chem Biol. 2015;11:639-659. doi:10.1038/nchembio.1893

[40] Menzella HG, Reid R, Carney JR, Chandran SS, Reisinger SJ, et al. Combinatorial polyketide biosynthesis by *de novo* design and rearrangement of modular polyketide synthase genes. Nat Biotechnol. 2005;23:1171-1176. doi:10.1038/nbt1128

[41] Conway KR, Boddy CN. ClusterMine360: a database of microbial PKS/NRPS biosynthesis. Nucleic Acids Res. 2013;41:D402-D407. doi:10.1093/nar/gks993

[42] Tremblay N, Hill P, Conway KR, Boddy CN. The use of ClusterMine360 for the analysis of polyketide and nonribosomal peptide biosynthetic pathways. Methods Mol Biol. 2016;1401:233-252. doi:10.1007/978-1-4939-3375-4_15

[43] Starcevic A, Zucko J, Simunkovic J, Long PF, Cullum J, et al. ClustScan: an integrated program package for the semi-automatic annotation of modular biosynthetic gene clusters and *in silico* prediction of novel chemical structures. Nucleic Acids Res. 2008;36:6882-6892. doi:10.1093/nar/gkn685

[44] Diminic J, Zucko J, Ruzic IT, Gacesa R, Hranueli D, et al. Databases of the thiotemplate modular systems (CSDB) and their *in silico* recombinants (r-CSDB). J Ind Microbiol Biotechnol. 2013;40:653-659. doi:10.1007/s10295-013-1252-z

[45] Ichikawa N, Sasagawa M, Yamamoto M, Komaki H, Yoshida Y, et al. DoBISCUIT: a database of secondary metabolite biosynthetic gene clusters. Nucleic Acids Res. 2013;41:D408-D414. doi:10.1093/nar/gks1177

[46] Hadjithomas M, Chen IA, Chu K, Ratner A, Palaniappan K, et al. IMG-ABC: a knowledge base to fuel discovery of biosynthetic gene clusters and novel secondary metabolites. mBio. 2015;6:e00932-15. doi:10.1128/mBio.00932-15

[47] Kellner F, Kim J, Clavijo BJ, Hamilton JP, Childs KL, et al. Genome-guided investigation of plant natural product biosynthesis. Plant J. 2015;82:680-692. doi:10.1111/tpj.12827

[48] Hur M, Campbell AA, Almeida-de-Macedo M, Li L, Ransom N, et al. A global approach to analysis and interpretation of metabolic data for plant natural product discovery. Nat Prod Rep. 2013;30:565-583. doi:10.1039/c3np20111b

[49] Chae L, Kim T, Nilo-Poyanco R, Rhee SY. Genomic signatures of specialized metabolism in plants. Science. 2014;344: 510-513. doi:10.1126/science.1252076

[50] Dreher K. Putting the plant metabolic network pathway databases to work: going offline to gain new capabilities. Methods Mol Biol. 2014;1083:151-171. doi:10.1007/978-1-62703-661-0_10

[51] Naithani S, Preece J, D'Eustachio P, Gupta P, Amarasinghe V, et al. Plant Reactome: a resource for plant pathways and comparative analysis. Nucleic Acids Res. 2017;45:D1029-D1039. doi:10.1093/nar/gkw932

[52] Starcevic A, Wolf K, Diminic J, Zucko J, Ruzic IT, et al. Recombinatorial biosynthesis of polyketides. J Ind Microbiol Biotechnol. 2012;39:503-511. doi:10.1007/s10295-011-1049-x

[53] Weber T, Kim HU. The secondary metabolite bioinformatics portal: computational tools to facilitate synthetic biology of secondary metabolite production. Synth Syst Biotechnol. 2016;1:69-79. doi:10.1016/j.synbio.2015.12.002

[54] Medema MH, van Raaphorst R, Takano E, Breitling R. Computational tools for the synthetic design of biochemical pathways. Nat Rev Microbiol. 2012;10:191-202. doi:10.1038/nrmicro2717

[55] Weber T, Blin K, Duddela S, Krug D, Kim HU, et al. antiSMASH 3.0—a comprehensive resource for the genome mining of biosynthetic gene clusters. Nucleic Acids Res. 2015;43:W237-W243. doi:10.1093/nar/gkv437

[56] Lee I, Ambaru B, Thakkar P, Marcotte EM, Rhee SY. Rational association of genes with traits using a genome-scale gene network for *Arabidopsis thaliana*. Nat Biotechnol. 2010;28:149-156. doi:10.1038/nbt.1603

[57] Caspi R, Billington R, Ferrer L, Foerster H, Fulcher CA, et al. The MetaCyc database of metabolic pathways and enzymes and the BioCyc collection of pathway/genome databases. Nucleic Acids Res. 2016;44:D471-D480. doi:10.1093/nar/gkv1164

[58] Le Fèvre F, Smidtas S, Combe C, Durot M, d'Alché-Buc F, et al. CycSim—an online tool for exploring and experimenting with genome-scale metabolic models. Bioinformatics. 2009;25:1987-1988. doi:10.1093/bioinformatics/btp268

[59] Yamanishi Y, Hattori M, Kotera M, Goto S, Kanehisa M. E-zyme: predicting potential EC numbers from the chemical transformation pattern of substrate-product pairs. Bioinformatics. 2009;25:i179-i186. doi:10.1093/bioinformatics/btp223

[60] Chou CH, Chang WC, Chiu CM, Huang CC, Huang HD. FMM: a web server for metabolic pathway reconstruction and comparative analysis. Nucleic Acids Res. 2009;37:W129-W134. doi:10.1093/nar/gkp264

[61] Kearse M, Moir R, Wilson A, Stones-Havas S, Cheung M, et al. Geneious basic: an integrated and extendable desktop software platform for the organization and analysis of sequence data. Bioinformatics. 2012;28:1647-1649. doi:10.1093/bioinformatics/bts199

[62] Johnston CW, Skinnider MA, Wyatt MA, Li X, Ranieri MRM, et al. An automated Genomes-to-Natural Products platform (GNP) for the discovery of modular natural products. Nat Commun. 2015;6:8421. doi:10.1038/ncomms9421

[63] Kanehisa M. KEGG bioinformatics resource for plant genomics and metabolomics. Methods Mol Biol. 2016;1374:55-70. doi:10.1007/978-1-4939-3167-5_3

[64] Law PJ, Claudel-Renard C, Joubert F, Louw AI, Berger DK. MADIBA: a web server toolkit for biological interpretation of *Plasmodium* and plant gene clusters. BMC Genomics. 2008;9:105. doi:10.1186/1471-2164-9-105

[65] de Klein N, Magnani E, Banf M, Rhee SY. microProtein Prediction Program (miP3): a software for predicting microProteins and their target transcription factors. Int J Genomics. 2015;2015:734147. doi:10.1155/2015/734147

[66] Rocha I, Maia P, Evangelista P, Vilaça P, Soares S, et al. OptFlux: an open-source software platform for *in silico* metabolic engineering. BMC Syst Biol. 2010;4:45. doi:10.1186/1752-0509-4-45

[67] Moriya Y, Shigemizu D, Hattori M, Tokimatsu T, Kotera M, et al. PathPred: an enzyme-catalyzed metabolic pathway prediction server. Nucleic Acids Res. 2010;38:W138-W143. doi:10.1093/nar/gkq318

[68] Kutmon M, van Iersel MP, Bohler A, Kelder T, Nunes N, et al. PathVisio 3: an extendable pathway analysis toolbox. PLoS Comput Biol. 2015;11:e1004085. doi:10.1371/journal.pcbi.1004085

[69] van Iersel MP, Kelder T, Pico AR, Hanspers K, Coort S, et al. Presenting and exploring biological pathways with PathVisio. BMC Bioinformat. 2008;9:399. doi:10.1186/1471-2105-9-399

[70] Hanumappa M, Preece J, Elser J, Nemeth D, Bono G, et al. WikiPathways for plants: a community pathway curation portal and a case study in rice and *Arabidopsis* seed development networks. Rice. 2013;6:14. doi:10.1186/1939-8433-6-14

[71] Skinnider MA, Dejong CA, Rees PN, Johnston CW, Li H, et al. Genomes to natural products PRediction Informatics for Secondary Metabolomes (PRISM). Nucleic Acids Res. 2015;43:9645-9662. doi:10.1093/nar/gkv1012

[72] Carbonell P, Planson AG, Fichera D, Faulon JL. A retrosynthetic biology approach to metabolic pathway design for therapeutic production. BMC Syst Biol. 2011;5:122. doi:10.1186/1752-0509-5-122

[73] Planson AG, Carbonell P, Grigoras I, Faulon JL. A retrosynthetic biology approach to therapeutics: from conception to delivery. Curr Opin Biotechnol. 2012;23:948-956. doi:10.1016/j.copbio.2012.03.009

[74] Hoff KJ, Stanke M. WebAUGUSTUS - a web service for training AUGUSTUS and predicting genes in eukaryotes. Nucleic Acids Res. 2013;41:W123-W128. doi:10.1093/nar/gkt418

[75] Kelder T, van Iersel MP, Hanspers K, Kutmon M, Conklin BR, et al. WikiPathways: building research communities on biological pathways. Nucleic Acids Res. 2012,40:D1301-D1307. doi:10.1093/nar/gkr1074

[76] Kutmon M, Riutta A, Nunes N, Hanspers K, Willighagen EL, et al. WikiPathways: capturing the full diversity of pathway knowledge. Nucleic Acids Res. 2016;44:D488-D494. doi:10.1093/nar/gkv1024

[77] Durot M, Bourguignon PY, Schachter V. Genome-scale models of bacterial metabolism: reconstruction and applications. FEMS Microbiol Rev. 2009;33:164-190. doi:10.1111/j.1574-6976.2008.00146.x

[78] Feist AM, Herrgård MJ, Thiele I, Reed JL, Palsson BØ. Reconstruction of biochemical networks in microorganisms. Nat Rev Microbiol. 2009;7:129-143. doi:10.1038/nrmicro1949

[79] Shannon P, Markiel A, Ozier O, Baliga NS, Wang JT, et al. Cytoscape: a software environment for integrated models of biomolecular interaction networks. Genome Res. 2003;13:2498-2504. doi:10.1101/gr.1239303

[80] Overbeek R, Olson R, Pusch GD, Olsen GJ, Davis JJ, et al. The SEED and the Rapid Annotation of microbial genomes using Subsystems Technology (RAST). Nucleic Acids Res. 2014;42:D206-D214. doi:10.1093/nar/gkt1226

[81] Orth JD, Thiele I, Palsson BØ. What is flux balance analysis? Nat Biotechnol. 2010;28:245-248. doi:10.1038/nbt.1614

[82] Schellenberger J, Que R, Fleming RM, Thiele I, Orth JD, et al. Quantitative prediction of cellular metabolism with constraint-based models: the COBRA Toolbox v2.0. Nat Protoc. 2011;6:1290-1307. doi:10.1038/nprot.2011.308

[83] Garcia-Albornoz M, Thankaswamy-Kosalai S, Nilsson A, Väremo L, Nookaew I, Nielsen J. BioMet Toolbox 2.0: genome-wide analysis of metabolism and omics data. Nucleic Acids Res. 2014;42:W175-W181. doi:10.1093/nar/gku371

[84] Boele J, Olivier BG, Teusink B. FAME, the flux analysis and modeling environment. BMC Syst Biol. 2012;6:8. doi:10.1186/1752-0509-6-8

[85] Schilling CH, Covert MW, Famili I, Church GM, Edwards JS, Palsson BO. Genome-scale metabolic model of *Helicobacter pylori* 26695. J Bacteriol. 2002;184:4582-4593. doi:10.1128/JB.184.16.4582-4593.2002

[86] Oh YK, Palsson BO, Park SM, Schilling CH, Mahadevan R. Genome-scale reconstruction of metabolic network in *Bacillus subtilis* based on high-throughput phenotyping and gene essentiality data. J Biol Chem. 2007;282:28791-28799. doi:10.1074/jbc.M703759200

[87] Puchałka J, Oberhardt MA, Godinho M, Bielecka A, Regenhardt D, et al. Genome-scale reconstruction and analysis of the *Pseudomonas putida* KT2440 metabolic network facilitates applications in biotechnology. PLoS Comput Biol. 2008;4:e1000210. doi:10.1371/journal.pcbi.1000210

[88] Henry CS, Broadbelt LJ, Hatzimanikatis V. Thermodynamics-based metabolic flux analysis. Biophys J. 2007;92:1792-1805. doi:10.1529/biophysj.106.093138

[89] Asadollahi MA, Maury J, Patil KR, Schalk M, Clark A, Nielsen J. Enhancing sesquiterpene production in *Saccharomyces cerevisiae* through *in silico* driven metabolic engineering. Metab Eng. 2009;11:328-334. doi:10.1016/j.ymben.2009.07.001

[90] Finn RD, Coggill P, Eberhardt RY, Eddy SR, Mistry J, et al. The Pfam protein families database: towards a more sustainable future. Nucleic Acids Res. 2016;44:D279-D285. doi:10.1093/nar/gkv1344

[91] Blin K, Medema MH, Kottmann R, Lee SY, Weber T. The antiSMASH database, a comprehensive database of microbial secondary metabolite biosynthetic gene clusters. Nucleic Acids Res. 2017;45:D555-D559. doi:10.1093/nar/gkw960

[92] Röttig M, Rausch C, Kohlbacher O. Combining structure and sequence information allows automated prediction of substrate specificities within enzyme families. PLoS Comput Biol. 2010;6:e1000636. doi:10.1371/journal.pcbi.1000636

[93] Röttig M, Medema MH, Blin K, Weber T, Rausch C, et al. NRPSpredictor2: a web server for predicting NRPS adenylation domain specificity. Nucleic Acids Res. 2011;39:W362-W367. doi:10.1093/nar/gkr323

[94] Liu Y, Young K, Rakotondraibe LH, Brodie PJ, Wiley JD, et al. Antiproliferative compounds from *Cleistanthus boivinianus* from the Madagascar dry forest. J Nat Prod. 2015;78:1543-1547. doi:10.1021/np501020m

[95] Liu Y, Cheng E, Rakotondraibe LH, Brodie PJ, Applequist W, et al. Antiproliferative compounds from *Ocotea macrocarpa* from the Madagascar dry forest. Tetrahedron Lett. 2015;56:3630-3632. doi:10.1016/j.tetlet.2015.01.172

[96] Nyandoro SS, Munissi JJE, Gruhonjic A, Duffy S, Pan F, et al. Polyoxygenated cyclohexenes and other constituents of *Cleistochlamys kirkii* leaves. J Nat Prod. 2016. doi:10.1021/acs.jnatprod.6b00759. PMID: 28001067

[97] Prakash P, Gupta N. Therapeutic uses of *Ocimum sanctum* Linn (Tulsi) with a note on eugenol and its pharmacological actions: a short review. Indian J Physiol Pharmacol. 2005;49:125-131. PMID: 16170979

[98] Willis JC. A dictionary of the flowering plants and ferns. Cambridge: The University Press; 1919

[99] Khare CP. Indian medicinal plants: an illustrated dictionary. Heidelberg: Springer; 2007, p. 443

[100] Upadhyay AK, Chacko AR, Gandhimathi A, Ghosh P, Harini K, et al. Genome sequencing of herb Tulsi (*Ocimum tenuiflorum*) unravels key genes behind its strong medicinal properties. BMC Plant Biol. 2015;15:212. doi:10.1186/s12870-015-0562-x

[101] Ke Y, Ye K, Grossniklaus HE, Archer DR, Joshi HC, et al. Noscapine inhibits tumor growth with little toxicity to normal tissues or inhibition of immune responses. Cancer Immunol Immunother. 2000;49:217-225. PMID: 10941904

[102] Ye K, Ke Y, Keshava N, Shanks J, Kapp JA, et al. Opium alkaloid noscapine is an antitumor agent that arrests metaphase and induces apoptosis in dividing cells. Proc Natl Acad Sci USA. 1998;95:1601-1606. PMID: 9465062

[103] Zhou J, Gupta K, Yao J, Ye K, Panda D, et al. Paclitaxel-resistant human ovarian cancer cells undergo c-Jun NH_2-terminal kinase-mediated apoptosis in response to noscapine. J Biol Chem. 2002;277:39777-39785. doi:10.1074/jbc.M203927200

[104] DellaPenna D, O'Connor SE. Plant gene clusters and opiates. Science. 2012;336:1648-1649. doi:10.1126/science.1225473

[105] Battersby AR, Hirst M, McCaldin DJ, Southgate R, Staunton J. Alkaloid biosynthesis. XII. The biosynthesis of narcotine. J Chem Soc Perkin 1. 1968;17:2163-2172. PMID: 5691486

[106] Winzer T, Gazda V, He Z, Kaminski F, Kern M, et al. A *Papaver somniferum* 10-gene cluster for synthesis of the anticancer alkaloid noscapine. Science. 336:1704-1708. doi:10.1126/science.1220757

[107] Rischer H, Oresic M, Seppänen-Laakso T, Katajamaa M, Lammertyn F, et al. Gene-to-metabolite networks for terpenoid indole alkaloid biosynthesis in *Catharanthus roseus* cells. Proc Natl Acad Sci USA. 2006;103:5614-5619. doi:10.1073/pnas.0601027103

[108] Noble RL. The discovery of the vinca alkaloids-chemotherapeutic agents against cancer. Biochem Cell Biol. 1990;68:1344-1351. doi:10.1139/o90-197

[109] Dong HP, Wu HM, Chen SJ, Chen CY. The effect of butanolides from *Cinnamomum tenuifolium* on platelet aggregation. Molecules. 2013;18:11836-11841. doi:10.3390/molecules181011836

[110] Hoshino S, Wakimoto T, Onaka H, Abe I. Chojalactones A-C, cytotoxic butanolides isolated from *Streptomyces* sp. cultivated with mycolic acid containing bacterium. Org Lett. 2015;17:1501-1504. doi:10.1021/acs.orglett.5b00385

[111] Kim W, Lyu HN, Kwon HS, Kim YS, Lee KH, et al. Obtusilactone B from *Machilus thunbergii* targets barrier-to-autointegration factor to treat cancer. Mol Pharmacol. 2013;83:367-376. doi:10.1124/mol.112.082578

[112] Shen KH, Lin ES, Kuo PL, Chen CY, Hsu YL. Isolinderanolide B, a butanolide extracted from the stems of *Cinnamomum subavenium*, inhibits proliferation of T24 human bladder cancer cells by blocking cell cycle progression and inducing apoptosis. Integr Cancer Ther. 2011;10:350-358. doi:10.1177/1534735410391662

[113] Yang SY, Wang HM, Wu TW, Chen YJ, Shieh JJ, et al. Subamolide B isolated from medicinal plant *Cinnamomum subavenium* induces cytotoxicity in human cutaneous squamous cell carcinoma cells through mitochondrial and CHOP-dependent cell death pathways. Evid Based Complement Alternat Med. 2013,2013:630415. doi:10.1155/2013/630415

[114] Risinger AL, Mooberry SL. Taccalonolides: novel microtubule stabilizers with clinical potential. Cancer Lett. 2010;291:14-19. doi:10.1016/j.canlet.2009.09.020

[115] Lau W, Sattely ES. Six enzymes from mayapple that complete the biosynthetic pathway to the etoposide aglycone. Science. 2015;349:1224-1228. doi:10.1126/science.aac7202

[116] Rajniak J, Barco B, Clay NK, Sattely ES. A new cyanogenic metabolite in *Arabidopsis* required for inducible pathogen defence. Nature. 2015;525:376-379. doi:10.1038/nature14907

Chapter 11

Towards Metabolic Engineering of Podophyllotoxin Production

Christel L. C. Seegers, Rita Setroikromo and
Wim J. Quax

Additional information is available at the end of the chapter

http://dx.doi.org/10.5772/67615

Abstract

The pharmaceutically important anticancer drugs etoposide and teniposide are derived from podophyllotoxin, a natural product isolated from roots of *Podophyllum hexandrum* growing in the wild. The overexploitation of this endangered plant has led to the search for alternative sources. Metabolic engineering aimed at constructing the pathway in another host cell is very appealing, but for that approach, an in-depth knowledge of the pathway toward podophyllotoxin is necessary. In this chapter, we give an overview of the lignan pathway leading to podophyllotoxin. Subsequently, we will discuss the engineering possibilities to produce podophyllotoxin in a heterologous host. This will require detailed knowledge on the cellular localization of the enzymes of the lignan biosynthesis pathway. Due to the high number of enzymes involved and the scarce information on compartmentalization, the heterologous production of podophyllotoxin still remains a tremendous challenge. At the moment, research is focusing on the last step(s) in the conversion of deoxypodophyllotoxin to (epi)podophyllotoxin and 4′-demethyldesoxypodophyllotoxin by plant cytochromes.

Keywords: etoposide, podophyllotoxin, *Podophyllum hexandrum*, *Anthriscus sylvestris*, metabolic engineering

1. Introduction

The high demand of podophyllotoxin derivatives for chemotherapy gives a severe pressure on the natural sources, such as *Podophyllum hexandrum* and *Podophyllum peltatum* [1]. The highest concentration of podophyllotoxin is found in *P. hexandrum* roots, with reported yields up to 6.6% dry weight (d.w.) [2]. The excessive harvesting has resulted in inclusion of *P. hexandrum* in the Convention on International Trade in Endangered Species (CITES) [3]. Chemical synthesis of podophyllotoxin is difficult due to the presence of four contiguous chiral centers and the presence of a base sensitive *trans*-lactone moiety [4]. The shortest synthesis described contains five steps from the commercially available 6-bromopiperonal into (epi) podophyllotoxin [5]. As an alternative, cell suspension cultures have been explored, but these produce only low amounts (max. 0.65% d.w.) of podophyllotoxin [6, 7]. As neither chemical synthesis nor *in vitro* production of podophyllotoxin is economically competitive with the extraction of podophyllotoxin from *P. hexandrum* roots, other alternatives are being searched for. Metabolic engineering aimed at constructing the pathway in a heterologous host is very appealing, but for that approach, an in-depth knowledge of the biosynthetic pathway toward podophyllotoxin is necessary.

2. Lignans and their biological activities

In 1936, Haworth was the first to describe a group of phenylpropanoid dimers (C_6C_3) linked by the central carbon (C8) as lignans [8]. The Haworth's definition of lignan has been adopted by the IUPAC nomenclature recommendations in 2000 [9]. According to this nomenclature, lignans can be divided into eight subgroups based on the oxygen incorporation into the skeleton and the cyclization pattern [10]. In the lignan pathway toward podophyllotoxin, six subgroups of lignans can be defined in the order of occurrence: furofuran, furan, dibenzylbutane, dibenzylbutyrolactol, dibenzylbutyrolactone, and aryltetralin (**Figure 1**). The other two subgroups are arylnaphthalene and dibenzocyclooctadiene. Dibenzylbutanes are only linked by the 8,8′ bond. An additional oxygen bridge is found in furofurans, furans, dibenzylbutyrolactols, and dibenzylbutyrolactones. A second carbon-carbon link is found in aryltetralins, arylnaphthalenes, and dibenzocyclooctadienes [10, 11]. The majority of the lignans has oxygen at the C9 (C9′) carbon; however, some lignans in the dibenzylbutanes, furans, and dibenzocyclooctadiene subgroups are missing this oxygen [10]. Humans metabolize the furofurans pinoresinol and sesamin, the furan lariciresinol, the dibenzylbutane secoisolariciresinol, and the dibenzylbutyrolactone matairesinol. These lignans are phytoestrogens, which can be converted into enterolactone or enterodiol by intestinal bacteria [12, 13]. Enterolactone and enterodiol have antioxidant, estrogenic, and anti-estrogenic activities in humans; furthermore, they may protect against certain chronic diseases [14]. Several lignans have been described to have antiviral properties; however, therapeutic applications are limited due to the toxicity [15]. The extract, podophyllin, of *Podophyllum* roots and rhizome was included in the U.S. Pharmacopeia in 1820. In 1942, it was removed, because of its severe gastrointestinal toxicity [16]. However, Kaplan described in 1944, the successful treatment of venereal warts (*Condylomata acuminata*) in 200 members of the military by topically applied podophyllin [17]. The aryltetralin podophyllotoxin is the active ingredient in podophyllin, which has been commercialized as a treatment for warts caused by the human papilloma virus [18]. Semisynthetic derivatives of podophyllotoxin were designed as chemotherapy compounds for oral administration or for intravenous treatment [19, 20].

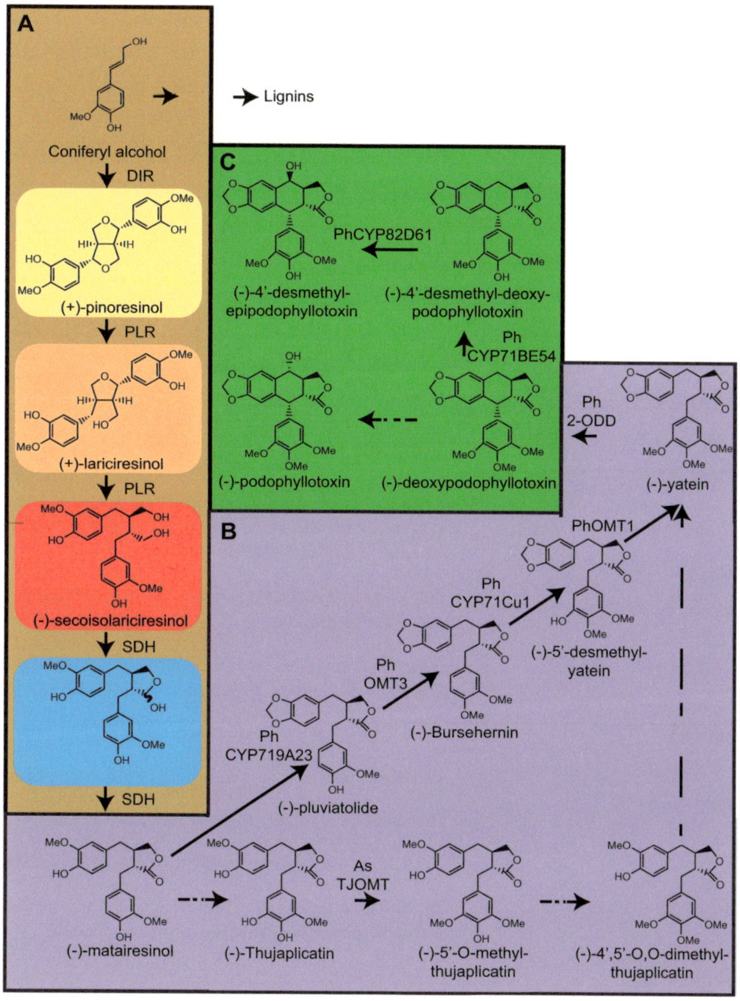

Figure 1. Lignan pathway in *Podophyllum hexandrum* and *Anthriscus sylvestris*. (A) Coniferyl alcohol toward matairesinol (brown box), (B) matairesinol toward deoxypodophyllotoxin (purple box), and (C) deoxypodophyllotoxin toward podophyllotoxin and demethyldesoxypodophyllotoxin (green box). Lignan subgroups are shown by various colors: yellow = furofuran, orange = furan, red = dibenzylbutane, blue = dibenzylbutyrolactol, purple = dibenzylbutyrolactone, and green = aryltetralin.

3. Importance of podophyllotoxin and derivatives for chemotherapy

Podophyllotoxin is a tubulin-interacting agent that inhibits mitotic spindle formation [21]. As podophyllotoxin is severely toxic if applied systemic, a number of less toxic derivatives have been generated and these are now widely used in cancer chemotherapy. Interestingly, the derivatives currently used in the clinic, etoposide, and teniposide, have a different mode of action than podophyllotoxin. They inhibit topoisomerase II by stabilizing its binding to DNA, which results in double-stranded breaks in the DNA and arrest of the cell cycle in the G2 phase [21]. Etoposide (VP-16, VePesid®) was synthesized in 1966 by Sandoz and was further developed by Bristol-Meyers from 1978 onwards. In 1983, it was approved by the FDA for the treatment of testicular cancer [22]. As etoposide is poorly soluble in water, the etoposide prodrug etoposide phosphate (Etopophos®) was designed by Bristol-Meyers Squibb, which was approved by the FDA in 1996 [23]. The prodrug is converted to etoposide within 30 min presumably by alkaline phosphatases. Furthermore, the pharmacokinetics and toxicity of etoposide phosphate are equal to etoposide [24, 25]. According to the National Cancer Institute and the Dutch government etoposide, phosphate should be used in combination therapy for various cancers (**Table 1**) [26–28]. Teniposide (VM-26, Vumon®) was synthesized in 1967 by

Cancer	Combination of drugs
Hodgkin lymphoma in children	Vincristine sulfate, etoposide phosphate, prednisone, doxorubicin hydrochloride
	Doxorubicin hydrochloride, bleomycin, vincristine sulfate, etoposide phosphate
	Doxorubicin hydrochloride, bleomycin, vincristine sulfate, etoposide phosphate, prednisone, cyclophosphamide
Non-hodgkin lymphoma	
- All	Rituximab, ifosfamide, carboplatin, etoposide phosphate
	Etoposide phosphate, ifosfamide, methotrexate
	Lomustine, etoposide phosphate, chlorambucil, prednisolone
- B-cell	Rituximab, etoposide phosphate, prednisone, vincristine sulfate, cyclophosphamide, doxorubicin hydrochloride
Malignant germ cell tumors	
- Nonbrain	Cisplatin, etoposide phosphate, bleomycin
- Ovarian/testicular	Bleomycin, etoposide phosphate, cisplatin
- Advanced testicular	Etoposide phosphate, ifosfamide, cisplatin
Acute myeloid leukemia	
- Children	Cytarabine, daunorubicin hydrochloride, etoposide phosphate
- Phase II	Cytarabine and amsacrine, etoposide or mitoxantrone
High-risk retinoblastoma in children	Carboplatin, etoposide phosphate, vincristine sulfate
Small cell lung cancer	Etoposide with cisplatin or carboplatin
	Cisplatin, cyclophosphamide, doxorubicin, vincristine, methotrexate
Relapsed Wilms tumor	Ifosfamide, carboplatin, and etoposide

Table 1. Cancer chemotherapy combination treatments with etoposide.

Sandoz and was further developed by Bristol-Meyers from 1978 onwards [22]. It is used in the treatment of acute myeloid leukemia and myelodysplastic syndromes in children and in acute lymphocytic leukemia [29, 30]. Toxicity problems are still an issue with etoposide; therefore, novel derivatives were designed and evaluated in preclinical and clinical studies [31]. The derivatives NK611, Gl-311, and TOP-53 were discontinued after phase I or II studies [22, 32, 33]. NK611, which is more water soluble than etoposide, shows similar toxic effects in humans as etoposide. However, only few patients showed efficacy in phase I studies [34–36]. No data of the phase I or II studies were found for GL-311 and TOP-53. Four newer derivatives are tafluposide, F14512, Adva-27a, and QS-ZYX-1-61 [31, 32]. Tafluposide (F-11782), a pentafluorinated epipodophylloid, inhibits topoisomerase I and II activity [37, 38]. In phase I study, stable disease was observed in 7 out of 21 patients with advanced solid tumors, such as choroid and skin melanoma [39]. Increasing the selectivity of anticancer agents is of great interest. As the polyamine transport system is upregulated in cancer cells, F14512 was designed to target the transport system by linking the epipodophyllotoxin core to a spermine chain [40]. Phase I study in adult patients with acute meloid leukemia showed clinical activity in relapsed patients, but limited activity in refractory patients [41]. F14512 will be tested in combination with cytarabine in a phase II study [41]. The minimal therapeutic effect of etoposide on dogs with relapsing lymphomas has resulted in a phase I study of F14512, which showed a strong therapeutic efficacy [42]. The derivative adva-27a, a GEM-difluorinated C-glycoside derivate of podophyllotoxin, is effective against multidrug resistant cancer cells [43]. Preparations are being made for a phase I study in pancreatic and breast cancer patients in Canada [44]. The derivative QS-ZYX-1-61 induces apoptosis by inhibition of topoisomerase II in human non–small-cell lung cancer [45]. Further investigations are necessary for this compound.

4. Overview of the lignan biosynthetic pathway

Podophyllotoxin is produced in the lignan pathway, which we will discuss in more detail in this section (**Figure 1**). Lignins and lignans are the major metabolic products of the phenylpropanoid pathway in vascular plants. Lignins are derived from coumaryl, coniferyl, and sinapyl alcohol, whereas lignans are derived from coniferyl alcohol [46].

4.1. Coniferyl alcohol toward matairesinol

The pathway toward podophyllotoxin starts with pinoresinol, lariciresinol, secoisolariciresinol, and matairesinol. Pinoresinol and lariciresinol are found in most vascular plants, such as *Arabidopsis thaliana*. Some species follow the lignan pathway toward podophyllotoxin until the branch point matairesinol, such as the *Forsythia* species. Lignans further downstream toward podophyllotoxin are found in more specialized plants. An interesting question is whether the capability of podophyllotoxin production is restricted to a limited number of plants, or that other closely related plants have cryptic pathways as shown in bacteria [47]. To answer this question, an in-depth discussion of the lignan pathway is necessary as we do below. Coniferyl alcohol is converted into matairesinol in five steps by three enzymes: dirigent protein, pinoresinol-lariciresinol reductase, and secoisolariciresinol dehydrogenase (**Figure 1A**).

4.1.1. *Dirigent protein*

In 1997, Davin and coworker showed that the dirigent protein (DIR) from *Forsythia suspensa* can couple two coniferyl alcohols stereospecific to (+)-pinoresinol after their oxidation by a nonspecific oxidase or nonenzymatic single-electron oxidant [48]. Davin and coworkers showed that the DIR protein lacks a detectable catalytic active (oxidative) center and that the rate of dimeric lignan formation is similar in the presence or absence of DIR protein; however, the DIR protein is necessary for enantioselectivity [48]. Both (+)- and (−)-pinoresinol-forming proteins were found in plants. The (+)-forming DIR protein is important for the lignan pathway in the direction of podophyllotoxin synthesis. (+)-Forming DIRs are the ScDIR protein from *Schisandra chinensis*, the *psd-Fi1* from *Frullania intermedia*, and PsDRR206 from *Pisum sativum* [49–51]. In *A. thaliana*, 16 DIR homologs were found of which four were characterized as follows: two formed (−)-pinoresinol (AtDIR5 and AtDIR6); the other two showed nonstereoselective coupling of coniferyl alcohols [49, 52]. On the other hand, *Linum usitatissimum* has (+)-forming and (−)-forming DIR proteins [53]. Kim and coworkers solved the crystal structure of the (+)-pinoresinol forming PSDRR206 of *P. sativum* to 1.95A [54]. Homology modeling of the (−)-pinoresinol forming AtDIR6 in the PSDRR206 crystal structure showed six additional residues in the longest loop of the (+)-forming DIR, which are present in all (+)-forming DIRs. Site-directed mutagenesis could be used to confirm whether one or more of these residues are responsible for the enantioselectivity of the DIR [54].

4.1.2. *Pinoresinol-lariciresinol reductase*

In 1996, Dinkova-Kostova and coworkers found the pinoresinol-lariciresinol reductase (PLR) in *F. intermedia*, which could reduce (+)-pinoresinol to (+)-lariciresinol and sequentially to (−)-secoisolariciresinol [55]. The (−)-secoisolariciresinol-forming PLRs are important for podophyllotoxin synthesis. These PLRs were found in *F. intermedia* (PLR-Fi1), *Linum album* (PLR-La1), *L. usitatissimum* (PLR-Lu2) and *Linum corymbulosum* (PLR-Lc1) [56–59]. A PLR with opposite enantioselectivity was found in *L. usitatissimum* (PLR-Lu1) [57, 58]. PLR can have selectivity or preference toward one of the enantiomers. The *Thuja plicata* PLRs accept both enantiomers of pinoresinol; however, they were selective for the lariciresinol substrate, as PLR-TP1 accepts only (−)-lariciresinol and PLR-TP2 only (+)-lariciresinol [60]. In *Linum perenne*, it was found that PLR_Lp1 can convert (±)-pinoresinol to (±)-lariciresinol and (±)-secoisolariciresinol, with a preference for (+)-pinoresinol and (−)-lariciresinol [61]. The *F. intermedia* (PLR-Fi1) and *L. usitatissimum* (PLR-Lu1) PLRs were found to convert (+)-lariciresinol to (−)-secoisolariciresinol before depletion of (−)-pinoresinol [56, 57]. On the other hand, *L. album* (PLR-La1) and *L. perenne* (PLR-LP1) PLRs first seem to convert all (+)-pinoresinol to (+)-lariciresinol before converting (+)-lariciresinol further to (−)-secoisolariciresinol [57, 61]. For *A. thaliana* proteins with strict substrate, specificity toward pinoresinol was found as weak or no activity toward lariciresinol was observed [62]. Therefore, these proteins are annotated as pinoresinol reductases (AtPrRs). AtPrR1 reduces both enantiomers, and AtPrR2 only reduces (−)-pinoresinol [62]. The crystal structures of PLR-Tp1 of *T. plicata* were resolved to 2.5 A, and a homology model of PLR-Tp2 with opposite enantioselectivity was deduced from the PLR-Tp1 structure [63]. Three residues in the substrate binding site were different, which could explain the enantioselectivity [63].

4.1.3. *Secoisolariciresinol dehydrogenase*

Secoisolariciresinol dehydrogenase (SDH) from *F. intermedia* and *P. peltatum* convert (−)-secoisolariciresinol into (−)-matairesinol, through the intermediary (−)-lactol. Neither of them was able to convert the opposite enantiomer [64]. Crystallization of *P. peltatum* SDH (1.6 A) showed that it is a tetramer. The ternary complex was obtained by the addition of cofactors and (−)-matairesinol. Based on the position of (−)-matairesinol, also (−)-secoisolariciresinol could be modeled into the crystal structure. Using the same constrains, (+)-secoisolariciresinol could not be modeled into the crystal structure, which could explain the enantioselectivity [64, 65].

4.2. Matairesinol toward deoxypodophyllotoxin

Plant feeding experiments performed by various groups have revealed the metabolites intermediate between matairesinol and podophyllotoxin, such as yatein and deoxypodophyllotoxin in *P. hexandrum* [66, 67]. This was followed by the identification of the enzymes in *P. hexandrum* (**Figure 1B**). Marques and coworkers found that pluviatolide synthases in *P. hexandrum* (CYP719A23) and *P. peltatum* (CYP719A24) can convert (−)-matairesinol into (−)-pluviatolide by formation of the methylenedioxy bridge [68]. Lau and Sattely used transcriptome mining in *P. hex``vandrum* to identify four additional biosynthetic enzymes in the lignan pathway, which convert (−)-pluviatolide into deoxypodophyllotoxin [69]. Pluviatolide 4-O-methyltransferase (PhOMT3) converts (−)-pluviatolide into bursehernin by methylation at C4′OH. Bursehernin 5′-hydroxylase (CYP71CU1) incorporates a molecular oxygen at C5′ in bursehernin, which results in (−)-5′-desmethyl-yatein. In the following step, 5′-demethyl-yatein O-transferase (OMT1) converts (−)-demethyl-yatein to (−)-yatein by methylation at C5′OH. In the last step, deoxypodophyllotoxin synthase (2-ODD) converts (−)-yatein to (−)-deoxypodophyllotoxin by ring closure between C2 and C7′ [69]. Sakakibara and coworkers suggest a different route toward deoxypodophyllotoxin for *Anthriscus sylvestris* (**Figure 1B**) [70]. Feeding experiments showed incorporation of matairesinol, thujaplicatin, 5-methylthujaplicatin, and 4,5-dimethylthujaplicatin into yatein [70]. This was followed by the discovery of the enzyme thujaplicatin O-methyltransferase (AsTJOMT), which methylates thujaplicatin to form 5-O-methylthujaplicatin [71]. Furthermore, they found incorporation of matairesinol and pluviatolide in bursehernin, but no further incorporation into yatein. No literature has been reported in the presence of 5-demethylyatein in *A. sylvestris*. However, feeding of 5-demethylyatein to *A. sylvestris* results in yatein formation [70]. In the transcriptome of *L. album*, genes related to OMT3 and CYP71CU1 were found; however, no gene related to CYP719A24 was found (**Figure 1B**) [72, 73]. The differences in the lignan pathways in *P. hexandrum, A. sylvestris*, and *L. album* indicate the possibility that the later part of the lignan pathway might have convergently evolved in the various species, which decreases the probability of the presence of a cryptic pathway in other species.

4.3. Conversion of deoxypodophyllotoxin into demethyldesoxypodophyllotoxin

The *P. hexandrum* enzyme that converts deoxypodophyllotoxin into podophyllotoxin has not been identified yet. Lau and Sattely, attempted to find this enzyme, presumably a cytochrome, by mining the publicly available RNA-sequencing data set from the Medicinal Plants Consortium.

Furthermore, they analyzed transcriptome data from *P. hexandrum* after upregulating the podophyllotoxin biosynthesis genes by wounding the leaves. Both methods were successful in identifying podophyllotoxin biosynthesis genes as described in the previous session; however, the enzyme converting deoxypodophyllotoxin into podophyllotoxin was not found (**Figure 1C**). They found two P450 cytochromes that can convert deoxypodophyllotoxin into 4′-desmethylepipodophyllotoxin [69]. In the first step, CYP71BE54 converts (−)-deoxypodophyllotoxin to (−)-4′-demethyldesoxypodophyllotoxin. In the second step (-)-4′-demethyldesoxypodophylltoxin is converted to (−)-4′-desmethylepipodophyllotoxin by CYP82D61.

5. Engineering approaches

In this part, we will focus on genetic engineering approach`es to produce podophyllotoxin in a heterologous system. In order to produce podophyllotoxin in *Escherichia coli* or *Saccharomyces cerevisiae,* the pathway from the easily available glucose toward coniferyl alcohol has to be implemented into these organisms.

5.1. Production of coniferyl alcohol in *E. coli* and *S. cerevisiae*

Coniferyl alcohol can be produced in *E. coli* by a co-culture system. Coumaryl alcohol is produced upon insertion of four phenylpropanoid pathway genes [74]. The production can be increased by addition of four key shikimate pathway genes to overproduce tyrosine [75]. Addition of the genes for methyltransferase and HpaBC in another strain resulted in the accumulation of 125 mg/L coniferyl alcohol after 24 h. Co-culturing was necessary as HpaBC converts tyrosine to an unwanted side product [74]. The full biosynthetic pathway toward coniferyl alcohol has not been tested for expression in *S. cerevisiae* yet. However, production of ±100 mg/L coumaric acid has been shown [76]. To convert coumaric acid to coniferyl alcohol in *S. cerevisiae,* four or five additional genes have to be expressed; therefore, in order to produce coniferyl alcohol levels similar to *E. coli,* further optimization of coumaric acid production is necessary.

5.2. Cellular localization of enzymes from the lignan pathway

In order to engineer the lignan pathway for podophyllotoxin production in a heterologous cell, knowledge about the localization of lignans and their corresponding enzymes is necessary. Localization to the wrong organelle might abolish or lower production, as was shown for penicillin production [77]. The monolignol coniferyl alcohol is synthesized in the cytosol and transported over the plasma membrane for incorporation into lignin or lignan by an ABC membrane transporter, whereas the glucosylated form (coniferin) for storage could only be transported over the vacuolar membrane possibly by another ABC membrane transporter or proton-coupled antiporter [78, 79]. Analyses of transmembrane helices by the TMHMM predictor [80] indicated that DIR has one transmembrane helix. Furthermore, the DIR protein is a glycoprotein with a secretory signal peptide [50]. This indicates that the DIR protein is membrane attached, which is consistent with the findings in *F. suspense* stems. Only the insoluble fraction was capable of stereoselective conversion of coniferyl alcohol to (+)-pinoresinol, whereas soluble enzyme preparations only form racemic pinoresinol [81, 82]. As the DIR protein was found primarily localized within the plant cell wall [83], it might be difficult to target DIR to its natural compartment in bacteria and yeast. However, there is strong indication that monolignol dimerization also occurs intracellular as shown by protoplast experiments in *A. thaliana* and the racemic pinoresinol formation in crude cell-free enzyme preparation of *F. suspense* stems [81, 84]. The disadvantage is the absence of stereoselectivity in the coupling of the two coniferyl alcohols. However, this should not be a problem, if the influx of coniferyl alcohol is large enough. The following proteins lack a transmembrane helix or signal peptide according to the TMHMM predictor and SignalP [85]: PLR, SDH, OMT3, OMT1, and 2-ODD. PLR and 2-ODD are localized to the cytoplasm, and SDH, OMT3, and OMT1 to the chloroplast according to the plant specific localization tool Plant-mPloc [86]. However, the specific chloroplast localization tools ChloroP and PCLR suggest no chloroplast localization, which was confirmed by the localization tools MultiLoc2-LowRes and LocTree3 [87–90]. Therefore, we think that the proteins PLR, SDH, OMT3, OMT1, and 2-ODD are all localized in the cytoplasm. The four cytochromes CYP719A23, CYP71CU1, CYP71BE54, and CYP82D61 contain a targeting peptide and one or two transmembrane helixes. They are probably located in the endoplasmic reticulum (ER) membrane (according to an analysis by Plant-mPloc and MultiLoc2) as most plant cytochromes are anchored in the ER membrane and face the cytosolic side [91]. Our hypothesis is that deoxypodophyllotoxin is converted to podophyllotoxin by a cytochrome that is ER bound (**Figure 2**). Production of podophyllotoxin in *E. coli* would be feasible assuming that PLR, SDH, OMT3, OMT1, and 2-ODD can be actively expressed in the cytosol. As coniferyl alcohol has been produced before in this organism and cytochrome P450 enzymes with modified N-terminus have also been expressed successfully [92], some of the major steps toward podophyllotoxin might be performed in *E. coli*. The disadvantage of *E. coli* is the lack of NAD(P)H P450 reductase, the redox partner of cytochromes necessary for the supply of electrons from the cofactor NAD(P)H [92]. The establishment of a renewable supply has been proven difficult in *E. coli*.

5.3. Conversion of deoxypodophyllotoxin to (epi)podophyllotoxin by engineering

In 2006, Vasilev and coworkers showed that the human liver cytochrome P450 3A4 (CYP3A4) together with human NADPH P450 reductase can convert deoxypodophyllotoxin stereoselectivity into epipodophyllotoxin [93]. The disadvantage of this system is the usage of frozen cells and therefore the need to supply a regenerative system, such as glucose-6-phosphate dehydrogenase and NADP. Changing the system to a resting cell assay or cell-free assay with the usage of a cheaper cofactor and increasing the electron transfer between cytochrome and reductase would greatly increase the usability of this system. As CYP3A4 is quite unspecific, an approach to find a dedicated cytochrome converting deoxypodophyllotoxin into podophyllotoxin could be provided by the systematic analysis of cytochrome encoding genes found by Kumari and coworkers, who analyzed the transcriptome of *P. hexandrum* cultivated at two temperatures. The expression of DIR protein, PLR and SDH were upregulated by at least a factor two at 15°C compared to 25°C [94], accompanied by an increase of podophyllotoxin accumulation at 15°C. Fifteen cytochrome transcripts were upregulated by at least a factor two at 15°C compared to 25°C. These fifteen upregulated cytochrome transcripts would be interesting candidates for future investigation.

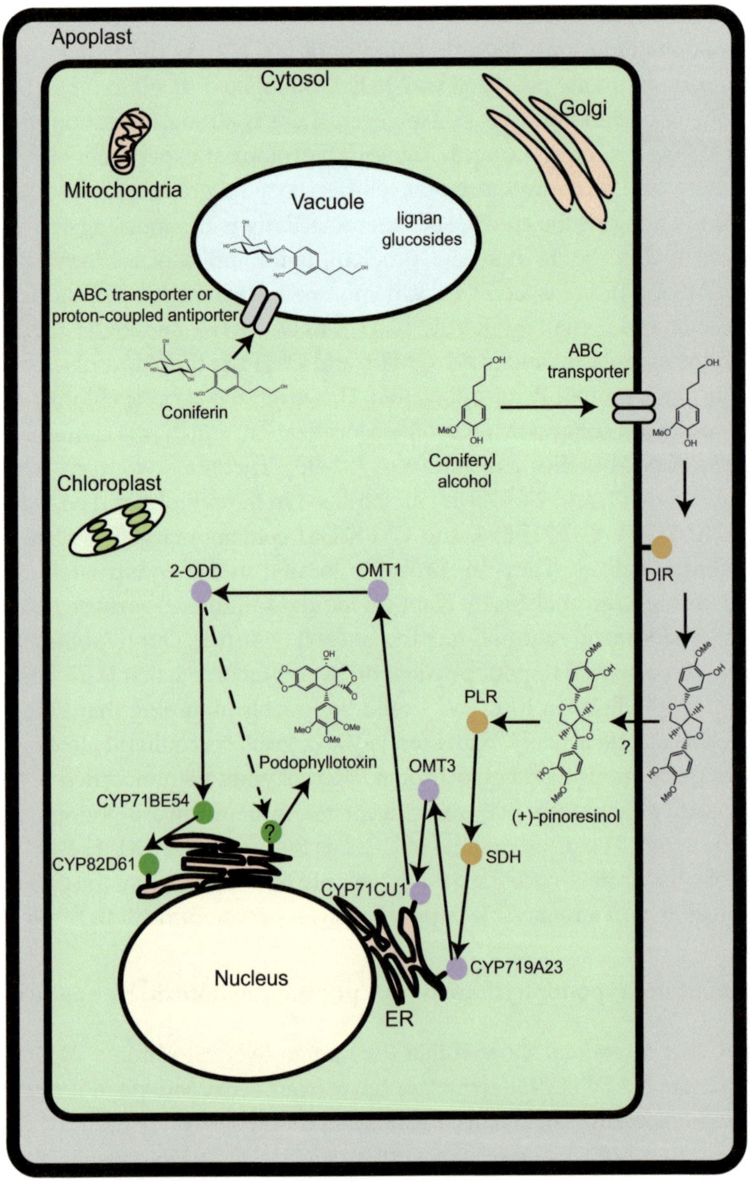

Figure 2. Schematic view of the proposed cellular localization of the enzymes in the lignan pathway in plant cells.

A cytochrome p450 system with high activity toward deoxypodophyllotoxin can form a very interesting production platform in conjunction with a sustainable source of this lignan, as is *A. sylvestris*, a common wild plant in Europe and temperate Asia, that can be cultivated easily [95, 96].

5.4. Production of etoposide

Industrially, podophyllotoxin is chemically converted to etoposide (**Figure 3**). Podophyllotoxin is converted to 4′-demethyl-epipodophyllotoxin by demethylation and epimerization in two steps with a yield of 52% followed by the protection of the phenolic group by conversion to

http://dx.doi.org/10.5772/67615

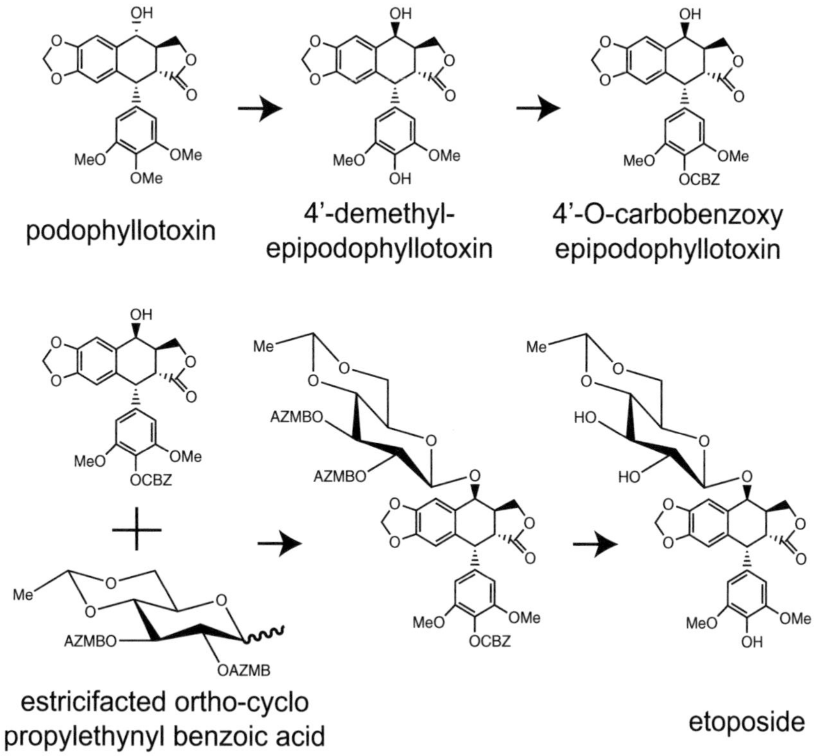

Figure 3. Conversion of podophyllotoxin into etoposide.

4′-O-carbobenzoxy-epipodophyllotoxin in one step with 89% yield [97]. 4′-O-carbobenzoxy-epipodophyllotoxin is then glycosylated to the esterification of *ortho*-cyclopropylethynylbenzoic acid, which is obtained in six steps from β-D-Glucose pentaacetate [98, 99]. After glycosylation, the protective groups are removed in one step with 90% yield [98]. As podophyllotoxin production from deoxypodophyllotoxin is not yet applicable on industrial scale, the chemical conversion of deoxypodophyllotoxin into epipodophyllotoxin is of interest, which can be performed in one step with a yield of 53% [100]. Epipodophyllotoxin can be converted chemically to etoposide in the same manner as podophyllotoxin. The chemical synthesis of etoposide from deoxypodophyllotoxin can be shortened by production of 4′-demethyl-epipodophyllotoxin from deoxypodophyllotoxin by CYP71BE54 and CYP82D61 from *P. hexandrum* (see Section 4.3). As only proof of concept has been shown, optimization is required to make this enzymatic conversion suitable for industrial application. Whether deoxypodophyllotoxin can be converted chemically directly to 4′-demethyl-epipodophyllotoxin still needs to be investigated.

6. Future perspectives

Recent insights in the lignan biosynthetic pathway by Lau and Sattely [69] have progressed the research in the lignan pathway enormously. Engineering of the lignan pathway in a heterologous host will become feasible, if the localization of the enzymes in the pathway has been determined. Depending on this localization, either *E. coli* or *S. cerevisiae* could be a suitable host for production of podophyllotoxin from glucose. The only missing step is the conversion of deoxypodophyllotoxin to podophyllotoxin. Finding this enzyme or replacing this step by the epipodophyllotoxin producing CYP82D61 (with or without CYP71BE54) will advance the development even more. Alternatively, deoxypodophyllotoxin can be chemically converted to etoposide. Considering the huge number of enzymes necessary for conversion of glucose to podophyllotoxin in *E. coli* or *S. cerevisiae*, commercial production in microbial hosts still has a long way to go. Until that time, an alternative approach can be the extraction of deoxypodophyllotoxin from the easy to cultivate *A. sylvestris* and converting this to (epi)podophyllotoxin. Enzymatic conversion needs to be optimized in order to obtain a system that can be used by the industry. Improvement should focus on engineering a cheap system, by usage of a resting cell assay or the usage of a cheap cofactor in a cell-free system. Furthermore, the deoxypodophyllotoxin conversion should be scaled up to industrial production.

Acknowledgements

This work was supported by EU regional funding. The PhytoSana project in the INTERREG IV A Deutschland-Nederland program: 34- INTERREG IV A I-1-01=193.

Author details

Christel L. C. Seegers, Rita Setroikromo and Wim J. Quax*

*Address all correspondence to: w.j.quax@rug.nl

Department of Chemical and Pharmaceutical Biology, Groningen Research Institute of Pharmacy, University of Groningen, Groningen, The Netherlands

References

[1] Guerram M, Jiang ZZ, Zhang LY. Podophyllotoxin, a medicinal agent of plant origin: past, present and future. Chin J Nat Med. 2012;10:161-9. doi:10.3724/SP.J.1009.2012.00161.

[2] Alam MA, Naik PK. Impact of soil nutrients and environmental factors on podophyllotoxin content among 28 *podophyllum hexandrum* populations of Northwestern Himalayan region using linear and nonlinear approaches. Commun Soil Sci Plant Anal. 2009;40:2485-504. doi:10.1080/00103620903111368.

[3] Convention of International Trade in Endangered Species of Wild Fauna and Flora. n.d. https://www.cites.org/eng/app/appendices.php#hash2 (accessed October 28, 2015).

[4] Canel C, Moraes RM, Dayan FE, Ferreira D. Podophyllotoxin. Phytochemistry. 2000;54:115-20. doi:10.1016/S0031-9422(00)00094-7.

[5] Ting CP, Maimone TJ. CH bond arylation in the synthesis of aryltetralin lignans: a short total synthesis of podophyllotoxin. Angew Chem Int Ed Engl. 2014;53:3115-9. doi:10.1002/anie.201311112.

[6] Petersen M, Alfermann W. The production of cytotoxic lignans by plant cell cultures. Appl Microbiol Biotechnol. 2001;55:135-42. doi:10.1007/s002530000510.

[7] Ionkova I, Antonova I, Momekov G, Fuss E. Production of podophyllotoxin in Linum linearifolium *in vitro* cultures. Pharmacogn Mag. 2010;6:180-5. doi:10.4103/0973-1296.66932.

[8] Turner EE, Hirst EL, Peat S, Haworth RD, Baker W, Linstead RP, et al. Organic chemistry. Annu Reports Prog Chem. 1936;33:228. doi:10.1039/ar9363300228.

[9] Moss GP. Nomenclature of lignans and neolignans (IUPAC Recommendations 2000). Pure Appl Chem. 2000;72:1493-523. doi:10.1351/pac200072081493.

[10] Umezawa T. Diversity in lignan biosynthesis. Phytochem Rev. 2003;2:371-90. doi:10.1023/b:phyt.0000045487.02836.32.

[11] Whiting DA. Ligans and neolignans. Nat Prod Rep. 1985;2:191. doi:10.1039/np9850200191.

[12] Heinonen S, Nurmi T, Liukkonen K, Poutanen K, Wähälä K, Deyama T, et al. *In vitro* metabolism of plant lignans: new precursors of mammalian lignans enterolactone and enterodiol. J Agric Food Chem. 2001;49:3178-86. doi:10.1021/JF010038A.

[13] Peñalvo JL, Heinonen SM, Aura AM, Adlercreutz H. Dietary sesamin is converted to enterolactone in humans. J Nutr. 2005;135:1056-62.

[14] Landete JM. Plant and mammalian lignans: a review of source, intake, metabolism, intestinal bacteria and health. Food Res Int. 2012;46:410-24. doi:10.1016/j.foodres.2011.12.023.

[15] Charlton JL. Antiviral activity of lignans. J Nat Prod. 1998;61:1447-51. doi:10.1021/NP980136Z.

[16] Ayres DC, Loike JD. Lignans: Chemical, Biological and Clinical Properties. vol. 30. Cambridge, NewYork, Port Chester, Melbourne, Sydney: Cambridge University Press; 1990.

[17] Culp OS, Kaplan IW. Condylomata acuminata: two hundred cases treated with podophyllin. Ann Surg. 1944;120:251-6.

[18] von Krogh G, Lacey CJN, Gross G, Barrasso R, Schneider A. European course on HPV associated pathology: guidelines for primary care physicians for the diagnosis and management of anogenital warts. Sex Transm Infect. 2000;76:162-8. doi:10.1136/sti.76.3.162.

[19] Kelly MG, Hart-Well JL. The biological effects and the chemical composition of podophyllin. a review. J Natl Cancer Inst. 1954;14:967-1010. doi:10.1093/jnci/14.4.967.

[20] Stähelin HF, von Wartburg A. The chemical and biological route from podophyllotoxin glucoside to etoposide: ninth cain memorial award lecture. Cancer Res. 1991;51: 5-15.

[21] Imbert TF. Discovery of podophyllotoxins. Biochimie. 1998;80:207-22. doi:10.1016/S0300-9084(98)80004-7.

[22] Liu YQ, Yang L, Tian X. Podophyllotoxin: current perspectives. Curr Bioact Compd. 2007;3:37-66. doi:10.2174/157340707780126499.

[23] Hande K. Etoposide: four decades of development of a topoisomerase II inhibitor. Eur J Cancer. 1998;34:1514-21. doi:10.1016/S0959-8049(98)00228-7.

[24] Senter PD, Saulnier MG, Schreiber GJ, Hirschberg DL, Brown JP, Hellström I, et al. Anti-tumor effects of antibody-alkaline phosphatase conjugates in combination with etoposide phosphate. Proc Natl Acad Sci U S A. 1988;85:4842-6.

[25] Thompson DS, Greco FA, Miller AA, Srinivas NR, Igwemezie LN, Hainsworth JD, et al. A phase I study of etoposide phosphate administered as a daily 30-minute infusion for 5 days. Clin Pharmacol Ther. 1995;57:499-507. doi:10.1016/0009-9236(95)90034-9.

[26] A to Z List of Cancer Drugs—National Cancer Institute. 2016. https://www.cancer.gov/about-cancer/treatment/drugs.

[27] Cytostatica | Farmacotherapeutisch Kompas. n.d. https://www.farmacotherapeutisch-kompas.nl/bladeren-volgens-boek/inleidingen/inl-cytostatica.

[28] Kalemkerian GP, Akerley W, Bogner P, Borghaei H, Chow LQ, Downey RJ, et al. Small cell lung cancer. J Natl Compr Canc Netw. 2013;11:78-98.

[29] PDQ Pediatric Treatment Editorial Board PPTE. Childhood Acute Myeloid Leukemia/Other Myeloid Malignancies Treatment (PDQ®): Health Professional Version. Bethesda: National Cancer Institute (US); 2002.

[30] Chemotherapy for acute lymphocytic leukemia. n.d. http://www.cancer.org/cancer/leukemia-acutelymphocyticallinadults/detailedguide/leukemia-acute-lymphocytic-treating-chemo therapy.

[31] Kamal A, Hussaini SMA, Rahim A, Riyaz S. Podophyllotoxin derivatives: a patent review (2012-2014). Expert Opin Ther Pat. 2015;25:1025-34.

[32] Liu YQ, Tian J, Qian K, Zhao XB, Morris-Natschke SL, Yang L, et al. Recent progress on C-4-modified podophyllotoxin analogs as potent antitumor agents. Med Res Rev. 2015;35:1-62. doi:10.1002/med.21319.

[33] Mizugaki H, Yamamoto N, Fujiwara Y, Nokihara H, Yamada Y, Tamura T. Current status of single-agent phase I trials in japan: toward globalization. J Clin Oncol. 2015;33:2051-61. doi:10.1200/JCO.2014.58.4953.

[34] Raβmann I, Schrödel H, Schilling T, Zucchetti M, Kaeser-Fröhlich A, Rastetter J, et al. Clinical and pharmacokinetic phase I trial of oral dimethylaminoetoposide (NK611) administered for 21 days every 35 days. Invest New Drugs. 1996;14:379-86. doi:10.1007/BF00180814.

[35] Raβmann I, Thödtmann R, Thödtmann R, Mross M, Hüttmann A, Berdel WE, et al. Phase I clinical and pharmacokinetic trial of the podophyllotoxin derivative NK611 administered as intravenous short infusion. Invest New Drugs. 1998;16:319-24. doi:10.1023/A:1006293830585.

[36] Pagani O, Zucchetti M, Sessa C, de Jong J, D'Incalci M, Fusco M De, et al. Clinical and pharmacokinetic study of oral NK611, a new podophyllotoxin derivative. Cancer Chemother Pharmacol. 1996;38:541-7. doi:10.1007/s002800050524.

[37] Perrin D, van Hille B, Barret JM, Kruczynski A, Etiévant C, Imbert T, et al. F 11782, a novel epipodophylloid non-intercalating dual catalytic inhibitor of topoisomerases I and II with an original mechanism of action. Biochem Pharmacol. 2000;59:807-19. doi:10.1016/S0006-2952(99)00382-2.

[38] Etiévant C, Kruczynski A, Barret JM, Perrin D, van Hille B, Guminski Y, et al. F 11782, a dual inhibitor of topoisomerases I and II with an original mechanism of action *in vitro*, and markedly superior *in vivo* antitumour activity, relative to three other dual topoisomerase inhibitors, intoplicin, aclarubicin and TAS-103. Cancer Chemother Pharmacol. 2000;46:101-13. doi:10.1007/s002800000133.

[39] Delord J-P, Bennouna J, Dieras V, Campone M, Lefresne F, Aslanis V, et al. First-in-man study of tafluposide, a novel inhibitor of topoisomerase I and II. Mol Cancer Ther. 2007;6:A138.

[40] Barret JM, Kruczynski A, Vispé S, Annereau JP, Brel V, Guminski Y, et al. F14512, a potent antitumor agent targeting topoisomerase II vectored into cancer cells via the polyamine transport system. Cancer Res. 2008;68:9845-53.

[41] Bahleda R, De Botton S, Quesnel B, Soria JC. 12th TAT congress 5-7 march 2014 Washington DC. Tackling Leuk. Phase I study F14512 relapsed or Refract. AML patients, 2014.

[42] Tierny D, Serres F, Segaoula Z, Bemelmans I, Bouchaert E, Pétain A, et al. Phase I clinical pharmacology study of F14512, a new polyamine-vectorized anticancer drug, in naturally occurring canine lymphoma. Clin Cancer Res. 2015;21:5314-23.

[43] Merzouki A, Buschmann MD, Jean M, Young RS, Liao S, Gal S, et al. Adva-27a, a novel podophyllotoxin derivative found to be effective against multidrug resistant human cancer cells. Anticancer Res. 2012;32:4423-32.

[44] Research programme: type II DNA topoisomerase inhibitors—Sunshine Biopharma—AdisInsight. n.d. http://adisinsight.springer.com/drugs/800032587.

[45] Chen MC, Pan SL, Shi Q, Xiao Z, Lee KH, Li TK, et al. QS-ZYX-1-61 induces apoptosis through topoisomerase II in human non-small-cell lung cancer A549 cells. Cancer Sci. 2012;103:80-7. doi:10.1111/j.1349-7006.2011.02103.x.

[46] Lewis NG, Davin LB, Sarkanen S. Lignin and lignan biosynthesis: distinctions and reconciliations. 1998; 697:pp. 1-27. doi:10.1021/bk-1998-0697.ch001.

[47] Rutledge PJ, Challis GL. Discovery of microbial natural products by activation of silent biosynthetic gene clusters. Nat Rev Microbiol. 2015;13:509-23. doi:10.1038/nrmicro3496.

[48] Davin LB, Wang HB, Crowell AL, Bedgar DL, Martin DM, Sarkanen S, et al. Stereoselective bimolecular phenoxy radical coupling by an auxiliary (dirigent) protein without an active center. Science (80-). 1997;275:362-7. doi:10.1126/science.275.5298.362.

[49] Kim KW, Moinuddin SGA, Atwell KM, Costa MA, Davin LB, Lewis NG. Opposite stereoselectivities of dirigent proteins in arabidopsis and schizandra species. J Biol Chem. 2012;287:33957-72. doi:10.1074/jbc.M112.387423.

[50] Gang DR, Costa MA, Fujita M, Dinkova-Kostova AT, Wang HB, Burlat V, et al. Regiochemical control of monolignol radical coupling: a new paradigm for lignin and lignan biosynthesis. Chem Biol. 1999;6:143-51. doi:10.1016/S1074-5521(99)89006-1.

[51] Seneviratne HK, Dalisay DS, Kim KW, Moinuddin SGA, Yang H, Hartshorn CM, et al. Non-host disease resistance response in pea (*Pisum sativum*) pods: biochemical function of DRR206 and phytoalexin pathway localization. Phytochemistry. 2015;113:140-8. doi:10.1016/j.phytochem.2014.10.013.

[52] Pickel B, Constantin MA, Pfannstiel J, Conrad J, Beifuss U, Schaller A. An enantiocomplementary dirigent protein for the enantioselective laccase-catalyzed oxidative coupling of phenols. Angew Chemie Int Ed. 2010;49:202-4. doi:10.1002/anie.200904622.

[53] Dalisay DS, Kim KW, Lee C, Yang H, Rübel O, Bowen BP, et al. Dirigent protein-mediated lignan and cyanogenic glucoside formation in flax seed: integrated omics and MALDI mass spectrometry imaging. J Nat Prod. 2015;78:1231-42. doi:10.1021/acs.jnatprod.5b00023.

[54] Kim KW, Smith CA, Daily MD, Cort JR, Davin LB, Lewis NG. Trimeric structure of (+)-pinoresinol-forming dirigent protein at 1.95 Å resolution with three isolated active sites. J Biol Chem. 2015;290:1308-18. doi:10.1074/jbc.M114.611780.

[55] Dinkova-Kostova AT, Gang DR, Davin LB, Bedgar DL, Chu A, Lewis NG. (+)-Pinoresinol/(+)-Lariciresinol Reductase from Forsythia intermedia: protein purrification, cDNA cloning, heterologous expression and comparision to isoflavone reductase. J Biol Chem. 1996;271:29473-82. doi:10.1074/jbc.271.46.29473.

[56] Katayama T, Davin LB, Chu A, Lewis NG. Novel benzylic ether reductions in lignan biogenesis in Forsythia intermedia. Phytochemistry. 1993;33:581-91. doi:10.1016/0031-9422(93)85452-W.

[57] von Heimendahl CBI, Schäfer KM, Eklund P, Sjöholm R, Schmidt TJ, Fuss E. Pinoresinol–lariciresinol reductases with different stereospecificity from Linum album and Linum usitatissimum. Phytochemistry. 2005;66:1254-63. doi:10.1016/j.phytochem.2005.04.026.

[58] Hemmati S, Heimendahl CBI von, Klaes M, Alfermann AW, Schmidt TJ, Fuss E, et al. Pinoresinol-Lariciresinol reductases with opposite enantiospecificity determine the enantiomeric composition of lignans in the different organs of *Linum usitatissimum* L. Planta Med. 2010;76:928-34. doi:10.1055/s-0030-1250036.

[59] Bayindir Ü, Alfermann AW, Fuss E. Hinokinin biosynthesis in Linum corymbulosum Reichenb. Plant J. 2008;55:810-20. doi:10.1111/j.1365-313X.2008.03558.x.

[60] Fujita M, Gang DR, Davin LB, Lewis NG. Recombinant pinoresinol-lariciresinol reductases from western Red Cedar (*Thuja plicata*) catalyze opposite enantiospecific conversions. J Biol Chem. 1999;274:618-27. doi:10.1074/jbc.274.2.618.

[61] Hemmati S, Schmidt TJ, Fuss E. (+)-Pinoresinol/(−)-lariciresinol reductase from Linum perenne Himmelszelt involved in the biosynthesis of justicidin B. FEBS Lett. 2007;581:603-10. doi:10.1016/j.febslet.2007.01.018.

[62] Nakatsubo T, Mizutani M, Suzuki S, Hattori T, Umezawa T. Characterization of *Arabidopsis thaliana* pinoresinol reductase, a new type of enzyme involved in lignan biosynthesis. J Biol Chem. 2008;283:15550-7. doi:10.1074/jbc.M801131200.

[63] Min T, Kasahara H, Bedgar DL, Youn B, Lawrence PK, Gang DR, et al. Crystal structures of pinoresinol-lariciresinol and phenylcoumaran benzylic ether reductases and their relationship to isoflavone reductases. J Biol Chem. 2003;278:50714-23. doi:10.1074/jbc.M308493200.

[64] Xia ZQ, Costa M a, Pelissier HC, Davin LB, Lewis NG. Secoisolariciresinol dehydrogenase purification, cloning, and functional expression. Implications for human health protection. J Biol Chem. 2001;276:12614-23. doi:10.1074/jbc.M008622200.

[65] Youn B, Moinuddin SGA, Davin LB, Lewis NG, Kang C. Crystal structures of apo-form and binary/ternary complexes of podophyllum secoisolariciresinol dehydrogenase, an enzyme involved in formation of health-protecting and plant defense lignans. J Biol Chem. 2005;280:12917-26. doi:10.1074/jbc.M413266200.

[66] Kamil WM, Dewick PM. Biosynthetic relationship of aryltetralin lactone lignans to dibenzylbutyrolactone lignans. Phytochemistry. 1986;25:2093-102. doi: 10.1016/0031-9422(86)80072-3.

[67] Jackson DE, Dewick PM. Biosynthesis of *Podophyllum lignans*—II. Interconversions of aryltetralin lignans in *Podophyllum hexandrum*. Phytochemistry. 1984;23:1037-42. doi:10.1016/S0031-9422(00)82604-7.

[68] Marques JV, Kim KW, Lee C, Costa M a, May GD, Crow JA, et al. Next generation sequencing in predicting gene function in podophyllotoxin biosynthesis. J Biol Chem. 2013;288:466-79. doi:10.1074/jbc.M112.400689.

[69] Lau W, Sattely ES. Six enzymes from mayapple that complete the biosynthetic pathway to the etoposide aglycone. Science (80-). 2015;349:1224-8. doi:10.1126/science.aac7202.

[70] Sakakibara N, Suzuki S, Umezawa T, Shimada M. Biosynthesis of yatein in *Anthriscus sylvestris*. Org Biomol Chem. 2003;1:2474-85.

[71] Ragamustari SK, Nakatsubo T, Hattori T, Ono E, Kitamura Y, Suzuki S, et al. A novel O-methyltransferase involved in the first methylation step of yatein biosynthesis from

matairesinol in *Anthriscus sylvestris*. Plant Biotechnol. 2013;30:375-84. doi:10.5511/plantbiotechnology.13.0527b.

[72] Weiss SG, Tin-Wa M, Perdue RE, Farnsworth NR. Potential anticancer agents II: antitumor and cytotoxic lignans from Linum album (Linaceae). J Pharm Sci. 1975;64:95-8. doi:10.1002/jps.2600640119.

[73] Shiraishi A, Murata J, Matsumoto E, Matsubara S, Ono E, Satake H, et al. De novo transcriptomes of *Forsythia koreana* using a novel assembly method: insight into tissue- and species-specific expression of lignan biosynthesis-related gene. PLoS One. 2016;11:e0164805. doi:10.1371/journal.pone.0164805.

[74] Chen Z, Sun X, Li Y, Yan Y, Yuan Q. Metabolic engineering of *Escherichia coli* for microbial synthesis of monolignols. Metab Eng. 2016;39:102-9. doi:10.1016/j.ymben.2016.10.021.

[75] Huang Q, Lin Y, Yan Y. Caffeic acid production enhancement by engineering a phenylalanine over-producing *Escherichia coli* strain. Biotechnol Bioeng. 2013;110:3188-96. doi:10.1002/bit.24988.

[76] Eichenberger M, Lehka BJ, Folly C, Fischer D, Martens S, Simón E, et al. Metabolic engineering of *Saccharomyces cerevisiae* for de novo production of dihydrochalcones with known antioxidant, antidiabetic, and sweet tasting properties. Metab Eng. 2016;39:80-89. doi:10.1016/j.ymben.2016.10.019.

[77] Gidijala L, Kiel JAKW, Douma RD, Seifar RM, van Gulik WM, Bovenberg RAL, et al. An engineered yeast efficiently secreting penicillin. PLoS One. 2009;4:e8317. doi:10.1371/journal.pone.0008317.

[78] Miao YC, Liu CJ. ATP-binding cassette-like transporters are involved in the transport of lignin precursors across plasma and vacuolar membranes. Proc Natl Acad Sci U S A. 2010;107:22728-33. doi:10.1073/pnas.1007747108.

[79] Tsuyama T, Kawai R, Shitan N, Matoh T, Sugiyama J, Yoshinaga A, et al. Proton-dependent coniferin transport, a common major transport event in differentiating xylem tissue of woody plants. Plant Physiol. 2013;162:918-26. doi:10.1104/pp.113.214957.

[80] Krogh A, Larsson B, von Heijne G, Sonnhammer EL. Predicting transmembrane protein topology with a hidden markov model: application to complete genomes. J Mol Biol. 2001;305:567-80. doi:10.1006/jmbi.2000.4315.

[81] Umezawa T, Davin LB, Yamamoto E, Kingston DGI, Lewis NG, Lewis NG, et al. Lignan biosynthesis in forsythia species. J Chem Soc Chem Commun. 1990;41:1405. doi:10.1039/c39900001405.

[82] Davin LB, Bedgar DL, Katayama T, Lewis NG. On the stereoselective synthesis of (+)-pinoresinol in Forsythia suspensa from its achiral precursor, coniferyl alcohol. Phytochemistry. 1992;31:3869-74. doi:10.1016/S0031-9422(00)97544-7.

[83] Burlat V, Kwon M, Davin LB, Lewis NG. Dirigent proteins and dirigent sites in lignifying tissues. Phytochemistry. 2001;57:883-97. doi:10.1016/S0031-9422(01)00117-0.

[84] Dima O, Morreel K, Vanholme B, Kim H, Ralph J, Boerjan W. Small glycosylated lignin oligomers are stored in arabidopsis leaf vacuoles. Plant Cell. 2015;27:695-710. doi:10.1105/tpc.114.134643.

[85] Petersen TN, Brunak S, von Heijne G, Nielsen H. SignalP 4.0: discriminating signal peptides from transmembrane regions. Nat Methods. 2011;8:785-6. doi:10.1038/nmeth.1701.

[86] Chou KC, Shen HB, Ehrlich J, Hansen M, Nelson W, Glory E, et al. Plant-mPLoc: a top-down strategy to augment the power for predicting plant protein subcellular localization. PLoS One. 2010;5:e11335. doi:10.1371/journal.pone.0011335.

[87] Emanuelsson O, Nielsen H, Heijne G Von. ChloroP, a neural network-based method for predicting chloroplast transit peptides and their cleavage sites. Protein Sci. 1999;8:978-84. doi:10.1110/ps.8.5.978.

[88] Schein AI, Kissinger JC, Ungar LH. Chloroplast transit peptide prediction: a peek inside the black box. Nucleic Acids Res. 2001;29:E82.

[89] Blum T, Briesemeister S, Kohlbacher O, Emanuelsson O, Brunak S, Heijne G von, et al. MultiLoc2: integrating phylogeny and gene ontology terms improves subcellular protein localization prediction. BMC Bioinformatics. 2009;10:274. doi:10.1186/1471-2105-10-274.

[90] Goldberg T, Hecht M, Hamp T, Karl T, Yachdav G, Ahmed N, et al. LocTree3 prediction of localization. Nucleic Acids Res. 2014;42:W350-5. doi:10.1093/nar/gku396.

[91] Schuler MA, Werck-Reichhart D. Functional genomics of P450s. Annu Rev Plant Biol. 2003;54:629-67. doi:10.1146/annurev.arplant.54.031902.134840.

[92] Gillam EMJ. Engineering cytochrome P450 enzymes. Chem Res Toxicol. 2007;21:220-31. doi:10.1021/tx7002849.

[93] Vasilev NP, Julsing MK, Koulman A, Clarkson C, Woerdenbag HJ, Ionkova I, et al. Bioconversion of deoxypodophyllotoxin into epipodophyllotoxin in *E. coli* using human cytochrome P450 3A4. J Biotechnol. 2006;126:383-93. doi:10.1016/j.jbiotec.2006.04.025.

[94] Kumari A, Singh HR, Jha A, Swarnkar MK, Shankar R, Kumar S. Transcriptome sequencing of rhizome tissue of Sinopodophyllum hexandrum at two temperatures. BMC Genomics. 2014;15:871. doi:10.1186/1471-2164-15-871.

[95] Magnússen SH. NOBANIS –Invasive Alien Species Fact Sheet -*Anthriscus sylvestris*. Database of the European Network on Invasive Alien Species. 2011.

[96] Hendrawati O, Woerdenbag HJ, Hille J, Quax WJ, Kayser O. Seasonal variations in the deoxypodophyllotoxin content and yield of *Anthriscus sylvestris* L. (Hoffm.) grown in the field and under controlled conditions. J Agric Food Chem. 2011;59:8132-9. doi:10.1021/jf200177q.

[97] Lee KH, Imakura Y, Haruna M, Beers SA, Thurston LS, Dai HJ, et al. Antitumor agents, 107. New cytotoxic 4-alkylamino analogues of 4′-demethyl-epipodophyllotoxin as inhibitors of human DNA topoisomerase II. J Nat Prod. 1989;52:606-13. doi:10.1021/np50063a021.

[98] Liu H, Liao JX, Hu Y, Tu YH, Sun JS. A highly efficient approach to construct (*epi*)-podophyllotoxin-4- *O* -glycosidic linkages as well as its application in concise syntheses of etoposide and teniposide. Org Lett. 2016;18:1294-7. doi:10.1021/acs.orglett.6b00216.

[99] Zong G, Barber E, Aljewari H, Zhou J, Hu Z, Du Y, et al. Total synthesis and biological evaluation of ipomoeassin F and its unnatural 11 *R* -epimer. J Org Chem. 2015;80:9279-91. doi:10.1021/acs.joc.5b01765.

[100] Yamaguchi Hi, Arimoto M, Nakajima S, Tanoguchi M, Fukada Y. Studies on the constituents of the seeds of Hernandia ovigera L. V Syntheses of epipodophyllotoxin and podophyllotoxin from desoxypodophyllotoxin. Chem Pharm Bull (Tokyo). 1986;34:2056-60. doi:10.1248/cpb.34.2056.